Basic Principles of Function: Science

Textbook, First Edition

Edited by Danik M. Martirosyan, PhD

Basic Principles of Functional Food Science

Textbook, First Edition

Functional Food Center Inc. / Functional Food Institute
4659 Texas St., Unit 15, San Diego, CA 92116, USA
Website: http://www.functionalfoodscenter.net

Printed and Edited in the United States of America

ISBN-13: 978-1721961290; ISBN-10:1721961291

For information regarding special discounts for bulk purchases, please contact Food Science Publisher Special Sales at 469-441-8272 or email ffc_usa@sbcglobal.net.

Important Notice:
This publication is neither a medical guide nor a manual for self-treatment. If you should suspect that you suffer from a medical problem, you should seek competent medical care. The reader should consult his or her health professional before adopting any of the suggestions in this book. Never disregard professional medical advice due to something you read in this textbook. This book only offers important information on functional foods and nutrition in overall health and wellness. Nonetheless, readers should be aware that nutrition and medicine are expanding fields and should continue to educate themselves on preventative measures. Their primary care provider and the patient are responsible for determining the best plan of care. The authors, editors, and publisher take no liability for any injury or illness that may arise by using the materials from this text

Food Science Publisher 2018
Edited by Danik M. Martirosyan, PhD

ACKNOWLEDGMENTS:

I would like to extend our warmest gratitude to each and every contributor of this book for having shared their articles with us. We include manuscripts authored by esteemed experts from many different countries, including Australia, Canada, United Kingdom, Italy, Japan, China, Denmark, Russia, India, Hong Kong, Hungaria, Indonesia, Malaysia, Brazil, Poland, Republic of Korea, Saudi Arabia, Taiwan, Thailand, Belarus, the USA and more.

It is our hope that those who read this book will become more knowledgeable about the role of functional foods and bioactive compounds in the prevention and management of chronic diseases.

I would like to thank all contributors, including Cara J. Westmark, Kasia Pisarski, Anju Dhiman, Vaibhav Walia, Arun Nanda, Daniel A. Abugri, Melissa Johnson, Callen Pacier, Ozge Kahraman, Swamy Gabriela John, Melvin Holmes, S. Sreelatha, Johanna Gur, Marselinny Mawuntu, Thomas Reynolds, and Marisol Ortiz.

Also, I would like to thank the Department of Pharmaceutical Sciences, Maharshi Dayanand University (India); Departent of Chemistry, Tuskegee University (USA); Center for Plant Biotechnology Research, Tuskegee University (USA); Functional Food Center/Functional Food Institute (USA); Department of Neurology, University of Wisconsin, Madison (USA); Università Politecnica delle Marche, Dipartimento di Scienze Agrarie (Italy); Department of Food Technology, Kongu Engineering College (India); Department of Food Science and Nutrition, University of Leeds (United Kingdom); Singapore-MIT Alliance for Research and Technology (Singapore); and University of San Fransisco (USA) for their support to contributors.

Danik M. Martirosyan, PhD, Founder of Functional Food Center/Functional Food Institute, Dallas, TX, USA

INTRODUCTION

Scientists, public health experts, food producers and consumers have united to generate research on functional food that allows the public to lessen pharmaceutical side effects and surgical costs in the treatment of serious illness.

This book presents not only innovative functional food ideas for managing chronic illnesses, but also the processes and scientific research which lead to these modern yet time-honored treatment methods. This issue not only preserves some of the wealth of contributions made in the field, but lays the foundation for a field of science that promises to expand in coming years, potentially changing modern society's relationship with medicine.

This cornerstone guide, written by internationally-recognized functional, medical, and bioactive food experts, covers the basics of functional food science. With more than 1,000 scientific references, this book provides scientists, medical doctors, nutritionists, food technologists, and students majoring in biology, nutrigenetic, and food science fields, as well as public health professionals with a comprehensive and up-to-date examination of functional foods.

This book provides modern information on functional food components, including antioxidants, dietary fibers, prebiotics, plant sterols, bioactive peptides, and flavonoids, and many other phytochemicals. This text presents some of the latest developments in nutrigenomics, molecular biology, and epidemiology, as well as the production, marketing, and distribution of functional foods.

In this textbook, our editorial board has included additional information and resources in order to enhance the learning experience of our readers. These additions include detailed editing of articles, new figures, tables, and pictures, end of chapter summaries for each chapter, test questions at the end of each chapter, and an updated glossary with new key words. We believe that this will help our readers to better understand the new material and concepts of functional food science.

In order to get the most out of this edition, it is recommended to read each chapter completely and to also review the summary paragraphs that conclude each chapter. These summaries lay out the main take-aways from the chapter and help to put the chapter as a whole into perspective. Also, the reader should complete the end of chapter questions after each chapter to make sure that the information is being retained and understood. Both of these components will assist the reader in studying and comprehending the material.

There are many new words in our glossary at the end of the textbook. These words can be found using the page numbers associated with them in order to find the chapter that contains them. These words have each been conveniently highlighted in the chapters so they may be easily located. It is to the readers' benefit to review these words in the glossary so that they may better understand the material in the chapters.

The book is collective work of 15 scientists, 9 universities, and other medical and food organizations across the globe.

Danik Martirosyan, PhD, Founder of Functional Food Center/Functional Food Institute, Dallas, TX, USA

CONTENTS

INTRODUCTION

CHAPTERS

1. **A New Definition for Functional Food by FFC: Creating Functional Food Products Using New Definition**
    Danik M. Martirosyan and Jaishree Singh   6

2. **Bioactive Compounds: Their Role in Functional Food and Human Health, Classifications, and Definitions**
    Danik M. Martirosyan and Kasia Pisarski   25

3. **Introduction to Functional Foods**
    Anju Dhiman, Vaibhav Walia, Arun Nanda   67

4. **Efficacy and Dose Determination**
    Daniel A. Abugri and Melissa Johnson   81

5. **Healthy, Functional, and Medical Foods. Similarities and Differences between these Categories. Bioactive Food Compounds**
    Cara J. Westmark   113

6. **Vitamin C: optimal dosages, supplementation and use in disease prevention**
    Callen Pacier and Danik M. Martirosyan   127

7. **Fortification of Foods with Micronutrients**
    Ozge Kahraman   147

8. **Functional Food Ingredients Market**
    Swamy Gabriela John and Melvin Holmes   167

9. **Sensory Evaluation of Functional Foods**
    S. Sreelatha   219

10. **Biotechnology and Functional Food**
    Thomas Reynolds and Danik M. Martirosyan   228

11. **Classification of "Healthy" Food by Quantification of Nutrient Content based on Functional and Therapeutic Effect on Human Health**
    Marisol Ortiz and Danik M. Martirosyan   239

12. **FFC's Advancement of Functional Food Definition**
    Johanna Gur, Marselinny Mawuntu, and Danik M. Martirosyan   257

CORRECT ANSWERS   272

GLOSSARY   278

AUTHOR INDEX   289

1

A New Definition for Functional Food by FFC: Creating Functional Food Products Using New Definition

Danik M. Martirosyan and Jaishree Singh

Functional Food Center/Functional Food Institute, 4659 Texas St., Unit 15, San Diego, CA 92116, USA

Introduction

Two thousand years ago, when Hippocrates said "Let food be thy medicine and medicine be thy food," he was on the right path. However, we may now revise this to "Let functional food be thy medicine." Accordingly, since 2006, we at the Functional Food Center (FFC) have incorporated this statement into our functional food-related books.

Functional food science arose out of public need, and is made possible through the collaboration of different sciences. This field of research incorporates food science, nutrition, and medicine to produce food products that are combinations of food and pharmaceuticals. Specifically, researchers study food components and their potentially-beneficial health effects. They first measure changes in health and homeostatic behavior using biomarkers or indicators in the body. Then, scientists determine the prominent health effects these functional foods have on the body as well as their optimal and safe dosages [1].

But while the steps to developing functional food are more or less consistent across the world, the definition of "functional food" is not [1]. For example, countries like Japan, the EU, and the United States do not have a single legislative definition for functional food, leading to numerous worldwide consequences. The lack of a globally consistent definition has encouraged unregulated publishing of health claims in some nations, restricting of functional food production in other countries, and an overall mistrust or unclear sense of what functional food is among government officials, public health professionals, and consumers [37]. While billions of dollars in sales have been generated through the development of functional food, these setbacks divert scientists from delivering functional food to chronically ill populations.

Consequently, in this chapter, we describe how functional food has been defined in the past, why a standard definition is necessary, and the rationale behind the FFC's new definition for functional food.

Challenges Due to the Absence of a Proper Definition

A standard definition for functional food is needed to facilitate greater communication between food experts, scientists, government officials, and the public, as well as to enable freer exchange of functional food products between countries.

There are several consequences of leaving the functional food definition open-ended. These include: the distortion of the meaning of functional food, ambiguous food labels, and the loss of scientific legitimacy among consumers and government officials. Thus, it is imperative that we clarify what we mean by "functional foods," "bioactive compounds," "nutraceuticals," and other terms.

As researchers discover more bioactive compounds in food, functional food science gains support from the scientific community. Accordingly, government support through research grants and health claim approval will become more crucial to creating new functional food products. The FFC believes that in order to fully inform and educate government officials and others about functional food and bioactive compounds, a new definition for functional food must be established [2, 37]. It is predicted that a new definition will have several benefits:

First, formalizing a definition for functional food will improve communication between food/nutrition scientists, policymakers, medical researchers and the public [7]. Increased communication will enable the implementation of better policies and food education among non-experts, which will also lead to greater funding for nutrition research and policy initiatives. Second, a definition will legitimize functional food science globally and allow for more progress in food, medical, and policy innovation. Finally, a formal definition will help dispel public misconceptions about functional food [38]. Due to the prevalence of functional food products in the world amongst numerous definitions, people harbor pre-existing notions about the legitimacy of functional food products. Moreover, due to their lack of knowledge or experience with functional food, media and non-experts spread false or misleading information, thereby planting seeds of doubt in the minds of consumers. Functional food scientists have a responsibility to properly educate the public about functional food because their products are relevant to the future of chronic disease care and prevention. Therefore, this new definition is a step that will, ideally, lead to greater use of functional food by chronically ill consumers. As a result of dedicated research, collaboration with fellow functional food scientists, and modern understanding of functional food, the FFC has developed a new definition for functional food.

Functional Food: Current Definition

In 2012 at the FFC's 10th International Conference in Santa Barbara, CA, a new definition for functional food was proposed: [3]

> *"Natural or processed foods that contain known or unknown biologically-active compounds; which provide a clinically proven and documented health benefit for the prevention, management, or treatment of chronic disease."*

Medical, research, and student participants accepted this definition at the conference, which has guided FFC's research and conferences since 2012. At the 17th international conference in

2014, which the U.S. Department of Agriculture (USDA) and Agricultural Research Service (ARS) jointly organized, a Panel Discussion was organized entitled, "The Definition of Functional Foods and Bioactive Compounds." Here, FFC's definition for **functional foods** was revised to:

> *"Natural or processed foods that contain known or unknown biologically-active compounds; which, in defined, effective, and non-toxic amounts, provide a clinically proven and documented health benefit for the prevention, management, or treatment of chronic disease."*

In this updated definition, the phrase "in effective non-toxic amounts" was added to highlight the importance of bioactive compound dosage in the consumption of functional food.

What Makes the FFC Definition "Unique?"

To clarify, FFC defines **food** as "components of a normal diet for optimized nutrition." This definition includes conventional foods, such as oranges or bran flakes, not pills or capsules.

Moreover, this definition of functional food highlights the importance of "bioactive compounds" within functional foods. Bioactive compounds are the backbone of functional food effectiveness. For almost 20 years, the FFC has collaborated with scientists who have studied the benefits of bioactive compounds in functional foods. Thanks to modern biochemical technology, food scientists can now separate food substances into fine chemical components and test these food extracts for biological behavior. As a result, researchers can run experiments on these compounds and draw causal relationships between bioactive compounds and health outcomes.

Because the new definition focuses on bioactive compounds, it provides an explanation for functional foods' ability to improve health and treat illness. This definition simplifies and explains how functional foods operate at biochemical and empirical levels. In other words, this definition helps navigate food scientists toward specific goals (e.g. identifying bioactive compounds and where they exist in a food, such as in the skin, pulp, or seeds) and provides directions for future functional food research (e.g. determining the health benefits of all bioactive compounds in a food and the mechanisms by which they produce effects).

According to Dr. Danik Martirosyan, founder of the Functional Food Center and Functional Food Institute, two important concepts within the topic of bioactive compounds are: the amount of bioactive compounds and ratio of bioactive compounds required to convert ordinary food into functional food. Different amounts of bioactive compounds are effective in different situations, and sometimes too much of a bioactive compound can be toxic. In general, consuming physiologic levels of bioactive compounds is safe, while higher levels of bioactive compounds (e.g. supra-physiological or therapeutic doses) require testing for health benefits and safety. Therefore, it is crucial to have a thorough discussion on the use and control of bioactive compounds in functional foods.

Another feature of the current definition is the use of biomarkers in functional food studies. **Biomarkers** are indicators in the body that give off signals in tissues, organs, or systems. Scientists often use biomarkers to determine the rate or effectiveness of a biological process in its natural state and after functional food administration. Biomarkers can be protein, blood sugar, cholesterol, triglyceride levels, or hormone levels. Like bioactive compounds, biomarkers are a diverse group of compounds and processes. As each and every bodily process triggers countless biological responses, there are numerous ways to measure the rate or effectiveness of a process.

Biomarkers are highly useful in functional food research. Firstly, when scientists theorize that a bioactive compound will have certain benefits, changes in biomarker activity confirm or deny these benefits. Secondly, biomarkers can indicate the mechanism by which bioactive compounds prevent or treat illness. Biological pathways are often long, convoluted processes; therefore, researchers may undergo years of research to confirm details about a pathway. Biomarkers are often integral parts of biological pathways. Analyzing these are excellent ways of determining reaction mechanisms, particularly the order of each process and the roles that each enzyme, protein, and molecule play. Thirdly, observing biomarkers in a specific process can clarify the role that a bioactive compound plays in the body on several levels. For example, scientists may measure proteins levels in the liver and hormonal stimulation in the stomach while administering lactose (milk sugar) to a patient. In this case, scientists measure biomarkers involved in disparate processes in order to observe how a bioactive compound (lactose) affects both their activity levels. Functional food scientists try to choose the most efficient, accurate, and easily measured biomarkers in their studies.

In total, with the addition of bioactive compounds and the implicit role of biomarkers, the new functional food definition is complete. While previous definitions simply stated that functional foods improve health and mitigate disease, the current definition provides a reason—activity by bioactive compounds—and implies the use of biomarkers, essential tools for gauging functional food effectiveness.

How New Definition Will Help Create New Functional Food Products

Establishing a definitive meaning for functional food will not only bring about a consensus between scientists and governmental officials; it will also help to formally introduce functional foods to global markets.

By 1997, Japan, Europe, and the United States each generated $3 billion in sales with a projected $130 billion dollars in global sales by 2015 [4, 5, 9]. However, food industrialists have made claims based on differing definitions. As a result, their health claims are not always based upon strong scientific research and experimentation. Therefore, as more functional food products enter the market, public health risks rise.

Functional food scientists would like to revise this process by establishing a new definition for functional food, which would allow food industrialists to base their health claims on supported research. Bringing legitimate functional foods to markets would benefit billions suffering from chronic diseases and general health problems.

Expanding Worldwide Consumer Acceptance

As the functional food market gains momentum, manufacturers increasingly recognize the need for consumer acceptance [6-10]. A 1999 study found that knowledge and beliefs about functional food play significant roles in determining whether individuals purchase or consume functional food [11]. Important beliefs about functional foods include "one's own impact on personal health, health benefit belief, perception of health claims, belief in the food-disease prevention concept, belief in the disease-preventative nature of natural foods, and opinions of the relationship between food and health" [13, 12-16].

As of now, consumer attitudes toward functional foods differs greatly between the EU and the United States. While Americans want to eat healthier food and consider themselves capable of doing so, they have, overall, not made that lifestyle shift [17]. More interestingly, while Americans have had a positive perception of functional foods since 1998, they are unfamiliar with the meaning of "functional food" [18]. In contrast to Americans, Northern Europeans are skeptical and Danish consumers consider functional foods to be ''unnatural and impure'' [19, 20].

Researchers also found that consumers who reported that they had "high knowledge" about functional foods were less likely to accept functional foods. This finding probably resulted from flaws in consumer self-research, and is significant because it suggests that consumers receive misinformation about functional food from unreliable sources, such as the internet, television, and other media sources. In contrast, a standardized definition and professional scientific marketing could properly educate consumers.

Measuring consumer attitudes towards functional foods worldwide is a complex process, taking into consideration consumers' trust of scientific claims, government agencies, and new foods in general. However, one can deduce that consumers in some Western countries want to pick healthy foods, but have inaccurate information and misplaced biases toward functional food.

Studies have shown that a person's belief in a food's health benefits is a powerful motivator towards their acceptance of the new food [8]. Hence, educating consumers about the health benefits of functional food may eradicate doubts in the minds of Western consumers [38]. While a formal standard definition alone cannot resolve all public doubts, functional food scientists, if given the opportunity and legislative legitimacy, can do so.

Steps to Bringing Functional Foods to the Market

According to the Institute of Food Technologists (IFT), an organization that distributes knowledge about food, nutrition, technology, and policy, bringing functional food to the mass market requires a series of steps involving research, communication with government agencies, and effective public marketing [21, 38].

The FFC agrees with IFT's general progression from research to marketing. However, we have created our own cycle of steps (Figure 1). In Step 1, we examine the link between a particular food and health benefits. Then, in step 2 we run in vitro and in vivo studies with non-living and animal specimens respectively. We run human studies in step 3. This involves administering human-appropriate dosages of bioactive compounds and testing for adverse side effects. In Step 4, we develop appropriate food vehicles for our bioactive compounds (e.g. fig, celery, or apple with a special yoghurt coating), and in Step 5, we market to the public and educate them about the health benefits of functional food. We run studies on populations to test for long-term effects and overall product effectiveness in step 6. Finally, in Step 7, we measure public attitudes toward functional food. Four additional research-related steps toward bringing functional foods to markets will be focused on in this chapter.

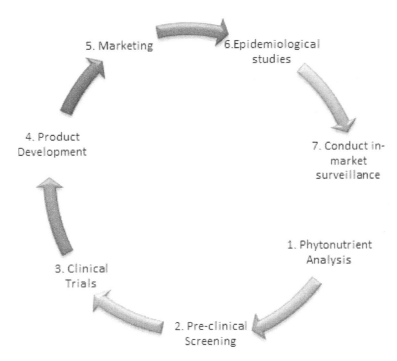

Figure 1. Steps for bringing functional foods to markets (FFC-2015)

Step 1: Identify the relationship between the food component and the health benefit.

First and foremost, scientists must prove their food has some link to health promotion. Functional foods are like drugs in that they can prevent, manage, and treat illness. Because bioactive compounds are vast and diverse, their modes of action fall within a wide range. For instance, compounds can be "mediators, anti-inflammatory agents, modulators of inflammatory cells, cytokines, and gene expression…or free radicals scavengers" [22].

Scientists have also found that phytochemicals can mimic hormones to produce a response or activate non-specific immune cells [23-28].

Some phytochemicals or bioactive compounds in functional foods act in biochemical enzymatic reactions as substrates and cofactors. This phenomenon, often seen in pharmacology, can speed up or slow down chemical reactions by aiding or inhibiting the enzymes involved. Phytochemicals may bind "to specific constituents to enhance absorption, transport or excretion, and scavenging and eliminating reactive or toxic chemicals and species" [21, 29-31]. As a result, bioactive compounds affect biochemical pathways and may alter inflammatory, fat storage, or energy storage processes. These results contain implications toward preventing obesity, cancer, and other chronic diseases.

Overall, bioactive compounds use their biological and chemical attributes, such as: "acidic, basic, chelating, hydrophobic and hydrophilic properties, as well as their amphipathic properties", to bind to "proteins, enzymes, free radicals, glycolipids and membranes of" microbial cells. Specifically, this binding slows or prevents microbes from replicating their genetic material which thereby slows the movement or progression of an infection. Phytochemicals can help kill microbes by changing or affecting microbial proteins, a process which may inhibit microbial gene replication.

There are innumerable in vitro and clinical studies that illustrate how functional foods benefit health and prevent, manage, or treat illness (21, 32-39).

Studying Bioactive Compounds with Biomarkers

The physiological effects of functional food are varied and are increasing as research progresses. However, certain categories of functional food effects have been identified [38]:

- Physical performance
- Cognitive, behavioral, and psychological function
- Organ or system function (gastrointestinal, genitourinary, bone)
- Chronic disease (heart disease, peripheral vascular disease, diabetes, hypertension, obesity, cancer, degenerative and inflammatory arthritis)

Measuring bioactive compounds activity can be challenging when the chemical structure or identity of the compound is unknown. In that case, researchers must examine the activity of biomarkers, like metabolites or surrogate compounds, in order to assess the health effects of a functional food.

Biomarkers or substitute biomarkers must illuminate the relationship between a functional food (and its bioactive compounds) and one or more biological functions. Ideal biomarkers should remain stable over a long period of time [38]. Below (Table 1) are examples of biomarkers that can be used in functional food studies.

Table 1: Biomarkers for Measuring Physiological Effects

Physiological Category	Biomarker Category	Biomarkers
Gastrointestinal	Digestive symptoms	Release of amylase, peristalsis, stomach churning, absorption
	Digestive rates	Gastric emptying time, intestinal transit times
	Digestive hormones	Insulin, cholecystokinin changes
Bone	Bone density	Bone mineral density by dual x-ray absorptiometry
Genitourinary	Symptom recurrence rates	Rates of fracture
	Levels of osteo compounds in serum/blood	Serum levels of osteocalcin, bone-specific alkaline phosphatase, vitamin D (hydroxyproline, pyridinium cross links, or cross-linked N-telopeptides of type 1 collagen)

Determining Causality

Determining causality, the relationship in which certain events (causes) lead to another set of events (effects), is a premier scientific activity [36]. While establishing causality is difficult (as it requires independent and dependent variables, control for confounding variables, and sufficient participants), the process can generate worthwhile results. For instance, scientists use existing causal relationships to understand new phenomena. Causality is a stronger link than correlation, which merely establishes a relationship between two events or variables. In other words, scientists strive to find causal links in order to better understand worldly phenomena. Functional food science is no different. In fact, the IFT believes that establishing causality is a key process to bringing functional foods to market [37].

There are several existing models of causality. One of the most well-known models was created by Bradford Hill in 1971 [38]. Hill's criteria helps determine the strength of proposed causal relationships [39]:

1. Strength of Association: There must be a strong correlation or relationship between the independent and dependent variables.
2. Temporality: The cause must precede the proposed effect.
3. Consistency: The result must be reproducible with different tests, experimenters, conditions, and instruments.
4. Theoretical Plausibility: A hypothesis regarding a particular cause-effect relationship should have some previously established research or theoretical reasoning behind it.
5. Coherence: The hypothesis should align somewhat with existing knowledge or theories about the variables of interest. It should not oppose existing knowledge unless the researcher has probable cause to do so.
6. Specificity in the causes: Ideally, the effect should only have one cause.
7. Dose Response Relationship: The relationship between an independent variable (e.g. amount of bioactive compound ingested) and dependent variable (e.g. cancer cell differentiation) is direct or dose-dependent. In other words, as the amount of bioactive compound ingested increases, the level of cancer cell differentiation also increases.
8. Experimental Evidence: Existing experimental or causal studies related to one's study will bolster one's claim.
9. Analogy: A researcher may use ideas from other scientific paradigms to formulate hypotheses or interpret results.

Step 2: Demonstrate efficacy, determine the intake level necessary to achieve the desired effect, and demonstrate that the functional food/bioactive compound(s) is not toxic at the efficacy level.

How well do bioactive compounds and functional foods work at promoting health? How much does the average adult need in order to stay healthy or reduce their risk of contracting an illness? These questions are essential to bringing functional foods to mainstream markets.

Researchers know that bioactive compounds and phytochemicals are diverse in their structures and modes of action, although scientists have determined how certain bioactive compounds function. For example, phytochemicals that help relieve symptoms of chronic disease may act as antioxidants. To do this, phytochemicals disrupt free radical reactions by donating their "hydroxyls, methoxylated, carboxylic, and methyl functional groups." Bioactive compounds could also act as antioxidants using "their hydrophilic, hydrophobic, acidic, basic, and charge to size properties" to inhibit enzymes propagating free radical synthesis. Finally, phytochemicals are capable of slowing bacterial and/or virus replication by blocking microbial invasion into "DNA, RNA, [or] protein synthesis" in cells [22].

When trying to determine the efficacy and/or proper dosage level of a bioactive compound, several factors must be considered, such as the bioactive compound's "class" (e.g. carbohydrates, proteins, lipids, vitamins, minerals, etc.), metabolism (e.g. absorption, transport, metabolism and excretion), analysis (e.g. analytical, chromatographic, genetic, combination, etc.), laboratory and clinical evaluation (e.g. in vivo, in vitro, epidemiological, etc.) and assessment of intake levels (e.g. recommended, upper and lower levels, toxicity) [22].

Thus, evaluating efficacy and intake levels of bioactive compounds requires both level approaches, from cellular to organismal, and multidimensional scientific approaches, from nutrition to genetics.

Measuring efficacy

Traditional medics of various cultures can attest to the success of plants as medicines and herbs. However, in order for these testimonies to be accepted in modern medicine, plants and their bioactive compounds must be tested through rigorous in vitro and in vivo studies [22].

Prior to running either in vitro or in vivo studies, researchers must decide on appropriate experimental methods. Efficacy testing requires accurate, sensitive, specific, and reliable experimental methods. When choosing testing method(s), scientists should consider the following questions [37]:

1. What is being studied and analyzed? Is it one entity or a collection of entities?
2. Is the entire entity of interest or only the bioactive component?
3. What are the lower and upper amounts of analyte that must be ascertained?
4. Does the compound of interest demonstrate varying levels of effectiveness depending on its chemical form?
5. Does the functional food matrix affect the compound's effectiveness?
6. Does food processing affect the compound of interest and/or experimental analysis?

Testing methods should measure the bioactive or harmful compound at the amount at which a certain effect is expected. Note that different bioactive compounds may have different "peak" levels, which then requires multiple efficacy tests.

In vitro studies

In order to study phytochemical effectiveness at fighting disease, researchers may begin with **in vitro** studies or inanimate lab-based studies. Often fibroblast (connective) or HeLa (cancer) cells are prepared in a pH and temperature-appropriate medium. Cells are usually "incubated at 37°C at 5% CO_2" while researchers measure cell growth with a light microscope. Researchers may also measure cell proliferation by dyeing the cells with trypan blue, adding trypsin, and counting the cells with a cell counter. Researchers can then measure growth by dyeing cells, allowing them to become chromophores, and measuring sample absorbance in a spectrophotometer. Afterwards, researchers prepare bioactive compounds in concentrations that either cause 50%, 90%, and 100% inhibition or cell death. These concentrations help determine a bioactive compound's inhibitory effectiveness.

Finally, researchers add the various concentrations of bioactive compound to cell lines containing microbes. Cell growth can be measured every 24 or 72 hours. Normal biological pathways suggest that parasites will attempt to multiply by infiltrating the healthy cells. The bioactive compound can stop the spread of infection by inhibiting cell growth and killing infected cells.

Using a light microscope, cell counter, or spectrophotometer, researchers can measure the cell growth that follows infection. If bioactive compounds successfully inhibit cell growth, researchers may use "immunological assays, cloning, and PCR techniques" to determine the mechanism(s) or pathway(s) by which the bioactive compound operates.

In vivo studies

In vivo studies involve living subjects, such as animals or humans. If researchers are conducting clinical or human research, they must get informed consent from participants. Participants must understand the experimental procedures; the "potential benefits, adverse effects, outcomes, and handling of the information collected from participants" [22]. Obtaining consent allows for ethical experimentation and protects researchers from legal charges if an experiment is unsuccessful.

Afterwards, researchers screen participants for certain requirements, such as age or symptoms of an illness. Researchers then conduct physical examinations of the participants, such as analyses of "blood, serum, plasma, urine, saliva, and sweat" [22].

Next, researchers prepare various concentrations of the bioactive compound in question in a tablet or syrup form. The bioactive compounds are administered to participants, animal or human, orally or via injection. Oftentimes, participants serve as their own experimental and control groups. For instance, researchers may administer the drug via injection to a participant's one arm or leg (experimental) and leave the other arm or leg alone (control). In this way, researchers obtain more accurate data and twice the amount of information than if they split the group into two treatments.

Depending on the study, researchers may measure levels of "proteins, lipids, fatty acids, gene expression, and certain enzymes" using "electrophoresis, high performance/thin layer chromatographic, and gas-liquid chromatography or gas chromatography-mass spectrometer (GC-MS)". Finally, researchers may use immunoassays to measure "antigen-antibody interactions and protein expression" [22]. After one month, researchers should conduct follow-up treatment to test for any adverse effects from the bioactive compound.

To reiterate, when conducting in vivo clinical studies, researchers must get informed consent from all participants and make sure that the condition and concentrations of the administered bioactive compounds are safe.

Use of Epidemiological Studies

Epidemiological studies are useful since they examine how chronic diseases develop in entire populations over long periods of time. In terms of functional food research, epidemiological studies can draw strong conclusions about the relationships between diet, biomarkers, and illness. Researchers should use epidemiological studies to identify populations affected by a certain disease as well as dietary behaviors and/or risk factors that contribute to disease progression [38].

Effects of Bioavailability on Effectiveness

Bioavailability is the quality of food by which its nutrients can be absorbed and reach the necessary tissues. Functional food can vary in its bioavailability based on its physical form, chemical form, and the other foods in an individual's diet. For example, "when a food component is coated, microencapsulated, emulsified, or altered in some way from its original state, its absorption and utilization may be affected." Food elements' chemical state may affect bioavailability. For instance, iron's ferrous form is better absorbed than its ferric form [40]. Some foods can affect the level of absorption of other foods. "For example, a high level of zinc in the diet decreases copper absorption [41], while dietary vitamin C increases iron absorption [42]." As a result, researchers should carefully document and analyze the form in which they prepare bioactive compounds.

Determining proper intake/dosages

Functional food professionals cannot prescribe bioactive compounds and specific dosages to treat illnesses. However, researchers understand that bioactive compounds have "optimal levels" as well as "upper limits of tolerance" in humans [22].

A bioactive compound's optimal and upper limits depend on a variety of factors, including the compound's structure, food source, illness in question, and a patient's sex, age, height, and weight [43]. Moreover, scientists need to examine the eating behavior of a target population; specifically, how much the target population consumes the bioactive compound naturally. For example, if the proposed food vehicle is a radish and the target population (say American diabetes patients, ages 60-80 do not consume radishes regularly), researchers may find it wise to change their food vehicle to a food consumed to a greater extent by their target population. Likewise, the entire diet of the target population must be examined in order for researchers to balance the amount of nutrients being supplied through their functional food with nutrients supplied through other foods. As previously stated, bioactive compounds consumed at high levels can become toxic.

Absolute and Relative Intake

The first step to determining proper dosages for a bioactive compound involves measuring humans' absolute and relative intake of the compound [44].

The **absolute intake** of a bioactive compound measures how much of the compound an average person consumes per day; to do this, researchers must compile nutrition information/content of mass-consumed food and then calculate how much of a particular nutrient an individual consumes.

Relative intake is the amount of a bioactive compound an individual consumes compared to the amount of other nutrients an individual consumes. To measure this, researchers should monitor the breadth of food that their target population consumes and analyze the nutrient levels found in the most commonly consumed foods.

Optimal vs. Toxic Intake levels: Bioactive compounds work best when taken in certain dosages. Researchers attempt to find these optimal levels when comparing experimental dosages with dosages consumed naturally in the world. Conversely, bioactive compounds should not be overused, as they can be dangerous at high levels. Specifically, when compounds are consumed at "**toxic levels**," they switch from being beneficial antioxidants, to harmful pro-oxidants. As a result, these once-helpful compounds can promote oxidation, leading to the organ/tissue damage and chronic disease [22, 45].

Allergen Safety

A final but important safety consideration is food allergies. **Food allergies** are medical conditions in which one's immune system reacts abnormally to the ingestion of particular foods [38, 46]. In individuals with food allergies, immune systems react adversely to certain food proteins. These "bad" proteins could either be naturally occurring or added during processing. Regardless, allergic symptoms range from "mild and annoying to severe and life threatening" [38, 47]. Considering the seriousness of food allergies in humans, functional food scientists should screen their products for allergens. There are indexes of existing protein allergens, but new proteins should also be tested for allergenic potential.

Quality of Scientific Evidence

Over time, the scientific community has compiled features of noteworthy literature, indicative of strong experimental evidence:

1. Double-blind experiments controlled for confounds
2. Long-term studies demonstrating consistent results and little to no adverse side-effects
3. Identified dose-response relationship
4. Identified biochemical mechanism and/or relevant biomarkers
5. Statistical significant results (e.g. $p < .05$)
6. Meaningful results to public health and wellness

Experimental contexts can greatly affect results from study to study. Confounding variables may include: "differences in dosage, the form of administration, the population tested, non-dietary factors such as smoking, and environmental contaminants or conditions..." [38]. Regardless, researchers should be able to explain inconsistencies between studies.

Step 3: Make approved health claims

Obtaining approval for food claims in Japan:

Japan, the birthplace of functional foods, acts as a pseudo-model for the FFC's steps for bringing functional foods to market. The Japanese government approves health claims and admission into the legislative category of FOSHU (Foods for Specific Health Uses) using an application process. The FFC supports the overall process by which Japan approves functional food. Japan is also noteworthy because it has a formal definition for functional food, enables greater understanding amongst its citizens, and acts as a leader in food sales.

Obtaining Approval for Food Claims in the U.S.

In contrast to Japan, the United States has not formally defined "functional food." While sales are strong in the U.S., functional food manufacturers exploit the concept of functional food for the sake of profit, thereby weakening scientists' motivation to create good products. This vicious cycle prevents quality functional foods from getting on the market and reaching chronically ill populations.

FDA Functional Food Approval

Currently, the Food and Drug Administration (FDA) evaluates functional foods in the same way they do conventional food. As a result, functional food manufacturers cannot make claims stating functional foods have the ability to prevent, manage, or treat illness, because that would classify functional foods as drugs or pharmaceuticals. Drugs undergo much more scrutiny than foods; FDA drug approval requires the completion of a "new drug application," which involves enormous testing and funding [38].

As for food health claims, the FDA only allows manufacturers to state that their food's health benefits are derived from the food's "nutritive value" or growth promotion, replacement of nutrient loss, and energy provision [47]. Besides the definition for "nutritive value" being vague, it does not accurately reflect how functional food provides health benefits, which restricts the range of permissible health claims [38].

Specifically, functional food manufacturers must avoid any language that indicates disease reduction. This leads to claims that are confusing, misleading, or even false. For example, instead of saying that a functional food reduces blood cholesterol (which implies that original blood cholesterol was high), food manufactures would have to say that their product "maintains normal cholesterol levels," a false statement if the food did lower cholesterol.

IFT adds that "scientific, regulatory, and business frameworks must be in place" in order to evaluate functional foods for efficacy and safety, prevent regulatory error, and improve consumer understanding of these products [38]. Finally, IFT agrees that "traditional definitions and arbitrary distinctions between food and medicine" is an issue that must be addressed in order to properly educate consumers and increase functional food access in markets [38].

Assessment of Functional Food Scientists

At the FFC, we are aware of the amount of time and resources needed to create safe, effective, and good quality functional foods. Scientists who are professional and invested in functional food creation must undergo:

1. Nutritional and biochemical education
2. Scientific research
3. Product development
4. Marketing and investment in all this steps

This process requires years of studies and multimillion dollar investments. We believe that government agencies, such as the U.S. FDA and EU FUFOSE should be wary of those seeking to manufacture and market functional foods. In other words, we believe that governments should not only judge a manufacturer's or scientist's research findings, but also his or her background and experience in this area [38]. Market research has shown that food manufacturers take advantage of legitimate scientific inquiry by, for example, utilizing a prior approved health claim tested by experienced scientists [38]. This process, of course, generates greater profits but compromises the potency of health claims and food research. Ideally, functional food researchers and manufacturers should be very experienced, professional, and demonstrate their commitment to creating safe, effective, and quality functional foods. As implied above, creating proper functional food is a highly involved and collaborative process, requiring intense dedication and respect for the scientific process. Therefore, government agencies should carefully weigh the intentions of prospective scientists who hope to market and sell functional foods.

Step 4: Get a special label for functional foods

Japan's functional food regulation is unique because each approved functional food is stamped with a FOSHU label. This designation separates functional food products from ordinary food products, allowing for greater clarity and accessibility to consumers. The FOSHU stamp also allows for greater legitimacy among consumers, because it implies that high quality research, funding, and regulation went into that food product. In this way, functional foods or FOSHU have a higher status in Japan than regular foods.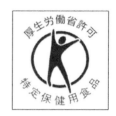

Bringing more legitimate functional foods to the market will be difficult. However, establishing a formal definition for functional foods is an important step. When governments and scientists agree on what makes a food "functional," laws and policies can be put in place that encourage research and greater dissemination of products. If the public (which is often guided by personal beliefs and self-education) is properly educated about functional foods, then they will naturally come to welcome functional foods. A standardized definition and legislative legitimacy will give functional food scientists the right and credibility to educate the public. As a result, world will exhort functional food production and research into the role of diet on health. Ultimately, a new definition for functional food is the first step to bringing quality functional foods to consumers all over the world.

SUMMARY

> ➢ Functional food originated in Japan in the 1980s. Food scientists submitted evidence that their foods had "advantageous physiological effects." Approved foods then acquired special FOSHU, or Food for Specific Health Uses, labels.
> ➢ Europe, the United States, other countries and various scientific organizations attempted to create their own definitions of functional food. This led to high sales worldwide, but confusion between countries and among the public on the meaning of functional food.

➢ The Functional Food Center (FFC) defines "functional food" as natural or processed foods that contains known or unknown biologically-active compounds; which, in defined, effective non-toxic amounts, provide a clinically proven and documented health benefit for the prevention, management, or treatment of chronic disease. This definition is unique because of its acknowledgement of "bioactive compounds"; or biochemical molecules that improve health through physiological mechanisms. Also, this definition notes that bioactive compounds must be taken in non-toxic amounts, because bioactive compounds have upper limits before they become dangerous.

➢ The FFC seeks to standardize the functional food definition in order to legitimize functional food science. We also want to formally bring functional foods to markets, improve international communication, and better population health.

REVIEW QUESTIONS

1. The following term is deemed to be somewhat synonymous with functional food:
   a. Dietary supplement
   b. Probiotics
   c. Nutraceutical
   d. Bioactive compounds

2. A food in a U.S. supermarket contains a claim that "it supports immune function and healthy cholesterol levels." This claim would be considered a:
   a. Structure/function claim
   b. Health claim
   c. Nutrient content claim
   d. Nutritional claim

3. The main difference between functional food and ordinary food is that:
   a. Functional food comes in the form of a pill or capsule
   b. Functional food is genetically modified
   c. Functional food can be consumed safely at any amount
   d. Functional food has some health benefit beyond basic nutrition

4. What is not a part of Hill's criteria?
   a. The relationship between an independent variable and dependent variable is direct or dose-dependent.
   b. The result must be reproducible with different tests, experimenters, conditions, and instruments.
   c. The result must be widely accepted by the general public
   d. There must be a strong correlation or relationship between the independent and dependent variables

5. What does not affect a bioactive compound's effect on the body?
   a. Patient's physiological properties
   b. The compound's structure
   c. Illness in question
   d. How long ago the compound has been consumed

6. Indicators in the body that give off signals in tissues, organs, or systems, and are often used to determine the rate or effectiveness of a biological process in its natural state and after functional food administration are called
    a. Biomarkers
    b. Dosage markers
    c. Functional Food
    d. Bioactive compounds

7. Strong experimental evidence is backed by
    a. A general consensus in the community without verified scientific evidence
    b. Long term studies where variables have been controlled to produce the most positive effect
    c. Long term studies that can only be applied in very specific conditions
    d. Long term studies with consistent results and little to no adverse side effects

8. Bioavailability varies based on
    a. The food's chemical form or state
    b. Other types of food that are consumed along with it
    c. The process used to prepare the food
    d. All of the above

9. All of the following are categories of functional food effects except
    a. Physical performance
    b. Genetic modification
    c. Organ or system function
    d. Cognitive, behavioral, and psychological function

10. Which country is considered the birthplace of functional foods?
    a. The United Kingdom
    b. The United States
    c. Japan
    d. Germany

Answers: 1. **(C)** 2. **(B)** 3. **(D)** 4. **(C)** 5. **(D)** 6. **(A)** 7. **(D)** 8. **(D)** 9. **(B)** 10. **(C)**

List of Abbreviations: Agricultural Research Service, ARS; Food and Drug Administration, FDA; Functional Food Center, FFC; Food for Specific Health Uses, FOSHU; Functional Food Science in Europe, FUFOSE; gas chromatography–mass spectrometer, GC-MS; Institute of Food Technologists, IFT; U.S. Department of Agriculture, USDA

Competing Interests: The authors have no financial interests or any other conflicts of interest to disclose.

Authors' Contributions: Danik Martirosyan, PhD: conceived and designed the study, analyzed and interpreted the data and actively involved in writing the manuscript; Jaishree Singh (intern student at FFC): collected the data, wrote the manuscript.

REFERENCES:

1. Dhiman, Anju, Vaibhav Walia, and Arun Nanda. "Introduction to the Functional Foods." Introduction to Functional Food Science: Textbook. 2nd ed. Richardson, TX: Functional Food Center, 2014.

2. O'Donnell, C.D. 2003 Ten trends in nutraceutical ingredients. Prepared Foods. 172: 89-92.

3. Functional Food Center, Dallas, Texas. Web. 3 Apr. 2015. [http://functionalfoodscenter.net].

4. Heasman M: The regulation of functional foods and beverages in Japan. In Proceedings of the first Vitafoods International Conference. Edited by Blenford DE. Copenhagen: Food Tech Europe; 1997.

5. Young J: A perspective on functional foods. Food Science and Technology Today 1996, 10: 18-21.

6. Gilbert, L. (1997). The consumer market for functional foods. Journal of Nutraceuticals, Functional and Medical Foods, 1(3), 5–21.

7. Bredahl, L. (2000). Determinants of consumer attitudes and purchase intentions with regard to genetically modified foods – results of a cross-national survey. MAPP working paper, Aarhus School of Business.

8. Grunert, K. G., Bech-Larsen, T., & Bredahl, L. (2000). Three issues in consumer quality perception and acceptance of dairy products. International Dairy Journal, 10, 575–584.

9. Verbeke, Wim. "Consumer acceptance of functional foods: socio-demographic, cognitive and attitudinal determinants." Food quality and preference 16.1 (2005): 45-57.

10. Weststrate, J. A., van Poppel, G., & Verschuren, P. M. (2002). Functional foods, trends and future. British Journal of Nutrition, 88 (Suppl. 2), S233–S235.

11. IFIC (1999). Functional foods: Attitudinal research (1996–1999).Washington: IFIC, International Food Information Council Foundation.

12. Hilliam, M. (1996). Functional foods: the Western consumer viewpoint. Nutrition Reviews, 54 (11), S189–S194.

13. Childs, N. M. (1997). Functional foods and the food industry: consumer, economic and product development issues. Journal of Nutraceuticals, Functional and Medical Foods, 1 (2), 25–43.

14. Bech-Larsen, T., & Grunert, K. (2003). The perceived healthiness of functional foods: a conjoint study of Danish, Finnish, and American consumers' perception of functional foods. Appetite, 40, 9–14.

15. Wrick, K. L. (1995). Consumer issues and expectations for functional foods. Critical Reviews in Food Science and Nutrition, 35 (1&2), 167–173.

16. Childs, N. M., & Poryzees, G. H. (1997). Foods that help prevent disease: consumer attitudes and public policy implications. Journal of Consumer Marketing, 14 (6), 433–447.

17. Gilbert, L. (2000). The functional food trend: what's next and what Americans think about eggs. Journal of the American College of Nutrition, 19 (5), 507S–512S.

18. IFIC (2002). The consumer view on functional foods: yesterday and today. Food Insight, 2002 (May/June), 5, 8.

19. Meakelea, J., and Niva, M., (2002). Changing views of healthy eating: cultural acceptability of functional foods in Finland. Paper presented at Nordisk Sociology Kongress, P_a Island Reykjavik, Iceland, August 2002.

20. Niva, M. (2000). Consumers, functional foods and everyday knowledge. Paper presented at Conference of nutritionists meet food scientists and technologists, Porto, Portugal, 2000.

21. "Bringing Functional Foods to Market." - IFT.org. Web. 9 Mar. 2015. [http://www.ift.org/knowledge-center/read-ift-publications/science-reports/scientific-status-summaries/functional-foods/bringing-functional-foods-to-market.aspx].

22. Abugri, Daniel A., and Melissa Johnson. "Efficacy of Bioactive Compounds and Determine Intake Level Necessary to Achieve Desired Effect." Print.

23. Chihara G, Maeda Y, Sasaki T, Fukuoka F. (1969). Inhibition of mouse sarcoma 180 by polysaccharides from Lentinusedodes (Berk.). Nature, 222:687–8.

24. Lindequist U, Niedermeyer THJ, J ülich W-D. (2005). The Pharmacological Potential of Mushrooms Review. eCAM 2(3)285–299.

25. Mizuno T. (1999). The extraction and development of antitumor-active polysaccharides from medicinal mushrooms in Japan (review). International Journal of Medicinal Mushrooms, 1:9–30.

26. Reshetnikov SV, Wasser SP, Tan KK. (2001). Higher basidiomycota as a source of antitumor and immunostimulating polysaccharides (review). International Journal of Medicinal Mushrooms; 3:361–94.

27. Waltner-Law ME, Wang XL, Law BK, Hall RK, Nawano M, and Granner DK. (2002). Epigallocatechin Gallate, a Constituent of Green Tea, Represses Hepatic Glucose Production. Journal of Biological Chemistry, 277, 34933-34940.

28. Wasser SP, Weis AL. (1999). Medicinal properties of substances occurring in higher Basidiomycetes mushrooms: current perspectives (review). International Journal of Medicinal Mushrooms; 1:31–62.

29. Dillard CJ, German JB. Phytochemicals: nutraceuticals and human health. J Sci Food Agr 2000; 80:1744-1756.

30. Liu RH. Health benefits of fruit and vegetables are from additive and synergistic combinations of phytochemicals. Am J Clin Nutr 2003; 78:517S-520S.

31. Wallig MA, Heinz-Taheny KM, Epps DL, Gossman T. Synergy among Phytochemicals within Crucifers: Does It Translate into Chemoprotection? J Nutr 2005; 135:2972S-2977S.

32. Habtemariam S. Natural inhibitors of tumor necrosis factor-alpha production, secretion and function. Planta Medica 2000; 66:303-13.

33. Gerritsen ME, Carley WW, Ranges GE, Shen CP, Phan SA, Ligon GF, Perry CA. Flavonoids inhibit cytokines- induced endothelial cell adhesion protein gene expression. American Journal of Pathology 1995; 147:278-292.

34. Middleton E. Jr. Effect of plant flavonoids on immune and inflammatory cell function. Advance Experimental Medicine and Biology 1998; 439:175-182.

35. Di Carlo G, Mascolo N, Izzo AA, Capasso F. Flavonoids: old and new aspects of a class of natural therapeutic drugs. Life Sciences 1999; 65:337-353.

36. "Causality." Web. 24 Mar. 2015 [http://sekhon.berkeley.edu/papers/causality.pdf].

37. Clydesdale, Fergus. "Functional foods: opportunities and challenges." Food Tech 58.12 (2004): 35-40.

38. Hill, A.B. 1971. Statistical evidence and inference. Chpt. in "Principles of Medical Statistics," 9th ed. pp. 309-323. Oxford University Press, New York, NY

39. "How Do Epidemiologists Determine Causality?" Web. 22 Mar. 2015. [http://www.southalabama.edu/coe/bset/johnson/bonus/Ch11/Causality%20criteria.pdf].

40. Fairbanks, V.F. 1994. Iron in medicine and nutrition. Chpt. In "Modern Nutrition in Health and Disease," 8th ed. M.E. Shils, J.A. Olson, and M. Shike. pp. 185-213. Lea and Febiger, Baltimore, MD.

41. Fosmire, G.J. 1990. Zinc toxicity. Am. J. Clin. Nutr. 51: 225-227. Friis, R.H. and Sellers, T.A. 1999. "Epidemiology for Public Health Practice," 2nd ed., Aspen Publishers, Inc., Gaithersburg, MD.

42. Olivares, M., Pizarro, F., Pineda, O., Name, J.J., Hertrampf, E., and Walter, T. 1997. Milk inhibits and ascorbic acid favors ferrous bis-glycine chelate bioavailability in humans. J. Nutr. 127:1407-1411.

43. Erdman JW, Balentine Jr. D, Arab L, Beecher G, Dwyer JT, Folts J,Harnly J, Hollman P, Keen CL, Mazza G, Messina M, Scalbert A,Vita J, Williamson G, and Burrowes J. (2005). Flavonoids and Heart Health: Proceedings of the ILSI North America Flavonoids Workshop, May 31–June 1, 2005, Washington, DC.

44. Mennen L I, Walker R, Bennetau-Pelissero C, Scalbert A. (2005). Risks and safety of polyphenol consumption. Am J Clin Nutr: 81(suppl):326S-9S.

45. Constantinou AI; Mehta R; Husband A.(2003). Phenoxodiol, a novel isoflavone derivative, inhibits dimethylbenz(a)anthracene (DMBA)-induced mammary carcinogenesis in female Sprague-Dawley rats. European Journal of Cancer, 39:1012-1018.

46. Taylor, S.L. and Hefle, S.L. 2001. Food allergies and other food sensitivities. Food Technol. 55(9): 68-83.

47. "CFR - Code of Federal Regulations Title 21." CFR - Code of Federal Regulations Title 21. Web. 23 Apr. 201.

2

Bioactive Compounds: Their Role in Functional Food and Human Health, Classifications, and Defintions

Danik Martirosyan and Kasia Pisarski

Functional Food Institute, 4659 Texas St., Unit 15, San Diego, CA, 92116, USA

Introduction

Bioactive natural products have been actively and seriously investigated since the mid-nineteenth century, after Louis Pasteur discovered that fermentation is caused by microorganisms [1]. Despite that compounds from leaves, roots, and stems have been used in medicine for thousands of years, the chemical nature of bioactive compounds remained a mystery [1]. Ancient documentation of medicinal plants was discovered in the Euphrates and Tigris region. Several clay plates found there had drawings and scripts of medicinal plants, known today as opium, thyme, and liquorice, and dated from approximately 4000 BC. Engravings found in rocks from Babylon indicated the use of cinnamon, coriander, garlic, saffron, and senna. Found in Luxor, among the Babylonians, 800 recipes and approximately 700 medicinal plants were discovered from at least 3000 BC, including aloe, absinth, peppermint, colocynth, Indian hemp (cannabis), garlic, opium, poppy, juniper, cumin, ricinus seeds, and Arabic gum" [2]. The Mayans treated intestinal ailments with "fungi grown on roasted green corn" nearly 3000 years ago [1]. Around the same time, Shen-nung, a Chinese emperor, left a medicinal document called the Pen-tsao, which provided descriptions of various plants, including ergot, gentian, liquorice, opium, poppy, rhubarb, and valerian, which indicated the medicinal use of these plants from his time period [2-4].

Hippocrates, considered to be "the father of medicine," described the plants that he used in 60 documents written throughout his lifetime (c. 460–360 BC). Hippocrates is known for his statement, "Let food be thy medicine and medicine be thy food." After Hippocrates, between 370-287 BC, the philosopher Theophrastus wrote "De Causis Plantarum," which consisted of 8 volumes of documents, of which 6 have survived. These documents describe plants and their medicinal uses [2]. "Historia Naturalis" was written by the Roman philosopher, Pliny the Elder (23–79 AD) and it describes the use of 250 medicinal plants. Aulus Cornelius Celsus (c. 25 BC – c. 50 AD) also described 250 medicinal plants in his work titled "De Medicina" [2]. Considered one of the earliest pharmacopeias, "De Materia Medica" was written by Pedanius Dioscordies (40–80 A.D.) [2]. It covers a range of herbal medicines, for example, the extract of mandragora plants which he used as an anesthetic [2].

Avicenna (980-1037 AD) was a Persian physician and philosopher known for his work, "The Canon of Medicine," describing the production of juices, tinctures, extracts of herbs, pills with coatings, and distillation of alcohol for pharmaceutical use. He created a system for pharmacies with remedies including aloe, camphor, mastix, rhubarb, and saffron. Avicenna also recognized the importance of nutrition [2].

One of the first to perform a clinical trial was the important medicinal reformer, Phillipus Aurelius Theophrastus Paracelsus Bombastus von Hohenheim (1493-1541), also known as Paracelsus. Before recommending any kind of treatment, he wanted to have proof that it was effective. Some of his theories include:

"The body is a conglomerate of chemical compounds that have to be in equilibrium with each other. If they are not, so the body is ill, and other chemical components must be added to get the body in balance again."
"The healing chemical products should be found in plants by extractions, alchemy, distillation and pyrolysis."
"Everything is poison; it is just the concentration that will decide if something is nontoxic."

His theory on toxicity is still valid today [2].

The fungus *Penicillium notatum* is the bacteria-killing compound discovered by Sir Alexander Fleming (1881-1955).

The first billion-dollar chemotherapy drug, taxol (paclitaxel), is a fungal endophyte yielded from the Pacific yew tree (Taxus brevifolia) [1, 2].

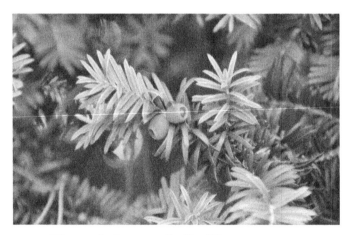

Figure 1: Image of a Pacific yew tree

Natural sources of bioactive compounds are now of interest to pharmaceutical, food, and pesticide industries, to name a few [5]. Over 50% of the latest drugs produced by pharmaceutical companies in the past two decades stem from plant origin. In the 20th century, pharmaceuticals primarily used alkaloids. Currently, the most studied bioactive compounds are flavonoids, a class of biophenols [5]. Plants contain the highest amounts of bioactive compounds, and most bioactive compounds have the ability to cause COX-2 inhibition in chemoprevention stages [6].

In defining the term "bioactive compounds," "bioactive" has the Greek root "bio" (life) and the Latin root "act" (drive, do). Bioactive compounds possess biological activity with the ability to modulate metabolic processes [7]. Plants produce bioactive compounds of either primary or secondary metabolite classifications. The primary metabolites are amino acids, carbohydrates, and lipids, which are essential for plant growth and the basic metabolism of the plant. Secondary metabolites are defined by their low abundance, composing less than 1-5% of the plant's dry weight, and are not needed for daily plant function [8]. However, secondary metabolites have important functions such as protection, attraction, and signaling [9]. Generally, the bioactive compounds of the secondary metabolites have pharmacological or toxicological effects on humans and animals [9]. Most plants have the ability to produce these compounds, while poisonous or medicinal plants contain higher concentrations of the more potent bioactive compounds [9]. Additionally, bioactive compounds are further classified into nutritive and non-nutritive ingredients, which possess significant benefits to maintain and promote health [7, 10]. According to Kris-Etherton et al., bioactive compounds are "extra-nutritional constituents that typically occur in small quantities in foods," which are believed to exert antioxidant, cardioprotective, and chemopreventive effects, beneficial in reducing the risks associated with the pathogenesis of certain diseases [6, 11]. As the scientific community continues to perform research on bioactive compounds found in functional foods, the latest definition of functional foods by the Functional Food Center (FFC) emphasizes "effective and non-toxic amounts." The advancement of research on the mechanisms of bioactive compounds and specific biomarkers drives the development of functional food products for health promotion and disease management. As functional foods research continues, the definition will continue to be refined. The FFC currently defines functional foods as "natural or processed foods that contain known or unknown biologically active compounds, which, in defined, effective, and non-toxic amounts, provides a clinically proven and documented health benefit utilizing specific biomarkers for the prevention, management, or treatment of chronic disease or its symptoms." [12].

New bioactive compounds are constantly discovered and identified. Generally, small molecules or bioactive compounds are found in the phytochemicals within functional foods. Bioactive compounds work together synergistically to benefit health and are also known as secondary metabolites [13]. Nutritive and non-nutritive bioactive compounds both have properties responsible for biological activity [7, 14]. Two of the most known properties are "cytostatic and antimitotic properties" found in numerous compounds [14]. These properties inhibit or arrest cell division, which are the essential properties of anti-carcinogens. The inability of the human body to synthesize many bioactive compound dictates that they must be obtained through the diet [6, 15].

Scientists have studied the health benefits of bioactive compounds found within foods. Through the use of biomarkers, scientists have determined specific health benefits associated with bioactive compounds. Biomarkers are molecules within the body that are tested or monitored to detect physiological changes and chronic diseases. These specific and sensitive biomarkers are associated with specific chronic diseases and their symptoms. As bioactive compounds prove their health benefits, a structural or functional claim can be introduced as supporting the specific chronic disease. This proof of claim initiates the ability to find natural or enriched foods with the bioactive compound specific to that biomarker and health claim. These natural and enriched foods are now functional foods. Scientists can then further provide the essential dose of functional foods to prevent and manage chronic disease and its symptoms [13]. A physiologic dose of bioactive compounds is achieved through the diet and will typically fall in the "characteristic range of plasma and tissue levels" [16]. A supra-physiologic dose, also referred to as a pharmacologic dose, exceeds the physiologic intake of bioactive compounds for extended periods of time and/or is an increased intake at 2-3 times the physiologic dose [16]. However, plasma levels do not reflect the cellular level of micronutrients where deficiencies can occur [16, 17]. Supra-physiologic doses may help provide nutrients at the cellular level, and help manage disease and its symptoms.

To obtain the "functionality" of a bioactive compound and receive its therapeutic benefit, a correct dosage is crucial. Bioactive compounds are not equal in the sense that the body absorbs some bioactive compounds better than it does others [13]. In the article, "A New Definition of Functional Food by FFC" (2015), two important concepts relating to bioactive compounds are: the amount of bioactive compounds and ratio of bioactive compounds to convert an ordinary food into a functional food. Different amounts of bioactive compounds are effective in different situations and at times, too much of a bioactive compound in a food can be toxic. In general, consuming physiologic levels of bioactive compounds is considered safe. Consuming higher levels of bioactive compounds (e.g. supra-physiological or therapeutic doses) must be tested for their safety and health benefits [13].

Nutritive Bioactive Compounds

Primary Metabolites

Nutritive bioactive compounds are classified as proteins, carbohydrates, lipids, vitamins, and minerals [7]. According to the article by the FFC, "The effects of bioactive compounds on biomarkers of obesity," vitamins are some of the most well-known bioactive compounds [10]. Nutritive bioactive compounds are added to enrich foods, providing numerous processed foods the known biologically active compounds necessary to make a functional food. Milk has been fortified with vitamin D for some time with recently added protein and omega fatty acids now being added to some brands of milk. Protein content has been increased in a variety of breads, and enriched grains provide added B vitamins and replaces fiber lost in the processing of grains.

Bioactive Lipids

Butyric acid a bioactive compound in milk lipids and is a main by-product of fiber fermentation [7]. Butyric acid induces regeneration and growth of cells in the large intestine, in addition to having anticancer properties in the colon, which are attributed to the induction of apoptosis in mutant colonic cells [7].

Polyunsaturated fatty acid (PUFA)

Bioactive compounds of polyunsaturated fatty acids (PUFAs) are essential nutritive compounds or essential fatty acids. Two classes of PUFAs are omega-3 and omega-6 (*n*-3 and *n*-6) fatty acids [20]. Linoleic acid, an omega-6 fatty acid, has 18 carbons and 2 double bonds [7]. Found mostly in plant glycosides, linoleic acid is essential for humans in the biosynthesis of prostaglandins [18]. The omega 3-fatty acid, alpha-Linolenic acid, elongates to docosahexaenoic acid (DHA) and eicosapentaenoic acid (EPA). DHA and EPA are essential for regulating metabolic processes, brain development, and heart health [7, 19, 20]. Bioactive compounds with pro-inflammatory and anti-inflammatory properties are formed through the hydrolysis process of fatty acids [19]. These bioactive compounds have demonstrated the ability to prevent atherosclerosis [20, 21, 22], regulate nuclear transcription factors involved in gene expression of inflammatory markers, and stimulate cognitive development [20, 23, 24].

Bioactive Proteins
Animal Protein Sources

The physiological activity of many proteins with biological functions occur in the gastrointestinal tract, where they "enhance nutrient absorption, inhibit enzymes, and modulate the immune system to defend against pathogens" [25]. Gelatin and fish proteins have bioactive compounds. First, gelatin has ACE (angiotensin converting enzyme) inhibitory peptides from bacterial collagenase. Fish protein also has ACE inhibitory peptides from pepsin, trypsin, and chymotrypsin [7].

In the animal protein beef, the animal feed determines the contents of bioactive components. Bioactive CLA (Conjugated linoleic acid) found in beef is a "collection of positional and geometrical isomers of cis-9, cis-12-octadecadienoic acids (C18:2) with a conjugated double bond system" [7]. The bioactive components of CLA, L-carnitine, and carnosine are affected and manipulated by what the animal is fed, with the richest natural source of CLA being found in milk fat [7, 26, 27]. Grass fed cattle provides higher levels of bioactive vitamin E, CLA, and omega-3 fatty acids, which are "higher in the intramuscular lipids of cattle" [26, 27]. Additional bioactive compounds found at different levels in different muscles are: coenzyme Q10, taurine, choline, anserine, and glutathione [26, 28-33]. Carnitine has hypocholesterolemic properties and carnosine antioxidant effects; coenzyme Q10 supports both cardiovascular and mitochondrial respiration; choline acts as a putative ergogenic agent; taurine has cardiovascular, hypolipidemic, and hypocholesterolemic properties; CLA has anti-carcinogenic, anti-obesity, anti-diabetic, anti-atherosclerosis, and immunomodulatory properties; anserine is an antioxidant and has buffering capacities; glutathione can increase the absorption of heme iron [7, 28]. Protein peptides are inactive until released within the gastrointestinal digestion [34].

Bioactive Milk Protein

The standard composition of milk is 3.5 percent protein, of which 80% is casein and 20% is whey proteins. These can be broken down into the following bioactive compounds: caseins (*a, B & k*) and whey (*B*-lactoglobulin, *a*-Lactalbumin, immunoglobulins (IgA, IgM, IgG), GMP, Lactoferrin, LPO, and Lysozyme) [7, 35]. The peptides' activity is determined by their sequences and inherent amino acid composition. A sequence can be 2 to 20 amino acids long and possesses multifunctional properties [35]. As an ion carrier for Ca, PO4 Fe, Zn, and Cu, caseins are precursors of bioactive peptides, immunopeptides, and phosphopeptides, are antihypertensive, and are opioid agonists and antagonists [7]. Furthermore, proteolyzation of phosphopeptides leads to the formation of ACE inhibitors during the ripening of cheese [35]. An opioid agonist found in whey, *B*-lactoglobulin, is fatty acid-binding and a retinol carrier. A calcium carrier also found in whey, *a*-Lactalbumin, has anti-carcinogenesis and immunomodulatory properties. Immune protection is furthered through the immunoglobulins IgA, IgM, and IgG, which are immunomodulatory and have anti-viral, carcinogenic, hypertensive, and thrombotic properties [7]. These bioactive milk peptides have been identified as potential ingredients in health-promoting functional foods [35].

Bioactive Egg Protein

The bioactive compounds found in eggs have determined eggs to be a functional food according to Andersen [36]. Several bioactive compounds in eggs can influence pro- and anti-inflammatory pathways [36]. Ovalbumin, ovotransferrine (conalbumin), ovomucoid, ovamucin, lysozyme, ovoinhibitor, ficin, ovoglycoprotein, ovomacroglobulin, and avidin are the bioactive egg proteins that can impact inflammation [7]. The predominant egg white protein composition is illustrated below in figure 2.

The roles of these specific bioactive egg proteins identified in figure 2 play in health include: Ovalbumin, a phosphoglycoprotein; Ovotransferrin (conalbumin), binds metal ions; Ovomucoid, inhibits trypsin; Ovomucin, a sialoprotein, viscous; Lysozyme, antimicrobial; and Avidin, binds biotin. Other bioactive egg proteins are: Ovoinhibitor, inhibits serine proteases; Ficin (cystatin) inhibitor, inhibits thioproteases; Ovoblycoprotein, a sialoprotein; Ovomacroglobulin, a strong antigenic; and Avidin, binds biotin [7, 36]. Other health benefits noted are: antibacterial, anti-inflammatory, gastric wall permeability, muscle wall thickening, and attenuated weight loss [36].

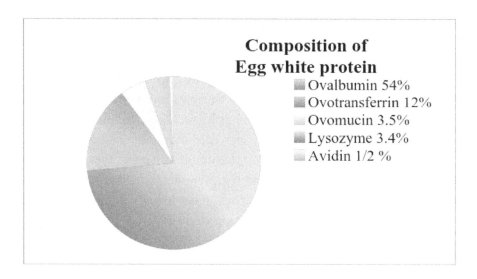

Figure 2: Martirosyan DM, Pisarski K. 2017. (Figure 2 created by Ref. 36 information)

Plant sources-bioactive protein

Plant sources, including corn, rice, wheat and soybean, consist of bioactive proteins, each bearing a specific main protein. The main protein present in corn is Alpha-zein protein with ACE inhibitory peptides by hydrolysis with thermolysine. Glutelin and prolamin are rice proteins with ACE inhibitory peptides. Wheat protein consists of Gliadin and glutelin proteins carrying opioid activity. Soybeans contain glycinins having anticarcinogenic properties and reduces high plasma cholesterol levels [7].

Lectins

Lectins are the major protein of lentils. These carbohydrate-recognizing proteins have a role in cell growth and death, immune function, regulation of body fat, repairing oxidative DNA damage, and protecting against cancer. They also have antimicrobial properties [7].

Bioactive proteins from glycoside, a carbohydrate fraction consists of galactose, N-acetyl-galactosamine, and N-neuraminic acid. Health benefits provided by these bioactive proteins include the ability to inactivate microbial toxins from *E. Coli* and *V. Cholerae*, promote bifidobacteria growth while suppressing gastric hormone growth, modulate immune system responses, and regulate blood circulation through antithrombotic and antihypertensive activities [7].

Bioactive Carbohydrates

Bioactive carbohydrates include dietary fiber as well as bioactive polysaccharides, oligosaccharides, and glycoproteins. Dietary fiber provides prebiotics and various oligosaccharides: Fructo-oligosaccharides, FOS (Inulins), Isomalto-oligosaccharides (Lactilol), Soy oligosaccharides (Pyrodextrins), Oligofructose, Transgalacto-oligosaccharides (TOS), Xylo-oligosaccharides, and Lactosucrose (Lactulose).

The bioactivities of polysaccharides found in medicinal plants are non-toxic with no known side effects. Additionally, bioactive polysaccharides are found in herbs, fungi, and seaweed, providing anti-cancer, anticoagulant, antioxidant, anti-tumor, anti-viral and immune-modulating activities [7, 37]. Both soluble and insoluble dietary fibers are non-digestible components of food. Health benefits from fiber include reducing rates of absorption of dietary fat and glucose and resorption of bile acids. Insoluble fiber is found in cereals, whole wheat bread, lentils, apples, and psyllium used as a dietary supplement in pill form to prevent constipation and reduce the risk of cancer [7].

Bioactive Vitamins

Essential in small amounts, bioactive vitamins are essential water or fat-soluble micronutrients. In high doses, such as supra-physiologic doses, bioactive vitamins can be toxic; therefore, adhering to non-toxic amounts is crucial.

Fat-soluble Bioactive Vitamins

Bioactive vitamin A supports vision in dim light. Bioactive vitamin E is essential for reproduction and has antioxidant activity. Bioactive vitamin K is essential for normal blood clotting and is produced in the gut. Bioactive vitamin D increases absorption, retention, and utilization of calcium and phosphorus in the body [7].

Bioactive vitamin A is can be toxic and even life threatening if taken in high doses or for extended periods. Excessive food sources of bioactive vitamin A may turn the skin orange or yellow without concern. However, supplementing 25,000 IU a day or more for extended periods can affect almost every part of the body, including the eyes, bones, blood, skin, central nervous system, liver, and genital and urinary tracts [38]. Beta-carotene provides protection against skin cancer; however, smokers who take beta-carotene supplements increase both their risk of lung cancer and death rate [16, 38]. Food sources appear to be safe [39]. Dizziness, headache, less frequent menses in women, mental problems, nausea, vomiting, and skin damage are all symptoms of overdosing bioactive vitamin A. In addition, blindness from severe toxicity can occur as well as an increased risk for gastric cancer, hip fractures, and osteoporosis. Children are at an increased risk of fluid on the brain and liver damage, along with the same complications [38]. Bioactive vitamin E includes 8 forms, with only the alpha-tocopherol form stored in the body [37]. Bioactive vitamin E plays a significant role in low-density lipoprotein (LDL) levels, "influencing the 'loading' of LDL" with bioactive vitamin E [16]. The bioactivity, which occurs in the liver, transports bioactive vitamin E into every LDL [16]. Abundant in food, bioactive vitamin K_1, phylloquinone is less bioactive than K_2 menquinones. Bioactive "vitamin K compounds undergo oxidation-reduction cycling within the endoplasmic reticulum membrane, donating electrons to activate specific proteins via enzymatic gamma-carboxylation of glutamate groups before being enzymatically reduced. Along with coagulation factors (II, VII, IX, X, and prothrombin), protein C and protein S, osteocalcin (OC), matrix Gla protein (MGP), periostin, Gas6, and other bioactive vitamin K-dependent (VKD) proteins support calcium homeostasis, inhibit vessel wall calcification, support endothelial integrity, facilitate bone mineralization, are involved in tissue renewal and cell growth control, and have numerous other effects" [40]. At very high doses, bioactive vitamin D can be very toxic. Excessive bioactive vitamin D can cause the intestines to absorb too much calcium, and high blood calcium levels and kidney failure can result from "long-term mega-doses" of bioactive vitamin D [38].

Water-soluble Bioactive Vitamins

Bioactive vitamins B and C are water-soluble vitamins. Niacin, folic acid, and bioactive vitamin B12 are part of bioactive vitamin B complex. Niacin is used and prescribed by physicians to aid in lowering blood cholesterol levels. Niacin deficiency can lead to a disease known as pellagra. The development of red blood cells requires an adequate supply of folic acid and is prescribed to women before or at conception to help prevent spine bifida. Bioactive vitamin B12 promotes energy and protects the cardiovascular system with food sources from animals, eggs, fish, plant sources, mushrooms, and/or fortified foods [7]. Essential for the formation and maintenance of cartilage, dentin, and collagen, therapeutic benefits of bioactive vitamin C can be reached at 200-300 mg per serving. However, toxicity due to bioactive vitamin C can occur when a supraphysiologic dose of 2000 mg or more is consumed daily and should only be administered in a clinical setting [41].

Bioactive Minerals

The structure and composition of body tissues includes several bioactive minerals, including: calcium (Ca), iodine, iron (Fe), iron chloride, magnesium (Mg), potassium (K), sodium (Na), selenium (Se), silicone, and zinc (Zn). Each of these bioactive minerals is an essential micronutrient and their bioactive activities provide specific functions.

The specific functions of these essential bioactive minerals are as follows: Calcium (Ca) is essential for the formation of bones and teeth. Iodine is an essential component of thyroid hormones. Iron (Fe) participates in oxygen transport and storage, electron transfer, and movement of oxygen from the environment to body tissues. Extra ellular volume and plasma osmolarity are bioactive activities of sodium (Na) and iron chloride (Cl). Magnesium (Mg) has a definitive role in nerve transmission, is an important mineral for the skeletal system, and affects blood pressure. Potassium (K) plays a role in both energy metabolism and membrane transport. Selenium (Se) has bioactive activities that are important functions for the thyroid, neural system, and immune system, and it additionally protects against oxidative stress, gastrointestinal disease, and cancer. Silicone supports healthy bone and mineral density. Zinc (Zn) performs catalytic, structural, and regulatory functions in protein, nucleic acid, carbohydrate, and lipid metabolism and is essential for eye health [7, 42].

Non-nutritive Bioactive Compounds

Non-nutritive bioactive compounds in food are health-promoting phytochemicals and natural antioxidants, which protect against DNA damage and modulate immune function. Important for plant growth, attraction, competition, defense, and signaling, these non-nutritive bioactive compounds are produced within plants besides the primary biosynthetic and metabolic routes [7] and used as the basis for various drugs [43]. Non-nutritive bioactive compounds are alkaloids, carotenoids, gluconsinolates, monoterpenes, organosulfur compounds, phytoestrogens, polyphenols, and saponins. Other non-nutritive bioactive compounds are enzyme inhibitors, phytic acid/phytates and phytosterols [7].

Secondary Metabolites

Phytochemicals

The "phyto" in the term phytochemical originates from the Greek root for "plant." Phytochemicals are plant chemicals and are defined as bioactive, non-nutritive plant compounds in fruits, vegetables, grains, and other plant foods that have been linked to reducing the risk of major chronic diseases" [15]. Synergistically, these compounds work in combination with each other to provide anti-proliferative properties that cannot be provided by one compound alone. According to the Journal of Nutrition (2004), clinical trials indicate that when combining four fruits (apple, blueberry, grape and orange), their antioxidant properties increase compared to when any one fruit is eaten alone. Additionally, particular bioactive compounds like essential fatty acids and chlorophylls are essential; the human body cannot synthesize these compounds and need to consume them through the diet [15].

Therefore, the essential bioactive compounds need to come from functional foods; they are the backbone of functional foods. Functional foods provide the compounds required to synergistically work together and provide optimal absorbability. Furthermore, it is estimated that one third of all cancer deaths in the United States could be avoided through appropriate dietary modification [15, 44-46]. Dietary recommendations suggest consuming adequate food sources of fruits and vegetables.

Polyphenols

Phenolic Compounds

The bioactive compounds known as phenolic compounds bear various chemical structures, each having their own physical properties. Phenolic compounds include 15 major structural classes comprised of over eight thousand naturally occurring phenolic compounds [47, 48]. Flavonoids, capsaicinoids, lignin, terpenoids, carotenoids, chlorophylls, vitamins, stilbene, phenolic acids, fibers, sterols, lipids, fatty acids, polysaccharides, and some plant-derived protein and peptides are the 15 major structural classes of phenolic compounds [6]. According to Obied in his article, "Biography of biophenols: past, present and future", the most studied biophenol classifications are: Flavonol (quercetin), Flavonoid glucoside (quercetin-3-O), rutinoside (rutin), Stilbene (Resveratrol), and Phenolic acid (caffeic acid and its quinic acid conjugate, chlorogenic acid).

Phenolic compounds are "produced as a response for defending an injured plant against pathogens." Their structure contains a minimum of one aromatic ring and one –OH group [47, 49]. The most basic phenol structure is shown in figure 3 below.

FIGURE 3. Phenol Structure

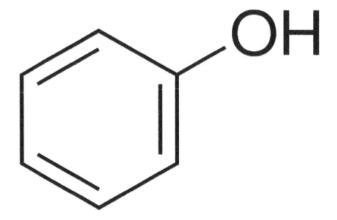

Image Source:
http://www.mpbio.com/images/product-images/molecular-structure/02194011.png

Table 1 provides a variety of examples of chemical structures of phenolic compounds and how the structures vary.

Table 1. Chemical structures of various phenolic compounds

Bioactive Compound	Chemical Structure
Flavonoid	
Capsaicinoid	
Lignin	 Lignin
Trepenoids	
Carotenoid	

The 15 major structural phenolic compounds are not found in all food sources. In fact, there are 11 major plant phenolic compounds. The table below provides carbon skeletons for these 11 major plant phenolic compounds [47, 50].

Additionally, many phenolic compounds are essential in protecting plants as well as humans. Phenolic compounds provide defense against herbivores, making the plant unpalatable and also defending the plant from microbial attacks [47, 50]. The fruit that is highest in total phenolic content and common in the American diet is the cranberry, followed by the apple, red grape, strawberry, pineapple, banana, peach, lemon, orange, pear, and grapefruit" [15, 56]. Broccoli has the highest phenolic content among vegetables, followed by spinach, yellow onion, red pepper, carrot, cabbage, potato, lettuce, celery, and cucumber [15, 57].

Table 2. Plant phenolics: major classes

Carbon Skeleton	Class name	Particulars
C6	Simple phenols	Catechol, phenol, hydroquinone, resorcinol and phloroglucinol
C6-C1	Benzoic acids	p-hydroxybenzoic acid, protocatechuic, vanillic, gallic, syringic, salicylic, o-pyrocatechuic and gentisic acids
C6-C2	Acetophenones ($C_6H_5C(O)CH_3$)	Found in chickory, used as a flavoring agent, additive to cigarettes
	Phenylacetic acids (Phenyl acetate) ($C_8H_8O_2$ or $C_6H_5CH_2CO_2H$)	Nitrogen binding agent and a carboxylic acid ester
C6-C3	The Phenylpropanoid Unit Hydroxycinnamic acids	Caffeic acid Cinnamic acids Coumarins
C6-C4	Hydroxyanthraquinones	Physcion
C6-C2-C6	Stilbenes	Resveratrol
C6-C3-C6	Flavonoids	Quercetin
(C6 –C3)2	Lignans	Matairesinol- $C20H22O6$ is found in asparagus, oil seeds, whole grains, fruits and vegetables. Regulates estrogen levels- escorts estrogen out- Flaxseed best source 1-2 T/day
(C6–C3–C6)n2	Bioflavonoids	Agathisflavone
(C6–C3)n	Lignins	Plant polymer- "strengthening material for the plant cell wall"
(C6–C3–C6)n	Proanthocyanidins Condensed tannins	Procyaxnidin

Table 2.0. References: [14, 47, 51-55]

Phytoesterogens

Isoflavones and lignans are the two groups of phytoesterogens. Soybeans and flaxseeds are the richest sources of these. These natural selected estrogen receptor modulators mimic the function of human estrogens and antiestrogens, providing protection against non-hormonal cancers, such as bowel cancer, cardiovascular diseases, and osteoporosis, as well as helping with menopausal symptoms [7]. Biological activities of phytoestrogens are highly variable, complex, and also species-specific. Isoflavones resemble oestradiol-17β and may act as an oestrogen agonist or antagonist through oestrogen receptor α and β" [58].

Alkaloids

Alkaloids are bitter compounds containing nitrogen-bearing molecules, and they are heterocyclic with anticholinergic activity. These secondary metabolites encompass a "broad variety of chemical structures," with over 20,000 compounds found in both plant and animal sources [59, 60]. Examples of alkaloids derived from amino acids (e.g. lysine, ornithine, and phenylalanine) are caffeine, ergots, LSD, morphine, quinine, reserpine, and strychnine [60].

The opium poppy (*Papaver somniferum*) is an opium alkaloid used as a painkiller and sedative medicinal plant containing 4 opium alkaloids. Opium alkaloids used in today's medicine are morphine, codeine, noscapine, and papaverine [2].

Saponins

Saponins are glycosides that have distinctive foaming characteristics and aid digestion. Saponins from oats and spinach can increase acceleration of the body's ability to absorb calcium, aiding in digestion [61]. Major sources of saponins are chickpeas and soybeans consisting of "lipid-soluble aglycone and water-soluble sugar residues, possessing anti-carcinogenic, hypocholesterolemic, and immune-stimulating properties" [7].

Monoterpenes

Monoterpenes are found in the essential oils of plants, herbs, mints, citrus fruits, cherries, and vegetables. Monoterpenes are naturally occurring hydrocarbons produced by the condensation of two isoprenes [62]. The anti-carcinogenic properties of limonene and perillyl alcohol effectively prevent and treat cancer "both in the initiation and promotion/progression stages" [62] as well as "decreasing the incidence of chemically induced tumors in the skin, liver, lung and breast" [7].

Glucosinolate and Isothiocyanates

Biologically active glucosinolates produce isothiocyanates, with a variety of these sulfur-containing glucosinolate compounds found in cruciferous vegetables. When hydrolyzed, different isothiocyanates are formed [61]. They reduce the risk of breast, esophagus, liver, lung, and stomach tumorigenesis, in addition to inhibiting carcinogen-induced formation and progression of cancer [7, 63].

Organosulfur compounds

Organosulfur compounds consist of water-soluble S-allylcysteine and S-allylmercaptocyteine compounds with antioxidant properties, and diallyl disulfide and diallyl sulfide compounds with anticarcinogenic effects. Found in garlic, the organosulfur compounds additionally provide a decreased risk of cardiovascular disease and reduce blood pressure, total and LDL cholesterol, and triglyceride levels [7].

Phytosterols

Structurally similar to cholesterol, the primary phytosterols are sitosterol, stigmasterol, and campesterol. Plants sources are of the unsaturated form; the saturated form, stanols, are more potent and are found in fruits, vegetables, and cereals. Phytosterols can reduce cholesterol serum levels [7].

Bioactive Carotenoids

Carotenoids are organic and known as "nature's most widespread pigments," imparting color and antioxidant properties. They are sourced from the chromoplast and chloroplast of many plants, fruits, vegetables, microorganisms, and even animals [7, 64]. The pigments are identified by their red, orange, and yellow colors, with over 750 natural occurring pigments identified [65]. Fats and other metabolic building blocks of phyto-synthetic organisms can produce carotenoids, and are produced in organisms such as fungi, certain bacteria, and algae [7]. The photo-oxidative damage is suggested to be involved in the pathology and biochemistry of several diseases affecting the skin and the eye, and carotenoids may protect light-exposed tissues" [64]. The bioactivities of the two predominant carotenoids, lutein and zeaxanthin, are photoprotectants preventing degeneration of the retina [64].

The structure and hydrogenation levels of carotenoids can vary. Either or both ends may be cyclized. Additionally, "oxygen-containing functional groups" may be present or a "40- carbon skeleton of isoprene units" [15]. The shape, chemical reactivity, and light-absorbing properties of carotenoids come from their long series of conjugated double bonds forming the central part of the molecule [15]. β-carotene is an example of a cyclic carotenoid, and lycopene is an example of an acyclic carotenoid [15].

A primary carotenoid in human blood and tissue is lutein [66]. Along with lutein, zeaxanthin is found within the xanthophyll class of carotenoids. Zeaxanthin is stored in the retina of the eye. Found in green vegetables such as broccoli, cabbage, and kale, lutein and zeaxanthin support eye health [67].

Carotenes form the second class of carotenoids. Carotenes have two categories: provitamin A and nonprovitamin A. Provitamin A has the ability to be converted to retinol in the body. Provitamin A carotenoids are: α-Carotene, β-carotene, and β-cryptoxanthin. The nonprovitamin A carotenoids are lutein, zeaxanthin, and lycopene, which cannot be converted to retinol [65]. The bioavailability of lycopene and its ability to convert provitamin A into retinol is dependent upon the amount already stored within the body. Too much stored provitamin A will inhibit the ability to convert provitamin A into retinol. Additionally, these fat-soluble compounds require a minimum of 3 to 5 grams of fat for absorption [65, 68, 69]. The carotenoids discussed above are the most common found in the American diet out of the 50 carotenoids known [65, 70]. Orange and red fruits and vegetables are richest sources of carotenoids, with chlorophyll covering the carotenoids found in leaf green vegetables as well as many other greens.

Capsaicinoids

Found in chili peppers, capsaicinoids are a group of chemicals having bioactive properties [71]. The International Journal of Cancer Research and Treatment defines capsaicin (trans-8-methyl-Nvanillyl-6-nonenamide) as "a homovanillic acid derivative and the major spicy component in chili peppers" [72]. Furthermore, pharmacologically and physiologically, capsaicin has been shown to alter the expression of several genes involved in cancer cell survival, growth arrest, angiogenesis, and metastasis, as well as having analgesic, antioxidant, anti-inflammatory, and anti-obesity properties [71-78].   Ongoing research with anticancer research as well as other researchers recently found that capsaicin targets multiple signaling pathways, oncogenes, and tumor-suppressor genes in various types of cancer models [72]. Each variety of pepper has its own unique specific capsaicinoids. These specific and unique characteristics of each capsaicinoid, although similar in structure, provide specific biological properties. The pungent sensation is found within the capsaicinoids of the hot pepper; the capsinoids in sweet peppers are non-pungent. Other antioxidants, ascorbic acids, and carotenoids are part of the bioactive compound profile of peppers [73].

Capsaicinoids have anti-obesity properties. The anti-obesity effect of capsaicinoids results from an increase in energy expenditure and lipid oxidation and a decrease in appetite [71]. An approximate increase of energy expenditure is 50kcal/day [71]. Synergistically, capsaicin and resveratrol promote apoptosis, resulting from the elevation of NO (nitric oxide) [72, 79].

Stilbenes

Antifungal properties identified in stilbenes are being considered for development of natural fungicides found in *Vitis vinifera* (common grape vine) waste– cane, root, and wood. Eleven stilbenes are identified and quantified as follows: ampelopsin A, E-piceatannol, pallidol, E-resveratrol, hopeaphenol, isohopeaphenol, E-ε-viniferin, E-miyabenol C, E-ω-viniferin, r2-viniferin, and r-viniferin [80]. The highest antifungal properties were found in wood extract then root extract [80].

Flavonoids

Flavonoids, known as "nature's biological response modifiers," have the ability to protect against oxidative and free radical damage as well as prevent formation of oxidized cholesterol through antioxidant effects [81]. With over 4,000 identified species, particular flavonoids have been shown to modify eicosanoid biosynthesis (antiprostanoid and anti-inflammatory responses), protect LDL from oxidation (prevention of atherosclerotic plaque formation), and promote relaxation of cardiovascular smooth muscle (antihypertensive, antiarrhythmic effects) [47, 81]. In addition, flavonoids have been shown to have antiviral and anti-carcinogenic properties, with greater antioxidant effects than Vitamins C and E, selenium, and zinc [81]. Specific flavonoids can protect oxidization of LDL and prevent atherosclerosis. The intake of flavonoids is "inversely related to mortality from coronary heart disease and the incidence of heart attacks" [81]. Antibacterial, anti-inflammatory, antiallergic, antimutagenic, antiviral, antineoplastic, anti-thrombotic, and vasodilatory actions have been confirmed in various plant medicines [81]. Each flavonoid has its own chemical structure with 12 subclassifications; the top six are listed in Table 3.

A correlation is recognized between the antioxidant (AO) activity and its chemical structure. Three essential structural requirements for "high AO-activity" are (i) ortho-dihydroxy (catechol), (ii) the 2,3-double bond and (iii) presence of 3- and 5-OH groups" [47]. Aside from these structural requirements, the number of hydroxyl substituents on the flavonoid molecule, the position of these hydroxyls, the presence of glycosides (-OR) or aglycons (-OH), and the overall degree of conjugation are important in determining AO-activity [47, 82].

Additionally, dietary flavonoids and their effect on weight have been researched. In a study of 2,734 monozygotic female twins, aged 18-83 years, the results supported that a higher amount of flavonoids consumed correlated with lower fat mass, independent of shared genetic and common environmental factors [83]. Dietary flavonoids include anthocyanins, flavan-3-ols, flavonols, and proanthocyanidins, with a median intake of 1.1 g/d [83]. Apricots are the richest fruit source of catechins, the monomer form of flavanols, with green tea, chocolate, and red wine being the richest food sources [84].

Table 3: Flavonoids: Top Six Sub classifications

Flavonoid Subclass	Examples of Individual Names	Food Sources	Health Benefits
Flavonols	Quercetin, kaempferol, and myricetin – most abundant flavonoids	Richest in onions, blueberries, broccoli, parsley, spinach, and tea	Five out of seven cohort studies found protective role in cardiovascular disease or stroke
Flavones	Predominantly glycosides of lutein, apigenin	Celery, chili peppers, oregano, parsley, peppermint, and thyme	Anti-inflammatory, anti-carcinogenic
Flavanones	Naringenin and hesperetin	Highest concentration in citrus fruits; tomato, grapefruit, lemon, orange, and aromatic plants like mint	Protect arterial stiffness- RC crossover trial in 6 months grapefruit juice.
Isoflavones	Structurally similar to estrogen Daidzein and genistein	Soy, tofu, natto, black bean sauce, legumes	Lower risk of breast cancer in women in menopause and lower risk of prostate cancer in men. Multiethnic Cohort Study - a reduced risk of endometrial cancer
Flavan-3-ols (Proanthocyandins)	Condensed tannins	Grapes, peaches, kakis, pears	RCS* – type 2 diabetes support
Flavan-3-ols cocoa	Condensed tannins "produce the astringent character of fruit" and bitterness in chocolate Epicatechin and procyanidins	Apples, berries, wine, cider, tea and beer	Glycemic control, improve vascular endothelial function, Heart Health-RDB* control study 100 adults lipoprotein profile improved, lower B/P & reduced 10yr risk of CVD by 20-30%. "Inhibited platelet adhesion activation, and aggregation"
Anthocyanins Anthocyanin mixture (320mg/day)	Mostly found in the skin - increases as the fruit ripens. Cyanidin Delphindin Malvidin	Abundant in fruit, red wine, leafy and root vegetables	RCS* – support glycemic control RDB** –Results after 24 weeks 150 hypercholesterolemia individuals reduced circulating markers of inflammation, including C-reactive protein, interleukin-1B (IL-1B) and soluble vascular [adhesion molecule-1 (sVCAM-1)"

Table 3 References: [84-93]   *RCS randomized control study; **RDB randomized, double blind

Found in edible plants and foods, most flavonoids are bound to contain at least one sugar molecule, with the exception of flavan-3-ols. Flavan-3-ols, catechins, and proanthocyanidins catalyze the release of sugar molecules. Additionally, when fermented soy-based products are exposed to microbial β-glucosidases, sugar molecules will be released from the glycosylated isoflavones. Flavonoid glycosides are not affected by cooking or food processing.; they have the ability to be intact until reaching the small intestine [85, 94, 95].

The bioavailability of dietary flavonoids is affected by gut microbiota and dietary intake. For flavonoids to be absorbed or excreted, a molecular transformation must occur; processes such as dehydroxylation, demethylation, glycosylation, and ring fusion are examples of this, utilizing gut microbial enzymes in the large intestine to produce metabolites. The metabolites produced are determined by the diversity and activity of colonic bacteria [96-100]. Optimal bioavailability of dietary flavonoids is therefore influenced by colonic microbiota.

Peptides

Bioactive peptides are "specific protein fragments that have a positive impact on body functions and may ultimately influence human health" [101]. Whey protein is a significant source; however, bioactive peptides are synthesized in both plants and animals. Casein peptides have many bioactive properties within polypeptide chains of caseins [102]. Bovine casein consists of four components: as1-, $as2$-, b- and k-caseins [102-104]. Bioactive agents have further been discovered in the milk sugars such as lactoferrin and lactoperoxidase [104].

Plant Sterols

Plant sterol esters are the bioactive compound found in many plant-based foods such as grains, leaves, nuts, seeds, and vegetable oil. One of their beneficial effects, according to research, is "lowering LDL cholesterol, which is one of the most common complications that come with obesity" [10]. In an 8-week clinical trial that tested this effect, an "average weight loss of 4.7 kg" and "a significant decrease in plasma lipid concentration, specifically total cholesterol and LDL cholesterol" were observed [10]. This study gave young adults between 21 and 30 snack bars made of rice bran (RB) and rice bran plus plant sterols (RB+ PS). The plant sterols found in muesli "significantly reduced LDL cholesterol levels by 4.4 % in a 4-week period" [10]. The bioactive compound, Beta-glucan, is a water-soluble fiber and polysaccharide found in a variety of plant sources. Polysaccharides help lower cholesterol by their ability to convert cholesterol into bile. Nitric Oxide levels are increased due to the beta-glucans found in oat bread, which support the "potential to lower blood pressure" [10].

Bioactive compounds found in both rice and beans contain polyphenolic compounds. The polyphenolic compounds determine the seed color of beans. Flavonoids such as flavonol glycosides, anthocyanins, and condensed tannins (proanthocyanidins) are the main polyphenolic compounds [105]. Proanthocyanidins (6, 9, 10, 16, 17, 20) are the most common in beans, and they have been found in black and blue-violet colored beans. According to Reynoso-Camacho et al., colored beans provide higher antioxidant content than many common foods, including vegetables. Lower glucose levels were noted in Type 2 diabetes patients after they consumed kidney beans. Several studies have also tested the effects of various beans on rat models. In one such study, in which rats were fed pinto, black, zapata, and Ayocote Morado beans, tumor multiplicity decreased. When the rats were fed black or navy beans, there was a 54%-59% decrease in "total tumor incidence [105]. Anthocyanin, a polyphenol, is identified as the major contributor for the dark-purple color of black rice [106].

Bioactive Compounds in Specific Food Sources

Omega-3 and omega-6 fatty acids can be found in seeds and are known for their anti-inflammatory properties. Antioxidant activity and health benefits are determined by the total phenolic content (TPC) using the Folin-Ciocalteu method [107]. A 6-hour defatting process extracted oil using a Soxhlet apparatus. Each seed is composed of various fatty acids in a ratio specific to that particular seed, such as the *Nigella stavia* (NS) having the highest ratio of omega-6 to omega-3 fatty acids at 36:1. Flaxseed, from the *Linum usitatissimum* (LU) plant, has the lowest ratio at 0.36:1 (phyto-constituents of phytoestrogens to fiber to omega 3-fatty acids). The method used a gas chromatogram to test these ratios [107]. The methanolic extract of seeds provides the bioactive compounds, Thymoquinone Cymene-2, 5-dione, m-Thymol, o-Cymene, 3-(Prop-2-enoyloxy) dodecane *a*-Phellandrene, S-3-Carene, and Valencene, with most of these supporting anti-inflammatory properties [107].

Nuts are sources of bioactive protein and lipid compounds. In one particular study of ten varieties of nuts, each was found to have a unique composition of bioactive compounds, including plant proteins, fiber, and phytosterols. Phytosterol content was found to be highest in peanuts, a member of the legume family, at 62 mg. Pistachio nuts came in second at 61 mg. Cashews, pine nuts, almonds, macadamia nuts, black walnuts, and pecans followed, with hazelnuts being the lowest in phytosterol content at 27 mg [85]. Polyunsaturated (PUFA) and monounsaturated (MUFA) fats are bioactive compounds supporting cardiac health, in addition to bioactive vitamin E, folate, and potassium. In controlled clinical trials, a reduction in both LDL cholesterol and serum levels was demonstrated in subjects who regularly consumed nuts [85, 108-111]. Additionally, raw cashews were found to have a variety of bioactive compounds that support eye health, including β-carotene (9.57 μg/100 g of DM), lutein (30.29 μg/100 g of DM), zeaxanthin (0.56 μg/100 g of DM), α-tocopherol (0.29 mg/100 g of DM), γ-tocopherol (1.10 mg/100 g of DM), thiamin (1.08 mg/100 g of DM), stearic acid (4.96 g/100 g of DM), oleic acid (21.87 g/100 g of DM), and linoleic acid (5.55 g/100 g of DM) [112]. Nuts have been further studied for their benefits toward cardiovascular health due to their supply of unsaturated fat, plant sterols, phytochemicals, vitamin E, folate, selenium, copper, and magnesium [86, 113].

Bioactive compounds are found in grasses, and these compounds are often particular to each grass. Research has confirmed that the bioactive compounds in wheatgrass and rice grass are different. Chlorophyll content is greater in wheatgrass, which is darker in color, whereas the lighter colored rice grass has a greater carotenoid content. Vitamin C is found at twice the amount in wheatgrass juice. Phenolic acid is found in higher levels in rice grass and includes pyrogallol, vanillic acid, and ferulic acid [114]. Due to these bioactive compounds in grasses, grass-fed cattle have higher levels of bioactive vitamin E, CLA, and omega-3 fatty acids [26].

Bioactive compounds can have antibiotic properties. A randomized clinical study in India recruited 60 women between the ages of 18-40, and its results supported that Proanthocyanidin, a compound found in cranberries (*Vaccinium macrocarpon*), can serve as antibiotic therapy against recurrences of urinary tract infections in women [6]. Furthermore, most berries, grapes, and red wine have bioactive compounds that have demonstrated efficacy as antioxidants, anti-tumors, anti-platelet aggregators, anti-inflammatory, as well as anti-aging compounds. The polyphenol resveratrol (found in grapes) and curcumin have been used to treat hepatitis, arthritis and colitis [6]. The anti-inflammatory property of resveratrol is the result of resveratrol's ability to increase adinopectin [10, 115].

Figure 4. Chemical Structure of Resveratrol

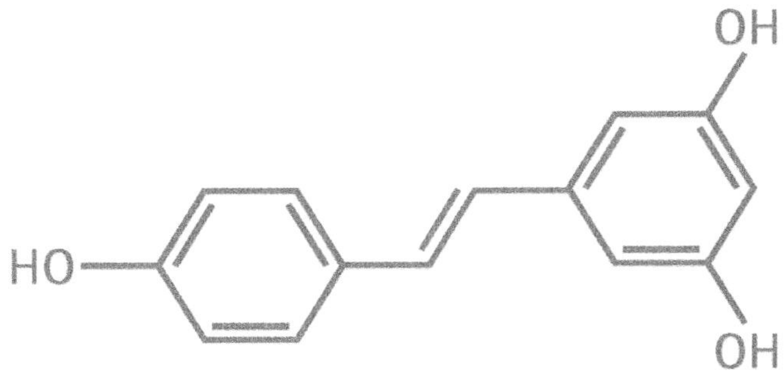

Figure 4 Image Source: http://www.evolva.com/resveratrol/request-info/

Potatoes are a significant source of protein with an amino acid profile greater than legumes or cereals. They contain several phenolic compounds, including p-coumaric, caffeic, chlorogenic, ferulic acid, and anthocyanins [116]. Drought-stress conditions were tested in a study of three potato varieties. All three amino acid profiles were enhanced in this two-year study with little effect on the bioactive compounds [116]. Both purple and red-fleshed potatoes were found to provide 3 to 4 times the concentration of phenolic acids and contain twice the flavonoid concentration of white-fleshed genotypes [117]. The antioxidant values (ORAC) of red-fleshed potatoes and purple-fleshed potatoes were 300% and 250% of the white-fleshed ORAC, respectively, and their peels provided 900 mg antioxidants in purple-flesh potatoes and 500 mg in red-fleshed potatoes [116, 117].

Sea cucumber extract is widely consumed in Asian countries and is also used in traditional Chinese medicine for its therapeutic bioactive compounds. It was found to have anticancer properties, namely against glioblastoma (GBM), the most common malignant astrocytic brain tumor [118]. The results of a recent study supported that the bioactive compounds found in sea cucumber extract included triterpene, glycosides, as well as sulfated polysaccharides, chondroitin sulfates, and glycosaminoglycans [118].

The bioactive compounds in rosehip, the fruit of the rose plant that is recognized as a pseudo-fruit, include cyclooxygenase inhibitors that may reduce the risk of cancer, heart disease, and various inflammatory conditions, such as anti-inflammatory galactolipid (2S)-1,2-di-O-[(9Z,12Z,15Z)-octadeca-9,12,15-trienoyl]-3-O-β-D-galactopyranosyl glycerol (GOPO), vitamin

C, phenolics, lycopene, lutein, zeaxanthin, and other carotenoids [119]. The chemical composition of rosehip can vary by region, cultivation method, climate, maturity, storage conditions, and the plant species. Antioxidant, anti-carcinogenic, and anti-mutagenic properties are provided by the abundant phenolics at 96 mg GAE/g dry weight and ascorbic acid ranging between 140-1100 mg/100 ml [84]. The richest source of phenolics and ascorbic acid is the *Rosa canina* species of rosehips, consisting of 880mg/100ml of ascorbic acid [120]. Anti-tumor and anti-inflammatory activity is found in the essential compound galactolipid GOPO, a compound in rosehips with no known toxicity. Various randomized clinical studies have supported that patients with chronic inflammatory disorders such as OA (osteoarthritis) and RA (rheumatoid arthritis) have benefited from rosehip supplements. Pain was significantly reduced and mobility increased in OA patients, while RA patients experienced moderately reduced pain and improved physical activity [120]. Tiliroside is a principal constituent of the rosehip seed, which exhibits anti-obese and anti-diabetes activities via the enhancement of fatty acid oxidation in the liver and skeletal muscle [120].

Bitter melon is a squash-like fruit used in cooking and widely consumed in Asia, Africa, South America, the West Indies, and Europe. The polypeptides found in the seeds and fruit are used for their medicinal properties of lowering blood sugar levels for Type II diabetes patients. The leaves and roots, on top of the fruit, are used for lowering blood sugar levels [121]. Antioxidant and anti-mutagenic properties are also noted in the extract of bitter melon. Further research is needed to confirm its chemo-preventative effects against carcinogenesis. Phenol contents were found to be higher when samples were oven-dried, compared to freeze-dried [81].

The bioactive compound tricin, an abundant flavonoid found in millet, wheat, and oats, has been shown to have anticancer effects in the lower gut. Additionally, tricin relaxes the smooth muscle of intestinal tissues, has powerful antioxidant and antihistaminic effects, and can inhibit malignant tumor cells of the breast and colon cells [81].

Bioactive Compounds Functioning Together

Scientists have studied the health benefits of components found within foods. Through the use of biomarkers, scientists have determined specific health benefits and the essential dosages of functional foods [13].

A physiologic dose of bioactive compounds is achieved through the diet and will typically result in levels that fall within the normal range of plasma and tissue levels [16]. Supra-physiologic doses, also referred to as pharmacologic doses, consist of exceeding the physiologic intake of bioactive compounds for extended periods of time and/or increasing intake to 2-3 times the physiologic dose [16]. Plasma levels are not reflective of the cellular levels of micronutrients, where deficiencies can still exist [16, 17].

Essential fatty acids, dietary fibers, antioxidants, bioactive vitamins, and bioactive minerals can have synergistic functional effects [6]. Plant sources have the highest composition of biochemical compounds, containing phenolic compounds, lipids, proteins/peptides, and carbohydrates [6]. Chemical structures and physical properties define their functional groups, and various classes of bioactive compounds are able to function and work together. Amounts of these compounds are usually small in their original dietary sources. Bioactive compounds are a wide category that encompasses flavonoids, capsaicinoids, lignin, terpenoids, carotenoids, chlorophylls, vitamins, stilbene, phenolic acids, fibers, sterols, lipids, fatty acids, polysaccharides, and some plant-derived proteins and peptides [6]. Numerous results of studies provide evidence that bioactive compounds, in combination, were more effective than when taken alone. At the molecular level, the combinations of curcumin plus *ar*-turmerone and curcumin plus coptisine synergistically attenuated TNR*a*-simulated NF-*K*B promoter activity [122].

Dietary fiber and polyphenols in carob fruits function together to treat diarrhea. In a study of young children 3 to 21 months in age, the duration of diarrhea was lessened by almost 2 full days among the children who were provided 1.5g/kg carob powder daily compared to the children treated with traditional oral rehydrating supplements like Pedialyte [123].

Antinutritional factors of bioactive compounds

Bioactive compounds can reduce or lessen the bioavailability and digestibility of certain nutrients [7]. Various health benefits can occur as these bioactive compounds create enzyme inhibitors, which can be helpful or poisonous. These molecules interact with the enzymes, causing the enzymes to not work normally. Amylase inhibitors can be therapeutic for diabetics by reducing the utilization of dietary starches. Inhibitors of the serine proteases trypsin and chymotrypsin inhibit chemically induced carcinogenesis [7].

Toxicity and Oxidation of Bioactive Compounds

Bioactive compounds, often secondary metabolites with various chemical properties from poisonous plants, can cause toxicity. When poisonous plants are ingested, the consequences can range from illness to "a departure from normal health" to death [124]. The severity of clinical signs varies widely; some as severe as having seizures, some can cause death, and some signs are unrecognized [124].

To determine upper limits (ULs), toxicologists look for adverse health effects that are most detrimental to the population [66]. There are three main steps developed to determine the UL of bioactive compounds. First, identify the "critical effect." Second, determine the "point of departure (POD) of the dose response curve." Thirdly, "apply the appropriate uncertain factors (UFs) to the POD" [66]. An overlap where benefit versus risk may also need to be assessed to determine the UL [66].

Therefore, to obtain the functional effects of a bioactive compound and receive its therapeutic benefit, taking the correct recommended dosage is crucial. Bioactive compounds are not equal in that the body absorbs some bioactive compounds better than others [13]. In the article, "A New Definition of Functional Food by FFD" (2015), two important quantities relevant to bioactive compounds are the amount and ratio of bioactive compounds to convert an ordinary food into a functional food. Different amounts of bioactive compounds are effective in different situations, and sometimes too much of a bioactive compound in a food can be toxic. In general, consuming physiologic levels of bioactive compounds is considered safe. Consuming higher levels of bioactive compounds (e.g. supra-physiological or therapeutic doses) must be tested from safety and health benefits [13].

Some toxic bioactive compounds that are produced in the plant are necessary to protect the plant from herbivores, insects, and microorganisms [49]. Solanine, a glycoalkaloid, a member of the steroidal toxic plant metabolites found in potatoes, increases when exposed to light and storage [49,125]. Mild clinical symptoms can occur at a level of 200 mg glycoalkaloids/mg potato, which is generally accepted as the highest tolerable limit has a zero safety margin [49, 126].

High intake levels of some bioactive compounds can be toxic to tissues and vital organs. Consideration of the compounds' original sources and binding sites are essential when determining safety and toxicity [6, 127]. Toxicity from a high concentration of bioactive compounds can cause growth retardation or inhibition, reduce food intake, promote anemia and patchy hyperplasia in the tubuli of the outer kidney medulla, and increase activity of several microsomal and cytoplasmic hepatic drug-metabolite enzymes. Low blood hemoglobin and kidney damage can be induced by a gallate concentration of 25,000-50,000 mg/kg or higher in the forms of either octyl or dodecyl [6, 128, 129]. For groups like young children and people on special diets, it is recommended to refrain from ingesting too much of certain compounds such as phototoxic furocoumarins found in celery and parsnips, goitrogenic glucosinolates in cabbage and mustard, oxalic acid in rhubarb, and phytic acid in grains and legumes [16, 130].

Toxicity of green tea extract is a risk when an excess of it is consumed. There are 34 adverse reports of liver damage and "abnormally high liver enzyme levels" in one study of 12 women according to a systematic review by the US Pharmacopeia (USP) Dietary Supplement Information Expert Committee [119]. Other studies of various green tea extracts indicated adverse effects such as gastrointestinal abdominal pain, upset stomach, nausea, muscle pain, and dizziness. Additional central nervous system symptoms may include restlessness, tremors, confusion, dizziness, agitation, and insomnia [119].

According to the University of Hawaii Department of Botany, these 8 categories are identified as the 8 toxic groups. Toxins in Groups I, II, and III will cause extensive cellular damage. Symptoms from these groups are delayed. Toxic damage has already occurred before symptoms appear, making toxicity no longer treatable. The toxins in Groups IV and V can "affect the autonomic system" with symptoms appearing shortly after consuming toxin [137]. The toxins in Groups VI and VII affect "the central nervous system" with symptoms such as hallucinations appearing shortly after consuming the toxin, for example, a mushroom [137]. The eighth category of toxic groups have unidentified toxins causing "gastrointestinal discomfort as soon as they are consumed" [137]. This eighth group is identified as gastrointestinal irritant(s). This eighth category consists of unrelated compounds producing similar symptoms, such as gastrointestinal irritation [137].

Oxidative stress and damage with an increased risk of disease can occur from excessive dietary supplementation of antioxidant molecules. An oxidative shift within the cellular environment can occur, causing pro-oxidants from the increased concentration of bioactive compounds [6]. Biophenols scavenge for free radicals, supporting antioxidant functions. "Oxidative stress happens when there is a serious imbalance between a biological system's ability to generate and detoxify reactive oxygen species (ROS)" [127].

Table 4 identifies toxic compounds contained in various categories of mushrooms. One example of each category is provided.

One Example of Mushroom Species	Toxic Compound	Reactions
Cyclopeptides Amanita phalloide	Amatoxins – highly toxic - Alpha- $C_{39}H_{45}N_{10}O_{14}S$ - Beta-$C_{39}H_{53}N_9O_{15}S$ Phallotoxins	- Amanita is the most common species - Amatoxins responsible for over 95% of mushroom fatalities - Liver, intestinal, and renal damage-possible death in 3-7 days - Alpha inhibits RNA polymerase II and protein synthesis
Gyromitrins Gyromitria	- Hydrazones Gyromitrin-$C_4H_8N_2O$ (n-methyl-N-formylhydrazone) - false morel (Gyromitra esculenta)	- Rapidly decomposes in stomach, forming acetaldehyde, N–methyl-N-formylhydrazine, monomethylhydrazine (MMH)* - Fruit in spring - Hepatotoxic, carcinogenic
Orellanin Cortinarius	Orellanine-tetrahydroxylated di-N-oxidized bipyridine-$C_{10}H_8N_2O_6$	- Longest delay for symptoms to appear - 3-20 days
Coprine Coprinus Atramentarius	Coprine N5-(1-hydroxycycloproyl) glutamine[142] $C_8H_{14}N_2O_4$	- Considered Group IV toxic mushroom - Antabuse-like - Toxic only when alcohol is consumed within 48 hours before or after mushrooms are ingested
Muscarine Clitocybe	Muscarine $C_9H_{20}NO_2$[146]	- Stimulates salivation, bladder cramping, diarrhea, vision problems
Muscarine Clitocybe	Miscimol $C_4H_6N_2O_2$	- Extremely toxic - Neurotoxic isoxazole isolated from species of Amanita - Central nervous system depressant - GABA agonists - Symptoms resemble alcohol intoxication appearing between 30-120 minutes

	Two major chemicals	- Hallucinogenic, LSD family
Psilocybin and Psilocin **Psilocybe cubensis** **Ralph Morales**	- Psilocybin-$C_{12}H_{17}N_2O_4P$ - Psilocin-$C_{12}H_{16}N_2O$ Other active chemicals - Baeocystin (10 mg entheogenic effect) - Norbaeocystin	- Effects central nervous system - Uncontrollable laughter, optical distortions, euphoria, disembodied experience and mystical experiences - Fruit in late summer through late autumn [128]
Gastrointestinal Irritants	- Unrelated compounds	- Gastrointestinal irritation

Table 4 References: [131, 133 – 148]

MMH is a water-soluble toxin that belongs in the Gyromitrin mushroom category and used in rocket fuel. Gastroenteritis, hepatorenal failure, hemolysis, methemoglobinema, seizures, and coma may result from MMH. The formation of MMH is caused by the conversion of acetaldehyde and N methyl-N-formylhydrazine [135].

Bioactive Compounds: Influence on Health

Health promotion and disease prevention are the primary potential benefits of functional foods. Epidemiological studies are used to determine the health benefits of particular micronutrients [88]. Bioactive compounds within functional foods, such as essential fatty acids, dietary fibers, antioxidants, vitamins, and minerals, all play a role in determining the functions of foods [6]. Optimal doses of specific compounds are required to achieve optimal health and prevent disease. However, the presence of certain disease states, metabolic disorders, and conditions may amplify or diminish the potential benefits of bioactive compounds [6]. The necessary intake to achieve a desired effect requires an integrative approach combining concepts and evidence from nutritional sciences, food science, molecular biology, biochemistry, plant science, genetics, epigenetics, genomics, proteomics, metabolomics, and other disciplines to determine the subcellular, cellular, tissue, and organismic outcomes [6].

The functions of these compounds in supporting health and wellness begin at the level of their specific biological targets. Each compound creates or inhibits chemical reactions with other specific constituents for detoxification, enhances absorption, and influences pathways for energy storage, inflammation, and adipogenesis. Some have chemopreventive, anti-inflammatory, anti-oxidative, anti-atherogenic, anti-carcinogenesis, cardioprotective, and anti-tumor properties. Harmful molecules such as bad cholesterol (LDL) can be decreased [6]. Potential health-promoting abilities have been discovered in *in vivo* studies with the bioactive compounds lycopene and *a*-tomatine, found in tomatoes [151].

The effects of numerous nutrients, including fatty acids, cholesterol, vitamin A, and vitamin D, on gene transcription are mediated by "nutrient sensors." These are specific transcription factors and nuclear proteins that largely determine the amount, timing, and cell specificity of gene expression [16]. In all metabolically active organs such as the liver, intestine, or adipose tissue, a group of ligand-activated transcription factors, members of the nuclear receptor superfamily, play a key role in the regulation and metabolism of nutrients and other food components, including biotransformation, energy metabolism, and nutrient transport [16, 152]. There are specific nuclear receptors for fatty acids called peroxisome proliferator activator receptors, which play an important role in lipid and carbohydrate metabolism [16, 153, 154]. Changes in gene expression can be measured by techniques such as Northern blotting, RNase protection assays, or real-time polymerase chain reaction, which is a recent promising addition to this list of tools. Most recently, the completion of the Human Genome Project has opened up a new area in gene expression study: now it is possible to look at all genes at once by using high-density microarrays [16, 155]. This allows us to get a complete picture of the nutrition-relevant transcriptome, one of the topics of the new field of nutritional genomics and nutrigenomics [16, 156].

The screening and enzymatic testing remedy for osteoarthritis (OA) has been proven to be effective with the use of flavocoxids [6]. Catechins and baicalin are flavonoids which have been documented to manage both the cyclooxygenase and 5-lipoxygenase pathways of arachidonic acid metabolism identified to be the underlying route for the pathological process of OA [6].

An animal study using a mouse model confirmed that the immune system can be up-regulated with an increase in regulatory T cells and improvement of intestinal epithelial cells in reducing the neutrophilic granulocyte numbers in the treated mice [6]. This implies that such compounds have the ability to up-regulate the immune system and help it fight infection and disease-causing agents [6]. Significant evidence confirms that the bioactive compounds resveratrol, curcumin, and simvastatin may be used to treat inflammatory bowel disease (IBD). However, geographical location, age, gender, height, weight, and body mass index are required to determine how much is essential to achieve optimal results [6].

Bioactive Compounds: Altered, Influenced, or Eliminated

The amount of bioactive compounds in a food can be increased, decreased, altered, influenced, or eliminated by a variety of processes. Environmental factors, fertilization, water supply, peeling, cooking, and processing methods all influence, change, add, or alter availability of bioactive compounds in foods. Furthermore, ripening fruit and increasing size will influence the concentration and quantity of compounds. The environmental factors that affect polyphenol content include factors relevant to how and where produce is grown: climate, temperature, soil type, fertilization, sunlight, rain, hydroponic versus biological cultures, and the use of fields vs. the greenhouse. Organically grown produce was found to be more nutrient dense, with 10-50% increase in secondary metabolites and bioactive vitamin C and less water, protein, nitrate, and bioactive vitamin A [157]. It has been noted that bioactive compounds increase when water supply is reduced [49, 84, 158]. Glucosinolate in cauliflower and broccoli are strongly influenced by the temperature they are grown in. Alkyl glucosinolates, glucoraphanin and glucoiberin, were highest when grown in temperatures $\leq 12°C$ and in increased radiation. Warmer temperatures and lower radiation produced indole glucosinolate glucobrassicin in broccoli [49]. Additionally, organic and sustainable agriculture has produced higher polyphenol content. Resveratrol was reduced by up to five times the amount when treated with fungicides [157]. Freezing, sterilization, or fermentation can influence acids that are not in free form but are created only by these processing techniques [84]. Steaming is the preferred method of cooking vegetables to avoid leaching. Quercetin was lost in tomatoes and onions: microwaving resulted in a 65% loss, boiling for 15 minutes resulted in a 75% loss, and frying resulted in a 30% loss. No phenolic acids were found in potatoes after freeze-drying or French-frying [84].

The highest concentrations of polyphenols are found in the outer part versus the inner part; therefore, peeling can "eliminate a significant portion of polyphenols" [84]. The concentration of polyphenols in corn increased when frozen. Researchers believe that the decrease in water when the corn is frozen causes an increase in polyphenols [159]. The polyphenol content in green vegetables stays relatively the same or increases [160]. However, this is not true for the other vegetables. Chart 1 provides details on various vegetables and the effect that cooking has on their total phenol content.

Bioactive compounds of chlorophyll a and b, total chlorophyll, and carotenoids were increased using fish protein hydrolysate (FPH) of 10 ppm. FPH, used as a liquid fertilizer, can increase antioxidant activity, nutritional value, and bioactive compounds. A significant increase was noted at 10 ppm and even at 5 ppm versus the controlled group. However, more is not better as the 15-20 ppm resulted in lower amounts [162].

Roasting alters bioactive compounds in both beneficial and non-beneficial ways, namely by adding or depleting compounds. Roasting and other cooking methods alter the amount of DPPH and ABTS radical scavenging activity in red peppers. Red peppers cooked by these methods confirm a significant decrease in radical scavenging activity. Stir-frying resulted in the least amount of DPPH, and ABTS radical activity decreased by 4 to 16%. The highest decrease of up to 60% occurred when the red pepper was boiled [86].

Figure 5. Phenol compounds increased and/or decreased - various vegetables and cooking methods

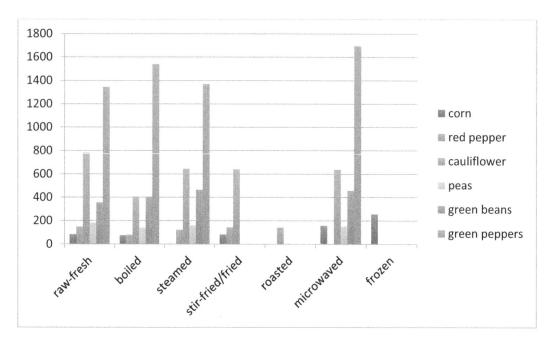

*values used median range(s)
Figure 5. Sources: [86, 160, 161]

Roasting canola oil, also known as Japanese rapeseed oil, has been demonstrated to increase health benefits. Traditional methods strip components in the oils, making the oil unhealthy, procarcinogenic, or prooxidant. However, during the roasting process of canola seeds, canolol was efficiently generated, increasing health benefits [113]. The potent scavenger of alkylperoxyl radical and peroxinitrate (ONOO) was created during the roasting and responsible for the increase in health benefits compared to oil using the traditional "hexane extraction" method [113]. These lipids can be further altered and enhanced after the addition of dried residue from both wine-fermented-waste and tomato-juice-waste, enhancing antioxidant components and turning previously low-functioning oils into function-enriching high grade oils [113]. The roasting of loquat leaves resulted in new bioactive phenolic compounds. In the traditional loquat tea made without roasting, the leaves contain flavonoids, but they do not provide the bioactive phenol compound. Tea is then made from the roasted leaves, providing antioxidant and anti-inflammatory benefits [164]. Black tea leaves contain monomer flavanols that are influenced by the heating of the leaves, causing the leaves to oxidize and create more complex condensed polyphenols from the initial monomer flavanols [84]. However, the processing of commercial teas alters flavonoid content, particularly decreasing flavanols and thearubigins in green and black teas [88].

Potatoes are the fourth most important crop; therefore, it is crucial to understand how cooking affects the bioactive compounds in this important crop. Additionally, potatoes are usually consumed after processing and cooking them, and not in their fresh form. Processing and cooking is responsible for eliminating up to 65-90% of the bioactive compounds in the potatoes [117].

Thermal cooking of black rice markedly reduced TPC (total polyphenol content) and TAC (total anthocyanin content). The TPCs were reduced by 67-80% and TACs were reduced between 45-54% [106].

Bioactive compounds can be influenced by biomarkers. Biomarkers are used to confirm whether the bioactive compound is beneficial or not [13]. Obesity biomarkers have been studied; research in clinical trials indicate that obesity may be counteracted by vitamins, a bioactive compound found in plant-based foods. A marked decrease was observed in waist circumferences, 3.9 cm in men and 10.7 cm in women, in addition to fasting glucose levels with Vitamin E as well as a significant decrease in weight and body fat with Vitamin D in a 12-month trial. Vitamin B-9 or folic acid reduced blood homocysteine levels by 15.8%. Decreasing blood homocysteine levels is important for obese people in lowering their risk of heart disease [10]. A multitude of bioactive compounds in green tea may fight obesity, specifically catechin epigallocatechin-3-gallate (EGCG), which has positive results especially with the addition of caffeine. An increase in energy expenditure, thermogenesis, and reducing fat oxidation and absorption all aid in weight loss. EGCG supplementation of between 800-856 mg has significantly reduced blood pressure as well as reducing abdominal fat by as much as 7.7% [10]. Exercise was combined with supplementation for the 7.7% reduction. The process occurs with the ability of catechins in green tea to fight the obesity biomarkers that increase energy expenditure and fat oxidation, reduce blood pressure, body weight, and cholesterol [10]. Other bioactive compounds found to affect biomarkers of obesity are apple polyphenols, quercetin flavonol, omega-3 fatty acids bioactive vitamin D, and prebiotics [10].

Weather and temperature may alter or enhance some vegetables. In a two-year study with 3 different potatoes grown under stressful drought conditions, the amino acid profiles of all three potatoes were enhanced with little effect on the bioactive compounds [116]. Phenol contents were found to be higher when samples of bitter melon were oven-dried versus freeze-dried [121].

The biochemical compounds in fruit further fight obesity. The extract of a small citrus peel consumed for 12 weeks improved body weight, waist circumference, and serum triglyceride levels [10]. The biomarkers IL-6 level and serum amyloid alpha levels, two highly substantial biomarkers of obesity, were decreased after consuming 4 cups of green tea a day [10]. Tea consumption in combination with exercise was shown to be 17% more effective in oxidizing fat than exercise alone [10]. Vitamin A was found to provide an uptake in metabolism, and in overweight children, bioactive vitamin C reduced oxidative stress: a biomarker of obesity linked to inflammation [10]. Inflammation may be reduced by the bioactive compounds found in grapes. Polyphenol resveratrol increases adinopectin, decreasing inflammation [10].

Extraction and Fingerprinting Bioactive Compounds

The process of extraction is of utmost significance, as it is important in determining the quality of the final extract. The proper solvent type, ratio of solvent to compound, temperature, and particle size are essential [6]. Numerous methods of extraction are dependent on the bioactive compound. The long extraction process requires simple methods to release the bioactive compound from the bonded membrane without the compound turning biologically inactive from either "contaminating or destroying their unique chemical or physical forms" [6]. The techniques employed are maceration, infusion, percolation, digestion, decoction, and hot continuous extraction (Soxhlet). Other techniques also include aqueous-alcoholic extraction by fermentation, counter current extraction, microwave-assisted extraction, ultrasound extraction (sonication), supercritical fluid extraction, and phytonic extraction (with hydrofluorocarbon solvents) [6, 128, 129]. Other techniques used are head space trapping, solid phase micro extraction, protoplast extraction, micro distillation, thermomicrodistillation, and molecular distillation [6, 164]. The consideration of using CO2 is highly recommended for the extraction process. This cost-effective recommendation is non-toxic as many can be toxic to humans as well as the environment [6].

Each extraction method can result in different levels of antioxidant properties. The acidic methanol extraction method provided markedly higher anthocyanin contents (TAC), from 285% to 730% more TAC in raw black rice than other extraction methods that used ethanol, acidic ethanol, or water. [128]. The hexane extraction method traditionally used when processing oils removes many of the functional compounds, the "peroxylradical-scavenging activities" of most oils, with the exception of extra virgin and unpurified or classic rapeseed-and sesame-seed oils [113].

Techniques to fingerprint bioactive compounds consist of several analytical, chromatographic and molecular techniques with a focus on high performance liquid chromatography/high performance thin layer chromatography (HPLC/HPTLC), Fourier-transform infrared spectroscopy (FTIR), and Immunoassay techniques" [6].

A chemical separation of bioactive compounds allows for identification using HPLC (high performance liquid chromatography). The identification and separation of bioactive compounds is achieved by using isocratic system (i.e. single unchanging mobile phase system). Solvent systems are either methanol or acetonitrile, or HPLC water at pH = 3.0 [6]. Gradient elution is the ideal technique to fingerprint bioactive compounds, consisting of several analytical, chromatographic and molecular techniques [6]. The essential focus is on high performance liquid chromatography/high performance thin layer chromatography (HPLC/HPTLC), Fourier-transform infrared spectroscopy (FTIR), and Immunoassay techniques [6]. An essential tool for fingerprinting bioactive compounds in plants, fungi, and marine functional food sources is high performance thin layer chromatography (HPTLC/HPLC) [6]. For proper identification of bioactive compounds via HPLC, two things are of vital importance: first, a detector of functionality must be properly selected, and second, optimal detection settings and an assay of separation must be properly established [6].

The unique characteristics of bioactive compounds allow an analytic tool known as the Fourier-transform spectroscopy (FTIR) to identify and characterize the bioactive compounds in functional foods in either a liquid or solid form. A comparison of bioactive compound spectrums is studied against an online library database. Qualitative and quantitative analyses use modern technique of the Immunoassay. The advantages of immunoassay techniques are (1) high specificity and sensitivity for receptor binding analyses, (2) high specificity and sensitivity for enzyme assays, and (3) high specificity and sensitivity for qualitative and quantitative analysis of bioactive compounds [6, 42, 165]. Enzyme-linked immunosorbent essay (ELISA) is more efficient and more sensitive than any conventional HPLC methods currently in use in bioactive compound extract mixture fingerprinting [6, 42, 165].

SUMMARY

> When we examine bioactive compounds from the point of functional foods, food bioactive compounds are primary and secondary metabolites of nutritive and non-nutritive natural components generating health benefits by preventing or managing chronic disease or its symptoms. Each bioactive compound is unique in its structure, with physiological mechanisms and concentrations dependent on the environment where it is sourced. Bioavailability varies on the extraction method used to pull the compounds out from their source. Cooking can alter and/or eliminate bioactive compounds. Synergistically, these compounds work together to impart beneficial health effects, with the best sources coming from food.

> To test the effectiveness a bioactive compound is, we use specific biomarkers, which are molecules utilized to identify changes that occur at the cellular level and are monitored to identify health or disease. Testing specific and sensitive biomarkers help to identify the health benefits of food bioactive compounds, which are the backbone of functional foods. Enriching food with these food bioactive compounds produces functional food where structural and functional statements on packaging can only occur after proven testing of the specific and sensitive biomarkers. The Functional Food Center (FFC) defines functional foods as natural or processed foods that contain known or unknown bioactive compounds; which, in defined, effective, and non-toxic amounts, provide a clinically proven and documented health benefit utilizing specific biomarkers for the prevention, management, or treatment of chronic disease or its symptoms".

> Excessive amounts of some bioactive compounds can be toxic; others are toxic by nature. Therapeutic doses may exceed the upper limit set the Food and Drug Administration (FDA); therefore, it is crucial to use the exact dose of the specific bioactive compound(s) for the specific disease and biomarker to avoid toxicity. The three steps to identify the upper limit and prevent toxicity are: identify the critical effect; determine the point of departure; and apply the unknown factors to the point of departure.

REVIEW QUESTIONS:

1. The definition of Functional Food includes:
   a. Natural or processed foods
   b. Contain known or unknown biologically-active compounds
   c. Clinically proven and documented health benefit
   d. Utilizing specific biomarkers for the prevention, management or treatment of chronic disease or its symptoms.
   e. A and B
   f. All of the above

2. What is true about bioactive compounds?
   a. They are the backbone of functional foods
   b. The term has root words meaning "life energy" – possessing biological activity
   c. They are always consistent
   d. A and B
   e. All of the above

3. Supra-physiologic or therapeutic doses of bioactive compounds:
   a. Can manage chronic diseases and its symptoms
   b. Make bioactive compounds available at the cellular level
   c. A and B
   d. None the of the above

4. The success of extracting bioactive compounds
   a. Will have no effect on the quality of compound
   b. Is of utmost importance
   c. Is dependent on only one extraction process
   d. Means that they perfectly retain antioxidant properties

5. Functionality of bioactive compounds is obtained when _____ is/are achieved to convert an ordinary food into a functional food.
   a. Consumed at higher levels
   b. The specific amount of the bioactive compound
   c. The ratio of bioactive compound
   d. A and B

6. Which of these choices is not a function provided by eggs?
   a. Inhibits certain proteases in the body
   b. Can have an effect on muscle wall thickening
   c. Known to prevent the spread of carcinogens
   d. Binds metal ions

7. _____ produce isothiocyanates.

a. Glucosinolates
b. Flavonoids
c. Saponins
d. Phenolic Compounds

8. All of the following are known classifications of bioactive compounds except
    a. Secondary Metabolites
    b. Non-nutritive ingredients
    c. Beneficiary supplements
    d. None of the above

9. A health benefit of consuming fiber is
    a. The reduction of rates of absorption of glucose
    b. The reduction of high levels of cholesterol
    c. The regulation of blood flow in the body
    d. The prevention of heart burn in the arteries

10. Specific protein fragments that have a positive impact on body functions and may ultimately influence human health are known as ____.
    a. Functional peptides
    b. Bioactive polysaccharides
    c. Bioactive compounds
    d. Bioactive peptides

11. Which of these are toxic compounds found in mushrooms?
    a. Amatoxins
    b. Muscarine
    c. Coprine
    d. All of the above

12. Which of these choices is a trait of non-nutritive bioactive compounds?
    a. Protect against DNA damage
    b. Regulate gene expression
    c. Modulate immune function
    d. A and C

13. What are nutrient sensors?
    a. Extra-nutritional constituents that typically occur in small quantities in foods
    b. Specific protein fragments that have a positive impact on body functions and may ultimately influence human health
    c. Specific transcription factors and nuclear proteins that largely determine the amount, timing, and cell specificity of gene expression
    d. None of the above

14. Which bioactive vitamin plays a significant role in low-density lipoprotein (LDL) levels, "influencing the 'loading' of LDL"?
    a. Bioactive vitamin E
    b. Bioactive vitamin A
    c. Bioactive vitamin K
    d. Bioactive vitamin B

Answers: 1. **(F)** 2. **(D)** 3. **(C)** 4. **(B)** 5. **(D)** 6. **(C)** 7. **(A)** 8. **(C)** 9. **(A)** 10. **(D)** 11. **(D)** 12. **(D)** 13. **(C)** 14. **(A)**

List of Abbreviations: AO antioxidant, ACE angiotensin converting enzyme, CLA Conjugated linoleic acid, DHA docosahexaenoic acid, EGCG epigallocatechin-3-gallate, ELISA Enzyme-linked immunosorbent essay, EPA eicosapentaenoic acid, FDA Food and Drug Administration, FFC Functional Food Center, FOS Fructo-oligosaccharides, FPH fish protein hydrolysate, FTIR Fourier-transorm infrared spectroscopy, GBM glioblastoma, HDL high-density-lipoprotein, HPLC/HPTLC high performance liquid chromatograpy/high performance thin layer chromatography, IBD inflammatory bowel disease, LDL low-density-lipoprotein, LU Linum usitatissinum, MMH monomethylhydrazine, MGP matrix Gla protein, MUFA monounsaturated fatty acid, NO nitric oxide, NS Nigella stavia, OA osteoarthritis, OC osteocalcin, POD Point of Departure, PS plant sterols, PUFA polyunsaturated fatty acid, RA Rheumatoid Arthritis, RB rice bran, RCS randomized control study, RDB randomized double blind, ROS reactive oxygen species, TAC total anthocyanin content, TOS Transgalacto-oligosaccharides, TPC Total polyphenol content, UF uncertain factors, UL Upper Limit(s), USP US Parmacopeia, VKD vitamin K-dependent

REFERENCES:

1. Strobel, Gary A. Microbe Mining. Natural History. Mar. 2014, 122(2):24-30.
2. Paulsen, B.S. Highlights through the history of plant medicine. The Norwegian Academy of Science and Letters. 2010. National Veterinary Institute. Oslo, Norway.
3. Hoeg, OA. ed. Vare medisinske planter. Trolldom, tradisjon og legekunst.1. ed. Oslo: Det Beste, 1984.
4. Nordal A. Forelesninger i farmakognosi. Oslo: Universitetsforlaget. 1960.
5. Hassan K. Obied. Biography of biophenols: past, present and future. Functional Foods in Health and Disease 2013; 3(6): 230-241.
6. Abugri, Daniel A, and Melissa Johnson, Ph.D. Efficacy of bioactive compounds and determine intake level necessary to achieve desired effect. *Introduction to Functional Food Science 3rd Edition.* 2014. Vol 1:72-95.
7. Singh, R. Bioactive Compounds in Foods and their role in health. Lecture Paper #16 An MHRD Project under its National Mission on Education through ICT (NME-ICT0 and University Grants Commission- Pathshaia Production of Courseware for Postgraduates. Advances in Food Science and Technology, E-Content for Post Graduate Courseware (http://epgp.inflibnet.ac.in), National Dairy Research Institute. India. 2015. Viday-mitra.
8. Lavecchia, T., Rea, G., Antonacci, A. and Giardi, M.T. Healthy and Adverse Effects of Plant-Derived Functional Metabolites: The Need of Revealing their Content and Bioactivity in a Complex Food Matrix. Crit Rev Food Sci Nutr. 2013. Jan;53(2):198-213.
9. Bernhoft, A. A brief review on bioactive compounds in plants. The Norwegian Academy of Science and Letters. 2010. National Veterinary Institute. Oslo, Norway:11-17.
10. Coats, Rebecca and Danik Martirosyan, Ph.D. The effects of bioactive compounds on biomarkers of obesity. Functional Foods in Health and Disease 2015; 5(11): 365-380.

11. Kris-Etherton PM, Hecker KD, Bonanome A, Coval SM, Binkoski AE, Hilpert KF, Griel AE, Etherton TD. Bioactive compounds in foods: their role in the prevention of cardiovascular disease and cancer. Am J Med 2002 Dec 30;113(9B):71-88.

12. Functional Food Center. www.functionalfoodenter.net. Updated August 2017.

13. Martirosyan, Danik and Jaishree Singh. A new definition of functional food by FFD: what makes a new definition unique? Functional Foods in Health and Disease 2015; 5(6):209-223.

14. Pereira David M., Patrícia Valentão, José A. Pereira and Paula B. Andrade. Phenolics: From Chemistry to Biology. Molecules 2009. 14: 2202-2211.

15. Rui Hai Liu, Potential Synergy of Phytochemicals in Cancer Prevention: Mechanism of Action: The Journal of Nutrition. Dec. 2004. 134(12):3479-85.

16. Biesalski, H.K., Dragsted, L.O., Elmadfa, I., Grossklaus, R., Muller, M., Schrenk, D., Walter, P. and Weber, P. Bioactive compounds: Safety and efficacy. Nutrition 25 (2009) 1206-1211.

17. Erhardt JG, Mack H, Sobeck U, Biesalski HK. b-Carotene and a-tocopherol concentration and antioxidant status in buccal mucosal cells and plasma after oral supplementation. Br J Nutr 2002; 87: 471–5.

18. National Center for Biotechnology Information. PubChem Compound Database; CID=5280450. https://pubchem.ncbi.nlm.nih.gov/compound5280450 (accessed Sept 12, 2017).

19. Balogun, K.A., Alber, C.J., Ford, D.A., Brown, R.J. and Cheema, S.K. Dietary Omega-3 Polyunsaturated Fatty Acids Alter the Fatty Acid Composition of Hepatic and Plasma Bioactive Lipids in C57BL/6 Mice: A Lipidomic Approach. PLOS One. November 21, 2013. https://doi.org/10.1371/Journal.pone.0082399.

20. Balogun KA, Albert CJ, Ford DA, Brown RJ, Cheema SK (2013) Dietary Omega-3 Polyunsaturated Fatty Acids Alter the Fatty Acid Composition of Hepatic and Plasma Bioactive Lipids in C57BL/6 Mice: A Lipidomic Approach. PLoS ONE 8(11): e82399. https://doi.org/10.1371/journal.pone.0082399.

21. Wassall, S.R., Stillwell, W, (2009) Polyunsaturated fatty acid-cholesterol interactions: domain formation in membranes. Biochim Biophys Acta 1788:24-32.

22. Riediger ND, Othman RA, Suh M, Moghadasian MH (2009) A systemic review of the roles of n-3 fatty acids in health and disease. J Am Diet Assoc 109:668-679.

23. Cottin SC, Sanders TA, Hall WL (2011). The differential effects of EPA and DHA on cardiovascular risk factors. Proc Nutr Soc 70: 215-231.

24. Banni S, Di Marzo V (2010) Effect of dietary fat on endocannabinoids and related mediators: consequences on energy homeostasis, inflammation and mood. Mol Nutr Food Res 54: 82-92.

25. Walther, B. and Sieber R. Bioactive proteins and peptides in foods. Int J Vitam Nutr Res. 2011 Mar;81(2-3): 181-92.

26. Purchas, RW. & Zou M. Composition and quality differences between the longissimus and infraspinatus muscles for several groups of pasture-finished cattle. Science Direct. January 2008. 470-9.

27. Purchas RW. Zou M, Pearce, P. & Jackson R. (2007). Concentrations of vitamin D3 and 25-hydroxyvitamin D3 in raw and cooked New Zealand beef and lamb. Journal of Food Coposition and Analysis, 2007. 20, 90-98.

28. Hathwar SC, Rai AK, Modi VK, Narayan B. Characteristics and Consumer Acceptance of Healthier Meat and Meat Product Formulations. A Review. Journal Food Science Technology. 2012 Dec; 49(6): 653-664.

29. Prates, JAM and Mateus CMRP. Functional foods from animal sources and their physiologically active components. Rev Med Vet. 2002; 3: 155-160.

30. Suh, JH, Shigeno ET, Morrow JD, Cox B, Rocha AE, Frei B, Hagen TM. Oxidative stress in the aging rat heart is reversed by dietary supplementation with ®-a-lipic acid. Faseb J. 2001;1 5: 700-706.

31. Zhou S and Decker EA. Ability of Carnosine and Other Skeletal Muscle Components to Quench Unsaturated Aldehydic Lipid Oxidation Products. J Agric Food Chem. 1999, 47(1):51-55.

32. Miguel L, Carlos MT, Irene L, Peter T, Jose R. Effect of histidine, cysteine, glutathione or beef on iron absorption in humans. Am Inst Nutr. 1984; 114: 217-223.

33. Arihara K. Strategies for designing novel functional meat products. Science Direct 2006. 74(1):219-229.

34. Swapna C. Hathwar, Amit Kumar Rai, Vinod Kumar Modi, and Bhaskar Narayan. Characteristics and consumer acceptance of healthier meat and meat product formulations – a review. *Journal Food Science Technology*. 2012 Dec; 49 (6):653-664.

35. Mohanty, D.P., Mohapatra, S., Misra, S. and Sahu, P.S. Milk derived bioactive peptides and their impact on human health – A review. Saudi J Biol Sci. 2016, Sept. 23(5):577-583.

36. Andersen, C.J. Bioactive Egg Components and Inflammation. Nutrients. 2015, Sep; 7(9); 7889-7913.

37. Brigelius, Flohe, R. Bioactivity of vitamin E. Nutr Res Rev. 2006 Dec; 19(2): 174-86.

38. Okamoto T, Kodoi R, Nonaka Y, Fukuda I, Hashimoto T, Kanazawa K, Mizuno M, Ashida H. Lentinan from shiitake mushroom (*Lentinus edodes*) suppresses expression of cytochrome P450 1A subfamily in the mouse liver. Biofactors. 2004, 21(1-4):407-409.

39. Wang J, Zhong M, Liu B, Sha L, Lun Y, Zhang W, Li X, Wang X, Cao J, Ning A, Huang M. Expression and functional analysis of novel molecule – Latcripin-13 domain from Lentinual edodes C91-3 produced in prokaryotic expression system. Gene. Jan 25 2015;55(2):469-475.

40. U., Reichrath, J., Holick, M.F. and Kisters K. Vitamin K: an old vitamin in a new perspective. Dermatoendocrinol. 2014. Jan-Dec; 6(1): e968490. Doi: 10.4161/19381972.2014.968490.

41. Ina K, Kataoka T, and Ando T. The use of lentinan for treating gastric cancer. Anticancer Agents Med Chem. 2013 Jun; 13(5):681-8.

42. Murray Michael, N.D.; and Joseph Pizzorno, N.D. The Encyclopedia of Natural Medicine 3rd Edition, 2012, Atria. New York: NY.

43. Rogerio, A.P., Sa-Nunes, A., and Faccioli, L.H. The activity of medicinal plants and secondary metabolites on eosinophilic inflammation. Pharmacol Res. 2010 Oct;62(4):298-307.

44. Willett, WC (2002) Balancing life-style and genomics research for disease prevention. Science 296:695-698.

45. Doll, R & Peto, R (1981) Avoidable risks of cancer in the United States, J. Natl. Cancer Inst. 66:1197-1265.

46. Willett WC (1995) Diet, nutrition and avoidable cancer. Environ. Health Perspect. 103:165-170.

47. Resat Apak, Kubilay Güçlü, Birsen Demirata, Mustafa Özyürek, Saliha Esin Celik, Burcu Bektaşoğlu, K. Işı Berker and Dilek Özyurt. Comparative Evaluation of Various Total Antioxidant Capacity Assays Applied to Phenolic Compounds with the CUPRAC Assay Molecules. 2007, 12(7): 1496-1547.

48. Balasundram N, Sundram K, Samman S. Phenolic Compounds in Plants and Agri-Industrial By-Products: Antioxidant Activity, Occurrence, and Potential Uses. Food Chem. 2006, 99: 191-203.

49. Hansen, M and Wold, A.B. Contents of bioactive compounds in food plants as affected by traditional breeding and environmental factors. The Norwegian Academy of Science and Letters, 2010. Bioactive compounds in plants-benefits and risks for man and animals:212-222.

50. Bennick, A. Interaction of Plant Polyphenols with Salivary Proteins. Crit. Rev Oral Biol. Med. 2002, 13: 184-196.

51. General Overview of Plant Phenolics. Available at: http://archive.lib.msu.edu.tic/thesdiss/mathias1976.pdf. On March 14, 2017.

52. National Center for Biotechnology Information. PubChem Compound Database; CID=7410. https://pubchem.ncbi.nlm.nih.gov/compound/7410 (accessed Aug 19, 2017).

53. National Center for Biotechnology Information. PubChem Compound Database; CID=119205, https://pubchem.ncbi.nlm.nih.gov/compound119205 (accessed Aug 19, 2017).

54. Murray Michael T. N.D. & Joseph Pizzorno, N.D. The encyclopedia of Natural Medicine 3rd Edition. 2012. Atria Books. New York.

55. National Center for Biotechnology Information. PubChem Compound Database; CID=119205, https://pubchem.ncbi.nlm.nih.gov/compound119205 (accessed Aug 19, 2017).

56. Sun, J. Chu, Y.-F., Wu X., & Liu R.H. Antioxidant and antiproliferative activities of fruits. A.J. Agric. Food Chem. 50:7449-7454.

57. Chu, Y.-F. Sun, J., Wu, X & Liu, R.H. (2002) Antioxidant and antiproliferative activities of vegetables. J.Agric. Food Chem. 50:6910-6916.

58. Madej, A., Lundh, T. Risk of adverse effects of phytoestrogens in animal feed. The Norwegian Academy of Science and Letters, 2010. Bioactive compounds in plants-benefits and risks for man and animals.

59. Boysen RI, Hearn M.TW. Comprehensive Natural Products II. 2010. (9): 5-49.

60. Dickerson, E. Alkaloids. J Natil Med Assoc 1913 Jul-Sep; 5(3): 157-158.

61. Cornell University. Saponins Department of Animal Science – Poisonous plants to livestock. 9/10/2015. Accessed August 20, 2017.

62. Gould, M.N. Cancer chmoprevention and therapy by monoterpenes. Environ Health Perspect. 1997 Jun.105(Suppl 4): 977-979.

63. Higdon J, Drake VJ, Delage B, Ho E. Isothiocyanaes. Linus Pauling Institute. Oregon State University. 2017. Accessed August 20, 2017.

64. Stahl, W. and Sies, H. Bioactivity and protective effects of natural carotenoids. Biochim Biophys Acta. 2005 May 30; 1740(2):101-7.

65. Higdon J, Drake VJ, Delage B, Johnson E.J. Carotenoids. Micronutrient Information. Linus Pauling Institute. Oregon State University. 2017.

66. Yates Allison A., John W. Erdman, Jr., Andrew Shao, Laurie C. Dolan, and James C Griffiths. Bioactive nutrients - Time for tolerable upper intake levels to address safety. March 2017. (84): 94-101.

67. Bhagwat S, Haytowitz DB., USDA Database for the Flavonoid, Content of Selected Food. November 2015. Release 3.2 www.ars.usda.gov/ARSUserFiles/80400525/Data/Flav/Flav3.2.pdf. Accessed August 17, 2017.

68. Nesheim JF, Sanjur AZ, Habicht JP. Serum retinol concentrations in children are affected by food sources of β-carotene, fat intake, and anthelmintic drug treatment. Am J. Clin Nutr. 1998;68(3):623-629.

69. Van Het Hof KH, West CE, Weststrate JA, Hautvast JG. Dietary factors that affect the bioavailability of carotenoids. J Nutr. 2000;130(3):503-506.

70. Wang XD. Carotenoids. In: Ross CA, Caballero B, Cousins RJ, Tucker KL, Ziegler TR, eds. Modern Nutrition in Health and Disease11th ed: Lippincott Williams & Wilkins; 2014:427-439.

71. Whiting S, Derbyshire E, Tiwari BK. Capsaicinoids and capsinoids. A potential role for weight management? A systematic review of the evidence. Appetite. 2012 Oct;59(2):341-8.

72. Clark, Ruth and Seong-Ho Lee, Anticancer Properties of Capsaicin Against Human Cancer. International Journal of Cancer Research. Anticancer Research (2016) 36:837-844.

73. Jayaprakasha GK, Haejin Bae, Kevin Crosby, John L. Jifon, Bhimanagouda S Patil. Bioactive Compounds in Peppers and Their Antioxidant Potential. November 15, 2012. doi: 10.1021/bk-2012-1109.ch004.

74. Simone DA, Baumann TK and LaMotte RH: Dose-dependent pain and mechanical hyperalgesia in humans after intradermal injection of capsaicin. Pain 38:99-107 189.

75. Brederson JD. Kym PR and Szallasi A: Targeting TRP channels for pain relief. Eur J Pharmacol. 2013. 716:61-76.

76. Galano A and Martinez A: Capsaicin, a tasty free radical scavenger: mechanism of action and kinetics. J Phys Chem. 2012. 116:1200-1208.

77. Kim CS, Kawada T, Kim BS, Han IS and Choe SY: Capsaicin exhibits anti-inflammatory property of inhibiting IkB-a degradation in LPS- stimulated peritoneal macrophages. Cell Signal. 2003. 15:299-306.

78. Kang JH, Kim CS, Han IS, Kawada T and Yu R: capsaicin, a spicy component or hot peppers, modulates adipokine gene expression and protein release from obese-mouse adipose tissues and isolated adipocytes, and suppresses the inflammatory responses of adipose tissue macrophages. FEBS Lett. 2007; 581:4389-96.

79. Kim MY, Trudel LJ and Wogan GN. Apoptosis induced by capsaicin and resveratrol in colon carcinoma cells requires nitric oxide production and caspase activation. Anticancer Res. 2009. 29:3733-3740.

80. Costet FC, Tristan R, Merillon JM. Stilbene from Vitis vinifera L. waste: a sustainable tool for controlling Plasmopara viticola. March 13. 2017. Doi:10.1021/acs.jafc.7b00241.

81. Nambiar VS, Sareen N, Daniel M, Gallego E. Flavonoids and phenolic acids from pearl millet (Pennisetum glaucum) based foods and their functional implications. Functional Foods in Health and Disease 2012, 2(7):251-264.

82. Tripoli E, Guardi ML, Giammanco S, Majo DD, Giammanco M. Citrus Flavonoids Molecular Structure, Biological Activity and Nutritional Properties: A Review. Food Chem. 2007. 104-446-479.

83. Jennings A, MacGregor A, Spector T, Aedin C. Higher dietary flavonoid intakes are associated with lower objectively measured body composition in women: evidence from discordant monozygotic twins. The American Journal of Clinical Nutrition. January 18, 2017. doi: 10.3924/ajcn.116.144394.

84. Manach C, Scalber A, Morand C, Remesy C, Jimenez L. Polyphenols: food sources and bioavailability. The American Journal of Clinical Nutrition. May 2004.79 (5):727-747.

85. Higdon J, Drake, VJ, Hu FB. Nuts. Linus Pauling Institute. Oregon State University. Micronutrient Information Center. 2017.

86. Hwang IG, Shin YH, Lee S, Lee J, and Yoo SM. Effects of Different Cooking Methods on the Antioxidant Properties of Red Pepper (*Capsicum annuum L.*). Preventive Nutrition and Food Science. 2012. Dec 17 (4): 286-292. doi: 10.3746/pnf.2012.17.4.286.

87. Wang L, Lee IM, Zhang SM, Blumberg JB, Buring JE, Sesso HD. Dietary intake of selected flavonols, flavones, and flavonoid-rich foods and risk of cancer in middle-aged and older women. The American Journal of Clinical Nutrition. January 21, 2009; 89(3). doi: 10.3945/ajcn. 2008. 26913.

88. Beecher, GR. Overview of Dietary Flavonoids: Nomenclature, Occurrence and Intake. The Journal of Nutrition. 2003. (133)10:3248S-3254S.

89. Ollberding NJ, Lim U, Wilkens LR, et al. Legume, soy, tofu and isoflavone intake and endometrial cancer risk in postmenopausal women in the multiethnic cohort study. J Natl Cancer Inst. 2012; 104(1):67-76.

90. Zhu Y, Ling W, Guo H, Song F, Ye Q, Zou T, Li D, Zhang Y, Li G, Xiao Y, Liu F, Li Z, Shi Z, Yang Y. Anti-inflammatory effect of purified dietary anthocyanin in adults with hypercholesterolemia: a randomized controlled trial. Nutr Metab Cardiovasc Dis. 2013; 23(9): 843-849.

91. Hollman PCH. Evidence for health benefits of plant phenols: local or systemic effects? Journal of Science of Food and Agriculture 81:842±852*online: 2001) doi: 10.1002/jsfa.900.

92. Jiang N, Doseff AI, Grotewold E. Flavones: From Biosynthesis to Health Benefits. Plants (Basel) 2016 Jun; 5(2):27.

93. Habauzit V, Verny MA, Milenkovic D, Barber-Chamoux N, Mazur A, Dubray C, Morand C. Flavanones protect from arterial stiffness in postmenopausal women Consuming grapefruit juice for 6 mo: a randomized, controlled crossover trial. Am J Clin Nutr. 2015 Jul;102(1):66-74.

94. Williamson G. Common features in the pathways of absorption and metabolism of flavonoids. In: Meskin MS, R. BW, Davies AJ, Lewis DS, Randolph RK, eds. Phytochemicals: Mechanisms of Action. Boca Raton: CRC Press; 2004:21-33.

95. Nemeth K, Plumb GW, Berrin JG, Juge N, Jacob R, Naim, HY, Williamson G, Swallow DM, Kroon PA. Deglycosylation by small intestinal epithelial cell β-glucosidases is a critical step in the absorption and metabolism of dietary flavonoid glycosides in humans. Eur J Nutr. 2003; 42(1):29-42.

96. Monagas M, Urpi-Sarda M, Sanchez-Patan F, Llorach R, Garrido I, Gomez-Cordoves C, Andres-Lacueva C, Bartolome B. Insights into the metabolism and microbial biotransformation of dietary flavan-3-ols and the bioactivity of their metabolites. Food Funct. 2010 Dec; 1(3):233-53.

97. Roowi S, Stalmach A, Mullen W, Lean ME, Edwards CA, Crozier A. Green tea flavan-3-ols: colonic degradation and urinary excretion of catabolites by humans. J Agric Food Chem. 2010; 58(2):1296-1304.

98. Stechell KD, Brown NM, Lydeking-Olsen E. The clinical importance of the metabolite equol-a clue to the effectiveness of soy and its isoflavones. J Nutr. 2002;132(12):3577-3584.

99. Yuan JP, Wang JH, Liu X. Metabolism of dietary soy isoflavones to equol by human intestinal microflora—implications for health. Mol Nutr Food Res. 2007;51(7):765-781.

100. Martin L, Miguelez EM, Villar CJ, Lombo F. Bioavailability of dietary polyphenols and gut microbiota metabolism: antimicrobial properties. Biomed Res Int. 2015; 2015:905215.

101. Cabuk B, Okulu B, Stanciuc N, Harsa ST. Nanoencapsulation of Biologically Active Peptides from Whey Proteins. Journal of Nutritional Health and Food Science 2(3):1-4.

102. Nagendra P. Shah. Effects of milk-derived bioactivities: an overview. British Journal of Nutrition (2000), 84, Suppl. 1: 3-10.

103. Walstra P & Jenness R. (1984) Diary Chemistry and Physics. New York: John Wiley.

104. Maubois & Leonil. (1989) Peptides du lait a activebiologigue. Lait 69:245.

105. Reynoso-Camacho R, Ramos-Gomez M, and Loarca-Pina G. Bioactive components common beans (Phaseolus vulgaris L.). Advances in Agricultural and Food Biotechnology. 2006: 217-236.

106. Sassy Bhawamai, Shyh-Hsiang Lin, Yuan-Yu Hou, and Yue-Hwa Chen. Thermal cooking changes the profile of phenolic compounds, but does not attenuate the anti-inflammatory activities of black rice. Food and nutrition research. 2016; Sep 20. doi: 10.3402/fnr.v60.32941.

107. Naik AS, Lele SS. Functional Lipids and Bioactive Compound from Oil Rich Indigenous Seeds. Nutrition and Food Engineering. 2012. 6(9). Waste.org/Publication/15046

108. Kris-Etherton PM, Zhao G, Binkoski AE, Coval SM, Etherton TD. The effects of nuts on coronary heart disease risk. *Nutr Rev.* 2001; 59(4):103-111.

109. Segura R, Javierre C, Lizarraga Ma, Ros E. Other relevant components of nuts: phytosterols, folate and minerals. *Br J Nutr.* 2006; 96 Suppl 2:S36-44.

110. Willett WC. 2001. Eat, Drink and be Healthy: *The Harvard Medical School Guideto Healthy Eating.* New York: Simon & Schuster.

111. Coates AM, Howe PR. Edible nuts and metabolic health. *Curr Opin Lipidol.* 2007; 18(1): 25-30.

112. Trox J, Vadivel V, Vetter W, Stuetz W, Scherbaum V, Gola U, Nohr D, Biesalski HK. Bioactive Compounds in Cashew Nut (*Anacardium occidentale* L.) Kernels: Effect of Different Shelling Methods. Journal of Agricultural and Food Chemistry. 2010.58(9): 5341-5346.

113. Maeda H, Satoh T, Islam WM. Preparation of functional enhanced vegetable oils. Functional Foods in Health and Disease 2016; 6(1):33-41.

114. Chomchan R, Siripongvutikorn S, Puttarak P, Rattanapon R. Investigation of phytochemical constituents, phenolic profiles and antioxidant activities of ricegrass juice compared to wheatgrass juice. Functional Foods in Health and Disease 2016; 6(12):822-835.

115. Tome-Carniero J, Gonzalvez M, Larrosa M, Yanez-Gascon, MJ, Garcia-Almagro FJ, Ruiz-Ros JA, Tomas-Barberan FA, Garcia-Conesa MT, Espin JC. Grape resveratrol increases serum adiponectin and downregulates inflammatory genes in peripheral blood mononuclear cells: a triple-blind, placebo-controlled, one-year clinical trial in patients with stable Coronary Artery Disease. Cardiovasc Drugs Ther. 2013; 27: 37-48.

116. Wegener C, Gisela J, Jurgens HU. Bioactive compounds in potatoes: Accumulation under drought stress conditions. Functional Foods in Health and Disease 2015; 5(3): 108-116.

117. Alam MZ, Wang-Pruski G, Jodges M, Hawkins GR, Kubik MD, Fillmore SAE. Effect of Cooking and Reconsitiution Methods of the Loss of Bioactive Compounds in Pigmented and Unpigmented Potatoes. Food and Nutrition Sciences, 2017; 8:31-55.

118. Kant S, Chaithirayanon K, Vivithanaport P, Siangcham T, Poomtong PRJ, Nobsathian S, Sobhon P. Extract of the sea cucumber, Holothuria scabra, induces apoptosis in Human glioblastoma cell lines. Functional Foods in Health and disease 2016; 6(7): 452-468.

119. Higdon J, Drake VJ, Delage B, Crozier A. Flavonoids. Linus Pauling Institute. Oregon State University. Micronutrient Information. 2017. Lpi.orgeonstate.edu/mic (accessed August 2017).

120. Fan C, Pacier C, Martirosyan DM. Rose hip (Rosa canina L): A functional food perspective. Functional Foods in Health and Disease 2014; 4(11): 493-509.

121. Shahidul I, Jalaluddin M, Hettiarachchy NS. Bioactive compounds of bitter melon genotypes (Momordica charanta L.) in relation to their physiological functions. Functional Foods in Health and Disease 2011 1(2):61-74.

122. Wasser SP, Weis A. Medicinal Properties of Substances occurring in Higher Basidiomycetes Mushrooms: Current Perspectives. International Journal of Medicinal Mushrooms. 1999. Vol 1(1):47-50.

123. Wasser SP. Current findings, future trends, and unsolved problems in studies of medicinal mushrooms. Appl Microbiol Biotechnol (2011) 89: 1323-32.

124. Ingebrigtsen K. Main plant poisonings in livestock in the Nordic countries. The Norwegian Academy of Science and Letters. 2010. Norwegian School of Veterinary Science, Oslo, Norway:30-43.

125. Van Gelder WMJ, Vinke JH, Scheffer JJC. Steroidal glycoalkaloids in tubers and leaves of *Solanum* species used in potato breeding. *Euphytica* 1988; **S**:147-158.

126. Korpan YI, Nazaranko EA, Skryshevskaya IV, Martelet C, Jaffrezic-Renault N, El´skaya. Potato glycoalkaloids: true safety or false sense of security? Trends in Biotechnology. 2004; 22: 147-151.

127. Memorial Sloan Kettering Cancer Center. Shiitake Mushroom. December 31, 2015..

128. Enman J, Rova U, Berglund KA. Quantification of the bioactive compound eritadenine iselected strains of shiitake mushroom (Lentinus edodes). *J Agric Food Chem.* 2007 Feb 21;55(4):1177-80.

129. National Center for Biotechnology Information. U.S. National Library of Medicine.

130. De Vries J. Food safety and toxicity. Boca Raton, CRC Press; 1996.

131. Horowitz BZ. FACMT. Mushroom Toxicity. Dec. 29, 2015. Emedicine.medscape.com/article/167398-overview. (accessed August 2017).

132. Lee DS. Amatoxin Toxicity. Medscape. Jul 21, 2015. Emedicine.medscape.com/article/1008902-overview.

133. Horowitz BZ, Gossman W. Toxicity, Mushrooms, Amatoxin. 2017. In: State Pearls (Internet). Treasure Island (FL): State Pearls Publishing; 2017.

134. Arshadi M, Nilsson C, Magnusson B. Gas chromatography-mass spectrometry determination of the pentafluorobenzoyl derivative of methylhydrazine in false morel (Gyromitra esculenta) as a monitor for the content of the toxin gyromitrin. Journal of Chromatography A. 1 September 2006;1125(2):222-233.

135. Michelot D, Toth B. Poisoning by Gyromitra esculenta—a review. J Appl Toxicol. 1991 Aug;11(4):235-43.

136. National Center for Biotechnology Information. PubChem Compound Database; CID-9548611, https://pubchem.ncbi.nlm.nih.gov/compound/gyromitrin. (accessed September 13, 2017).

137. Poisonous Mushrooms. University of Hawaii, Botany. Lecture 18. (accessed www.botany.hawaii.edu/faculty/wong/BOT135/Lect 18.htm)

138. Shao D, Tang, S, Healy R, Imerman PA, Schrunk DE, Rumbeiha WK. A novel orellanine containing mushroom Cortinarius armillatus. Science Direct May 2016. Vol 114:65-74.

139. National Center for Biotechnology Information. PubChem Compound Database; CID=89579, https://pubchem.ncbi.nlm.nih.gov/compound89579 (accessed Aug 19, 2017).

140. Keller-Dilitz H, Moser M, Ammirati J. Orellanine and Other Fluorescent Compounds in the Genus Cortinarius, Section Orellani. Mycologia. Sept-Oct 1985. 77(5).

141. Frank H, Zilker T, Kirchmair M, Eyer F, Haberl B, Tuerkoglu-Raach G, Wessely M, Grone HJ, Heemann U. Acute renal failure by ingestion of Cortinarius species confounded with psychoactive mushrooms: a case series and literature survey. Clin Nephrol 2009 Jun;71(6):727.

142. Hatfield GM, Schaumberg, JP. Isolation and structural studies of coprine, the disulfiram-like constituent of Coprinus atramentarius. 01 Nov 1975;38(6):489-496.

143. National Center for biotechnology Information. PubChem Compound Database; CID=108079, https://pubchem.ncbi.nlm.nih.gov/compound108079 (accessed Aug 19, 2017).

144. Michelot D. Poisoning by Coprinus atramentarius. Natural toxins. 1992 Mar. 1;1(2):73-80.

145. Stallard D, Edes TE. Muscarinic poisoning from medications and mushrooms. A puzzling symptom complex. Postgrad Med 1989 Jan;85(1):341-5.

146. National Center for Biotechnology Information. PubChem Compound Database; CID=4266, https://pubchem.ncbi.nlm.nih.gov/compound4266. (accessed Aug 19, 2017).

147. Beaumont K, Chilton, WS, Yamamura HI, Enna SJ. Muscimol binding in rat brain: Association with synaptic GABA receptors. Science Direct. Brain Research.9 June 1978. 148(1):153-162.

148. Shirota O, Hakamata W, Goda Y. Concise Large-Scale Synthesis of Psilocin and Psilocybin, Principal Hallucinogenic Constituents of "Magic Mushroom". Journal of Natural Products. 2003;66(6):885-887.

149. National Center for Biotechnology Information. PubChem Compound Database; CID=10624, https://pubchem.ncbi.nlm.nih.gov/compound10624 (accessed Aug 19, 2017).

150. National Center for Biotechnology Information. PubChem Compound Database; CID=4980, https://pubchem.ncbi.nlm.nih.gov/compound4980 (accessed Aug 19, 2017).

151. Levy AM, Kita H, Phillips SF, Schkade PA, Dyer PD, Gleich GJ, Dubravec VA. Eosinophilia and gastrointestinal symptoms after shiitake mushrooms. J Allergy Clin Immunol. 1998 May;101(5);613-20.

152. Chawla A, Repa JJ, Evans RM, Mangelsdorf DJ. Nuclear receptors and lipid physiology: opening the X-files. Science 2001; 94:1866-70.

153. Desvergne B, Wahli W. Peroxisome proliferator-activated receptors: nuclear control of metabolism. Endocr Rev 1996; 20:649-88.

154. Kersten S, Desvergne B, Wahli W. Roles of PPARs in health and disease. Nature 2000; 405:421-4.

155. Gershon D. Microarray technology: an array of opportunities. Nature 2002; 416:885-91.

156. Elliott R, Ong TJ. Nutritional genomics. BMJ 2002; 324:1438–42.

157. Holmboe-Ottesen, G. Increased levels of bioactive compounds in organically World. 2015. Vol. 1.

158. Schreiner M. Vegetable crop management strategies to increase the quantity of phytochemicals. *Eur J Nutr* 2005; 44: 85-94.

159. Memorial Sloan Kettering Cancer Center. Maitake. April 2, 2015. https://www.mskcc.org/cancer-care/integrative-medicine/herbs/maitake (accessed September 13, 2017.

160. Adachi K, Nanba H, Kuroda H. Potentiation of host-mediated antitumor activity in mice by beta glucan obtained from Grifola Frondosa (maitake). Chem Pharm Bull. 1987; 35:262-70.

161. Kubo K, Aoki H, Nanba H. Anti-diabetic activity present in the fruit body of Grifola frondosa (Maitake). Biol Pharm Bull 1994; 17:1106-10.

162. Horio H, Ohtsuru M. Maitake (Grifola fondosa) improved glucose tolerance of experimental diabetic rats. J Nutr Sci Vitaminol 2001; 47:57-63.

163. Masuda Y, Murata Y, Hayashi M, Nanba H. Inhibitory effect of MD-Fraction on tumor metastasis: involvement of NK cell activation and suppression of intercellular adhesion molecule (ICAM)-1 expression in lung vascular endothelial cells. Biol Pharm Bull 2008 Jun;31(6):1104-8.

164. Zhao Y, J. Collier J, Huang EC, Whelan J. Turmeric and Chinese goldthread synergistically inhibit prostate cancer cell proliferation and NF-kB signaling. Functional Foods in health and Disease 2014; 4(7):312-339.

165. Obied HK. Biography of biophenols: past, present and future. Functional Foods in Health and Disease 2013; 3(6):230-241.

3

Introduction to Functional Foods

Anju Dhiman, Vaibhav Walia, Arun Nanda

Department of Pharmaceutical Sciences, Maharshi Dayanand University, Rohtak 124001, Haryana, India

Introduction

Healthy eating contributes to good health and well-being, but busy consumers lack time to access their optimal diet. Increased affluence and urbanization has led to modern lifestyles, which are linked to various mental health problems such as depression, poor concentration, loss of memory, etc. Therefore, industrialized countries are now facing major challenges:

1. Controlling health care cost
2. Offering better opportunities to prolong the population's lifespan
3. Providing healthy, processed, and ready-to-eat foods to busy consumers
4. Emphasizing the use of food to promote a state of well-being, better health, and reduced risk of diseases.

Links between food and health increase interest in the relationships between diet, health and well-being. Over the last decade and primarily in Japan and the United States, these challenges, together with new concepts in nutrition, have justified the development of "**functional food**." The importance of a healthy lifestyle, including diet and its role in reducing our risk of illness and disease, can increase the demand of functional foods.

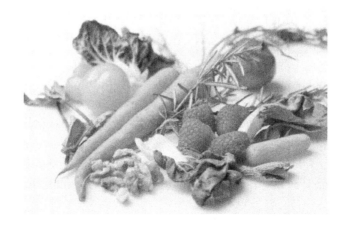

Functional Foods

A food can be called "functional" if it *contains a food component that targets one or a limited number of functions in the body, so as to have positive physiological or psychological effects beyond the traditional nutritional outcome.* The European Commision Concerted Action on Functional Food Science in Europe (FUFOSE) proposed a working definition of functional food: a food that improves the state of health and well-being and/or reduces the risk of disease beyond adequate nutritional effects. The component that makes the food "functional" can be either an essential macronutrient, if it has specific physiological effects, or an essential micronutrient, if its intake is above the daily recommendation. So, the term "functional food" should be considered for a food whose attraction lies in its health claims. Therefore, without an accompanying health claim, it cannot be called a functional food. According to the US Dietary Supplement Health and Education Act (DSHEA) of 1994, the term "**dietary supplement**" can be defined using several criteria, namely (a) a product intended to supplement a diet, that contains one or more of the following dietary ingredients: a vitamin, a mineral, an herb or other botanical organism, an amino acid, a dietary substance used to increase the total daily intake, or a concentrate, metabolite, constituent, extract, or a combination of these ingredients, (b) a product intended for ingestion in pill, capsule, tablet, or liquid form, (c) a product not represented for use as a conventional food or as the sole item of a meal or diet, (d) anything labeled as a "dietary supplement", and (e) a newly approved drug, certified antibiotic, or licensed biological products that were marketed as a dietary supplement or food before approval, certification, or license (unless this provision was waived by an authority such as Secretary of Health and Human Services, as in the USA). Many European countries have adopted the highly restrictive CODEX standards for dietary supplements, which eliminate the consumer's ability to purchase dietary supplements in therapeutic or meaningful preventive dosages. The major differences between dietary supplements and functional foods lie in the fact that dietary supplements are intended for ingestion in pill, capsule, tablet, or liquid form, not represented for use as a conventional food or as the sole item of a meal or diet, and are labeled as a dietary supplement. Functional foods, according to Zeisel, are not dietary supplements, but rather "consumed as part of a normal diet and deliver one or more active ingredients (that have physiologic effects and may enhance health) within the food matrix." [1]

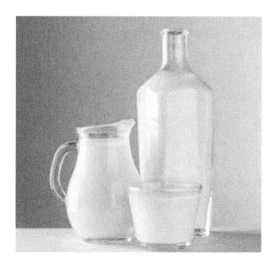

Types of Functional Foods

Prebiotics: A *prebiotic* is a selectively fermented ingredient that results in specific changes in the composition and/or activity of the gastrointestinal microbiota, thus conferring health benefits upon the host. They are generally oligomers made up of 4 to 10 monomeric hexose units. Their actions have been primarily directed toward the colon and they selectively stimulate beneficial microbes within the gut microbiota, directly stimulate immunity, protect against pathogens, and facilitate host metabolism and mineral absorption. The use of oligosaccharides selectively prevents the adhesion of certain bacterial species by mimicking binding sites. Prebiotics can act as a decoy for pathogen-binding cellular receptors in the gut. The addition of prebiotics in food may offer other benefits by improving host absorption of minerals (e.g. inulin type-fructans enhanced calcium absorption) primarily via the colonic mucosa in humans [2, 3].

Probiotics*: Probiotics* are live microorganisms that confer a health benefit on the host when administered in adequate amounts. The probiotic arsenal includes multiple mechanisms for preventing infection, enhancing the immune system, and providing increased nutritional value to food. Probiotics can enhance the host's defense system against pathogens by the promotion of mucin production or reduction of gut permeability. Promoting mucin production and reducing intestinal permeability may prevent penetration of pathogenic organisms and toxic substances, as well as the production of an array of antimicrobial compounds capable of inhibiting the growth of many food borne pathogens. In general, lactic acid bacteria produce organic acids, predominantly lactate and acetate, which create an acidic environment that is inhibitory to pathogens. The probiotic, *L. reuteri*, produces an antimicrobial agent, reuterin, which has a broad spectrum of activity against a variety of pathogens, including bacteria, fungi, protozoa and viruses [3].

Synbiotics are a combination of probiotics and prebiotics administered together.

Examples of functional foods:

Many functional foods now exist in various countries [4]. Some are:

Oat bran fiber: Fiber is the endogenous component of plant materials and is resistant to digestion by enzymes produced by humans. Consumption of soluble fiber has now been shown to lower LDL cholesterol levels through a series of processes that alter cholesterol and glucose metabolism. The mechanism of action is thought to involve increasing fecal bile acid excretion and interference with bile acid reabsorption. Specifically, this effect of fiber may be attributable to its binding and diluting actions on bile acids, and the lowering of intestinal pH. This inhibits the conversion of primary bile acids to secondary bile acids, thus resulting in a reduction in the absorption of fat and cholesterol. Consumption of about 25 g/day of oat-containing foods can reduce the risk of heart disease. The use of the soluble fiber oat bran in cardiovascular risk management was the first health claim allowed under the US Dietary Supplement Health Education Act (DSHEA) during the 1990s.

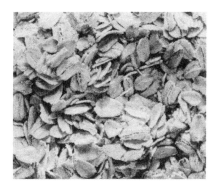

Soy protein: The consumption of soy protein is associated with a reduced risk of coronary heart disease, because it lowers the cholesterol concentrations through the activation of the LDL receptor pathway. The FDA concluded that soy protein is low in saturated fat and cholesterol, and may reduce the risk of coronary heart disease by lowering blood cholesterol levels. This could stem from its amino acid profile, which differs from those of animal proteins, resulting in a desirable lowering of circulating LDL cholesterol.

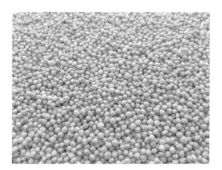

Fish oil fatty acids: The fatty acids found in fish and fish oils have gained publicity for their role in the prevention and management of cardiovascular disease. The recommended level of consumption of fish oil fatty acids with health benefits is 2–4 g/day. The scientific evidence about whether omega-3 fatty acids may reduce the risk of **coronary heart disease (CHD)** is suggestive, but not conclusive. It is not known what effect omega-3 fatty acids may have on the general population's risk of CHD [5].

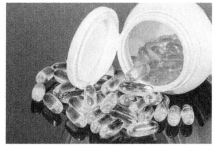

Functional Food Science

Designing and developing functional foods is a scientific challenge that should rely on the following [6]:

1. Basic scientific knowledge relevant to functions that pertain to modulation by food components, pivotal to maintenance of well-being and good health.
2. The exploitation of this knowledge in the development of markers, relevant to the key functions.
3. The generation of new hypotheses that will include the use of these validated, relevant markers and allow effective and safe intakes.
4. The development of advanced techniques for human studies that are minimally invasive and applicable on a large scale.

When researching and developing a functional food, the initial is the identification of a specific and potentially beneficial interaction between one or more components of the food and a genomic, cellular, biochemical or physiologic function in the organism. As such, a functional effect can then be defined. The conclusion of these experiments is a new hypothesis pertaining to the relevance of the functional effect to human health- tested in strictly designed nutritional studies.

Production of functional foods

A food product can be made functional in the following ways [7]:

1. Eliminating a component known to cause harmful effects when consumed (e.g., an allergenic protein).
2. Increasing the concentration of a component naturally present in food, to a point at which it will induce predicted effects [e.g., fortification with a micronutrient to reach a daily intake higher than the recommended daily intake, but compatible with the dietary guidelines for reducing risk of disease], or increasing the concentration of a nonnutritive component to a level known to produce a beneficial effect.
3. Adding a component that is not normally present in most foods and is not necessarily a macronutrient or a micronutrient, but for which beneficial effects have been shown (e.g., nonvitamin antioxidant or prebiotic fructan).
4. Replacing a component, usually a macronutrient (e.g. fats), whose excessive intake causes negative effects [e.g. chicory inulin such as Rafticream].
5. By increasing the bioavailability or stability of a component known to produce a functional effect, or to reduce the disease-risk potential of the food.

Selection criteria and characteristics of probiotics [8]: Before bacteria can be considered as a use for probiotics, it is recommended that they meet certain criteria and possess a number of intrinsic physico-chemical characteristics outlined in a joint report by the FAO and WHO in 2002. While probiotic bacteria, as a group, is **generally regarded as safe (GRAS)** organisms, safety tests should include the determination of antibiotic resistance profiles, evaluation of certain metabolic activities (such as D-lactate production and bile salt deconjugation), assessment of side effects in human trials, post-market epidemiological surveillance of adverse effects in consumers, toxin production, and finally haemolytic activity. Furthermore, animal trials should be undertaken, where possible and appropriate, before commencing human studies.

Motivation for the development of functional foods

The following are key points motivating the development of the functional foods [9]:

1. Consumers should be aware of the possible positive role in the management of disease risk. Increased education and overall heightening of interest in the general area of preventive health supports this fact.

2. Governments have become increasingly cognizant and supportive of the public health benefits of functional foods. For instance, Japan allows more than 200 functional foods to be marketed under existing FOSHU (Foods for Specialized Health Use) legislation, and the United States with the Food and Drug Administration (FDA) permits health claims to be made for about 15 categories of food.

3. Governments looking at regulatory issues for functional foods are more aware of the economic potential of these products as part of public health prevention strategies. The FDA now arranges a group of independent scientists to gather and weigh all the relevant clinical data for each health claim submission.

Development of Functional Foods

The development of new functional food products is increasingly challenging; products must be simultaneously palatable, healthy, and fulfill the consumer's expectations.

1. The primary aim of food science industries is to determine the optimum levels of key ingredients to obtain ideal sensory and physicochemical responses.

2. Then identify consumer expectation. The success of functional foods relies on a number of factors, including the level of concern about general health and different medical conditions; the belief that it is possible to influence one's own health; and awareness and knowledge of foods/ingredients that are supposed to be beneficial.

3. Afterward is the conception of hypotheses that include the use of these validated, relevant markers and allow effective and safe intakes.

4. The final step is the development of advanced techniques for human studies that, preferably, are minimally invasive and applicable on a large scale.

Functional foods supplier

1. In the mid 90's, several multinational food companies introduced functional food products into the EU and German market. This market of functional milk products was initiated by the market introduction of Nestlé's LC1 yogurt in 1995, followed by the Actimelline of Danone. Soon after, Japanese probiotic milk products were introduced, named ''Yakult'' in 1994 in the European market. Unilever introduced a specific functional variety of Becel-margarine (named ''Becel proactiv'') in the EU in 2000. It is supposed to lower the cholesterol level in the blood.

2. Another type of a functional food producer can be pharmaceutical or dietary product producing companies; e.g. Novartis Consumer Health, Glaxo SmithKline, Johnson & Johnson, or Abbott Laboratories. In particular, Novartis Consumer Health has launched a series of functional food products including biscuits, cereal, cereal bars and beverages

in different European countries, under the "AVIVA" brand in 1999. However, due to lower sales than expected, Novartis withdrew the AVIVA products from most markets after one year.

3. A third group of functional food producers are companies that specialize in a particular product category, which mostly belong to the market leaders on a national level. Examples for this type of company represent Molkerei Alois Muller (with its functional "ProCult" dairy products), Ehrmann ("DailyFit" dairy products), Bauer (with several probiotic dairy products), Eckes (ACE drinks) or Becker Fruchts (ACE fruit juice) in Germany.

Consumer acceptance of functional foods

1. Increasing the functionality of the food should not necessarily change its sensory quality. Bitter, acrid, astringent, or salty off-flavors often inherently result from enhancing food functionality with bioactive compounds or plant-based phytonutrients. The occurrence of off-flavors in juice decreased its acceptance and consumption, despite the presence of convincing health claims.

2. Another issue is whether consumers are willing to accept functional foods that taste worse than substitute conventional foods; and, if so, what their profile is and what the determinants of their willingness to compromise on taste are.

3. Women have been shown to be more reflective about food and health issues than men and they seem to have more moral and ecological misgivings about eating certain foods than men, who are more confident and demonstrate a rather uncritical and traditional view of eating.

4. Another relevant socio-demographic factor pertains to the presence of young children in the household. This factor may impact food choice because of its potential association with higher food risk aversion or higher quality consciousness, since parenting triggers a focus on nutrition- yielding a search for nurturing benefits through the provision of wholesome foods.

5. Middle-aged and elderly consumers are much more likely to be diagnosed with a lifestyle-related disease than younger consumers. Given the fact that prevention is a major motivation of the use of functional food, it can logically be hypothesized that experience with illnesses increases probabilities of functional food acceptance.

6. The use of functional foods may offer a new, less-demanding way of gaining an ethical reward through food choices: consumers feel that they can take care of themselves, and that making the "right" choices are socially acceptable. This rewarding feeling may be connected not only to the control over one's own health, but also to the positive impressions that an individual may want to evoke among other people.

Key Challenges in the development marketing research and acceptance of functional foods

1. What should be the dose of a probiotic? Market development. Market development is influenced by the degree of familiarity and acceptance of functional foods. According

to surveys in the United Kingdom, France, and Germany, up to 75% of the consumers have not heard the term ''Functional Food,'' but more than 50% of them agree to fortify functional ingredients in specific food products. Therefore, the acceptance to a specific functional ingredient is linked to the consumers' knowledge of the health effects of specific ingredients.

2. Functional ingredients that are in the mind of consumers for a relatively long period of time achieve considerably higher rates of consumer acceptance than ingredients that are used for a short period of time.

3. Consumers often do not know the health benefits of the specific groups of ingredients, and therefore are not able to assess the health effects.

4. Consumers are not willing to change their daily lifestyle or eating patterns for the consumption of a specific functional food product.

5. Due to limited consumer knowledge and awareness of the health effects of newly developed functional ingredients, there are strong needs for specific information and communication activities to consumers in this respect.

6. Functional food is positioned in a transitional zone between food and pharmaceuticals. In almost all European countries, as well as the European Union, these areas are traditionally regulated by separate institutions and are subject to different regulation regimes. A kind of ''grey zone'' emerges, with a high level of uncertainty.

7. Definition problems. These mainly exist for products with functions aimed to prevent nutrition-related diseases and/or to support health. In the EU and related national legislation, it is currently forbidden to use disease-related aspects in consumer information or product advertisement for functional foods.

8. The price for this functional food in comparison to ''conventional'' food products. Examples of recently launched functional food products indicate that consumers are only willing to accept limited price premia for such products.

9. Stating the type, viability, and number of bacteria contained in a probiotic product is important to both the consumer and health regulatory officials. To obtain a health claim for a probiotic product, food manufacturers will have to precisely define their microorganism. At the present time, there is little incentive for manufacturers to include this health information on their product; the costs for such quality assurance would be high. As regulations become clearer, manufacturers can expect that they will be required to state this information. Consumers are becoming more educated about probiotics, and they too will be pressuring food manufacturers for this information.

10. Identification of the biomarker that applies to all clinical trials involving probiotics because of the wide variety of diseases and conditions.

11. The amount and status of the bacteria that should be consumed to obtain a beneficial effect. There is still no consensus as to the minimum number of bacteria that need to be consumed to produce a beneficial effect on human metabolism and health.

12. The consumption of probiotics. Probiotics must be consumed every day because they do not colonize in the gut and are quickly flushed out of the GI tract when consumption is stopped. At this time, microbiological analyses of fecal material are the only way to

show that the probiotic bacteria have remained viable during their passage through the GI tract. This is a major limitation since the site of action of probiotics is the large intestine or even higher up the GI tract. Therefore, even if companies are able to report how many viable bacteria are contained in their product when consumed, they are not able to report how many bacteria actually produce the beneficial effect at the site of action.

13. *Lactococcus* and *Lactobacillus* are most commonly given the "generally recognized as safe" status, but some of the genera *Streptococcus* and *Enterococcus* and some other genera of LAB that could be potential probiotics contain opportunistic pathogens. Most LAB are considered safe for human consumption, and so their inclusion in probiotic products presents no problems. However, before any new probiotic microorganisms will be approved, data will have to be submitted clearly shows they are safe for human consumption.

14. One example is St John's wort, a popular herb utilized for treating mild depression. Hypericum extract from St. John's wort significantly increases the metabolic activity of liver cytochrome P_{450}. This enzyme inactivates several drugs, and thus would be expected to decrease their levels and activities in the body. Consuming St. John's wort has been shown to cause related decreases in plasma concentrations of theophylline, cyclosporine, warfarin and ethinylestradiol / desogestrel (oral contraceptives). Such data prompted the FDA to issue a Public Health Advisory about St. John's wort in February of 2000, as have Canadian authorities. In the United States, some consumer groups have lobbied the FDA to halt the sale of 75 functional foods enhanced with St. John's wort, as well as the following additional herbs: guarana, gotu kola, ginseng, ginkgo biloba, echinacea, kava kava and spirulina.

15. Develop and promulgate regulations or other guidance for industry on the evidence needed to document the safety of new dietary ingredients in dietary supplements.

16. Develop and spread regulations or other guidance for industry on the safety-related information required on labels for dietary supplements and functional foods.

17. Develop an enhanced system to record and analyze reports of health problems associated with functional foods and dietary supplements.

Future of functional foods

1. How functional foods and food ingredients might help prevent chronic disease or optimize health, thereby reducing healthcare costs and improving the quality of life for many consumers.

2. An emerging discipline that will have a profound effect on future functional foods research and development efforts, *nutrigenomics* investigates the interaction between diet and the development of diseases based on an individual's genetic profile. Interest in nutrigenomics was greatly augmented by the recent announcement that a rough draft of the complete sequence of the human genome has become available. Nutrigenomics will have a profound effect on future disease prevention efforts, including the future of the functional foods industry.

3. Another technology that will greatly influence the future of functional foods is **biotechnology**. Because biotechnology-derived crops have tremendous potential to improve the health of millions worldwide, including golden rice and iron-enriched rice, they are genetically engineered to provide enhanced levels of iron and β-carotene which could, in turn, help prevent iron deficiency anemia and vitamin A deficiency–related blindness worldwide.

4. The task of raising awareness and educating consumers is vitally important if functional foods are to fulfill their potential, but the question of who provides that education needs to be addressed. For many people, the media, especially television, is a major source of information about health and functional foods.

Research challenges for functional foods

- Defining the bioavailability of functional food ingredients.
- Identifying individual biological responses to functional foods.
- Developing appropriate biomarkers for a wider range of functional endpoints.
- Anticipating demand for personalized nutrition and the potential role of functional foods.
- Developing the potential utility of nutrigenomics, bioinformatics, proteomics, metabolomics and nanotechnology in the development of functional foods.
- Ensuring stability of functional food ingredients during manufacturing and passage through the GI tract to reach the target organ intact.
- Establishing Dietary Reference Intakes (DRIs) for a wider range of nutrients to enable commercial exploitation of more functional components.
- Identifying potential functional ingredients that could provide benefits in terms of health and well-being [13].

Functional foods in the treatment of the disorders

Arthritis: Arthritis involves the inflammation of the joints and the treatment generally focuses to reduce pain intensity, stiffness, and reduced non-steroidal anti-inflammatory drugs consumption. The supplementation with n-3 PUFAs for 3-4 months reduces pain intensity, stiffness, and also reduced non-steroidal anti-inflammatory drugs consumption in patients suffering from osteoarthritis.

Asthma: Fish oil containing more than 2% fat has been found to have a reduced risk of airway hyperresponsiveness. Children who regularly eat fish have a reduced risk of developing asthma than children who rarely eat fish. Supplementation of diet with n-3 fatty acids also confirmed benefit in the reduction of breathing difficulties and other symptoms, along with reduced drug doses required by asthma patients because of the results in the competitive inhibition of pro-inflammatory eicosanoid production and production of anti-inflammatory eicosanoids.

Neuroinflammation: A diet rich in EPA and DHA reduces neuroinflammation. Elderly people who eat fish or seafood (which is highly enriched in n-3 PUFAs) at least once a week have been shown to be at lower risk of developing dementia, including Alzheimer's disease. Evidence is also emerging which suggests that marine algae could possess therapeutic activities for combating neurodegenerative diseases associated with neuroinflammation. The *Ulva conglobata* extract almost completely suppressed the expression of the pro-inflammatory enzyme cyclooxygenase-2 (COX-2) and inducible nitric oxide (iNOS) in murine BV2 microglia. Similarly, the brown alga, *Ecklonia cava*, was reported to induce significant inhibition of NF-κB dependent cytokines as well as iNOS and COX-2, thus reducing inflammation. In addition, red alga *Neorhodomela aculeate* could be considered as a potential neuroprotective and anti-inflammatory agent to treat aging related neurological disorders [14].

Cardiovascular diseases: Reactive oxygen species (ROS) are involved in the pathogenesis of both acute and chronic heart diseases as a result of cumulative oxidative stress. In particular, oxidation of low-density lipoproteins (LDL) has a key role in the pathogenesis of atherosclerosis and cardiovascular heart diseases through the initiation of the plaque formation process. It has been shown that people consuming healthy diets, living active lifestyles, not smoking and not indulging in excessive alcohol consumption, tend to have a reduced risk of CVD. It is also known that diets leading to elevated serum total cholesterol, LDL-cholesterol, and triacylglycerol concentrations (while leading to reduced HDL-cholesterol concentrations), lead to reduced risk of coronary artery disease. As a result, treatment of hypercholesterolemia has focused on increasing fecal excretion of cholesterol and bile acids, and reducing hepatic cholesterol synthesis through diet modification are among the few optional strategies available. Consequently, a general nutritional plan to minimize hypertension risk includes attaining and maintaining a healthy body weight, consuming a diet rich in calcium, phosphorus, and magnesium, and consuming alcoholic beverages and sodium in moderation.

GIT disorders: The human gastrointestinal tract serves two main purposes: acting as a barrier to the external environment, and as the main entry portal for nutrients. The principal purported health-promoting effect of probiotics is their enhancement of mucosal immune defenses. These mechanisms include: increasing enzyme production, enhancing digestion and nutrient uptake, maintaining the host microbial balance in the intestinal tract by producing bactericidal substances that compete with pathogens and toxins for adherence to the intestinal epithelium, promoting intestinal epithelial cell survival, barrier function, protective responses, and regulating immune responses by enhancing the innate immunity, and preventing pathogen-induced inflammation. In the absence of microbes, there are profound deficiencies in intestinal epithelial and mucosal immunological development and functions, including the inability to generate proper immune responses to protect against infection and inflammation. In addition to nutritional functions, the intestinal epithelial cells are critical for maintaining normal intestinal homeostasis through several protective defense mechanisms. These include barrier functions formed by tight junctions, antibacterial substances synthesis, and active involvement in innate and adaptive immunity. Probiotics facilitate intestinal epithelial homeostasis through a number of biological responses, such as promoting proliferation, migration, survival, barrier integrity, antimicrobial substance secretion, and competition for pathogen interaction with epithelial cells. To enhance antibacterial and anti-inflammatory activities of the intestinal epithelium, probiotics stimulate cytoprotective protein synthesis and secretion, including heat shock protein, defensin, angiogenin, and mucin by intestinal epithelial cells [15, 16].

SUMMARY

- ➢ A food can be called functional if it contains a food component that targets one or a limited number of functions in the body, and has physiological or psychological effects beyond the traditional nutritional outcome.
- ➢ The major differences between dietary supplements and functional foods lie in the fact that dietary supplements are intended for ingestion in pill, capsule, tablet, or liquid form. They are not represented for use as a conventional food or as the sole item of a meal or diet, and are labeled as a dietary supplement.
- ➢ Biotechnology-derived crops have tremendous potential to improve the health of millions worldwide, including gold rice and iron-enriched rice. They are genetically engineered to provide enhanced levels of iron and beta-carotene.

REVIEW QUESTIONS

1. A selectively fermented ingredient that results in specific changes in the composition and/or activity of the gastrointestinal microbiota
   a. Probiotics
   b. Fiber
   c. Prebiotics
   d. Synbiotics

2. The following are all acceptable definitions of dietary supplements except
   a. a product intended for ingestion in pill, capsule, tablet, or liquid form
   b. a product not represented for use as a conventional food or as the sole item of a meal or diet
   c. consumed as part of a normal diet and deliver one or more active ingredients
   d. a newly approved drug, certified antibiotic, or licensed biological products that were marketed as a dietary supplement or food before approval, certification, or license

3. Which of the following is not a major challenge that industrialized countries are currently facing in relation to health?
   a. Controlling health care cost
   b. Offering better opportunities to prolong the population's lifespan
   c. Providing healthy, processed, and ready-to-eat foods to busy consumers
   d. Promoting the use of food to generate profit to be used in future treatment of chronic diseases.

4. Inflammation of the joints is known as
   a. Osteoarthritis
   b. Coronary Heart Disease
   c. Arthritis
   d. Osteoporosis

5. Which of the following could possibly be considered a functional food?
    a. Cornflakes that are fortified with bioactive compounds
    b. Naturally occurring vegetables found to help lower cholesterol
    c. Both a and b
    d. None of the above

6. Oxidation of ___ has a key role in the pathogenesis of atherosclerosis and cardiovascular heart diseases
    a. low-density lipoproteins (LDL)
    b. high-density lipoproteins (HDL)
    c. neutral-density lipoproteins (NDL)
    d. All of the above

7. Which one of the following reasons is a key motivator for the development of functional foods?
    a. The unification of society towards a more standard diet
    b. The management of the risk of disease
    c. The spread of localized ingredients across the rest of the world
    d. None of the above

8. How do you make a food product not originally classified as "functional" into such?
    a. Eliminate unnecessary components known to cause no harm when consumed
    b. Increasing the concentration of a component to the point at which ny higher dosage would cause detrimental effects to the human body
    c. Replacing a component previously causing negative effects with a component that causes less detrimental effects.
    d. Increasing bioavailability or stability of the component known to produce a functional effect

9. Designing and developing functional foods is a scientific challenge that should rely on which of the following?
    a. The exploitation of this knowledge in the development of markers, relevant to the key functions
    b. Basic scientific knowledge relevant to functions that pertain to modulation by food components
    c. The development of advanced techniques for human studies that are minimally invasive and applicable on a large scale
    d. All of the above

10. Which of the listed foods is not an example of a known functional food?
    a. Fish oil fatty acids
    b. Soy protein
    c. Becel-margarine
    d. Oat bran fiber

Answers: 1. **(C)** 2. **(C)** 3. **(D)** 4. **(C)** 5. **(C)** 6. **(A)** 7. **(B)** 8. **(D)** 9. **(D)** 10. **(C)**

REFERENCES:

1. Halsted CH. Dietary supplements and functional foods: 2 sides of a coin? Am J Clin Nutr. 2003 Apr; 77 (4 Suppl):1001S-1007S.

2. Vyas U, Ranganathan N. Probiotics, Prebiotics, and Symbiotics: Gut and Beyond. Gastroenterol Res Pract. 2012; 2012: 872716.

3. Delphine M, Saulnier A, Jennifer K, Glenn SR, Versalovic J. Mechanisms of Probiosis and Prebiosis: Considerations for Enhanced Functional Foods. Curr Opin Biotechnol. 2009; 20(2): 135–141.

4. Peter J. Jones. Clinical nutrition: 7. Functional foods — more than just nutrition. CMAJ. 2002; 166(12): 1555–1563.

5. Wijnkoop IL, Jones PJ, Uauy R, Segal L, Milner J. Nutrition economics – food as an ally of public health. Br J Nutr. 2013; 109(5): 777–784.

6. Roberfroid MB. Concepts and strategy of functional food science: the European perspective. *Am J Clin Nutr. 2000; 71(6): 1660-1664.*

7. Culligan EP, Hill C, Sleator RD. Probiotics and gastrointestinal disease: successes, problems and future prospects. Gut Pathog. 2009; 1:19.

8. Jones PJ. Clinical nutrition: 7. Functional foods — more than just nutrition. CMAJ. 2002; 166(12): 1555–1563.

9. Daniel Granato, Gabriel F. Branco, Adriano Gomes Cruz, Jose de Assis Fonseca Faria, and Nagendra P. Shah. Probiotic Dairy Products as Functional Foods. Vol. 9, 2010 _ ComprehensiveReviews in Food Science and Food Safety 455-470.

10. Istvan Siro, Emese Kapolna, Beata Kapolna, Andrea Lugasi. Functional food. Product development, marketing and consumer acceptance - A review. Appetite 51 (2008) 456–467.

11. Clare M. Hasler. Functional Foods: Benefits, Concerns and Challenges—A Position Paper from the American Council on Science and Health. *J. Nutr.* December 1, 2002 vol. 132 no. 12 3772-3781.

12. P.J.A. Sheehy and P.A. Morrissey, Nutritional Aspects of Food Processing and Ingredients, Chapter 3 - Functional Foods: Prospects and Perspectives, P.J.A. Sheehy and P.A. Morrissey, pp 45-65. Eds. C.J.K. Henry & N.J. Heppell (1998). Gaithersburg, Aspen Publishers.

13. Sinéad Lordan, R. Paul Ross, and Catherine Stanton. Marine Bioactives as Functional Food Ingredients: Potential to Reduce the Incidence of Chronic Diseases. Mar Drugs. 2011; 9(6): 1056–1100.

14. Avrelija Cencic and Walter Chingwaru. The Role of Functional Foods, Nutraceuticals, and Food Supplements in Intestinal Health.

15. Fang Yan and David Brent Polk. Probiotics: progress toward novel therapies for intestinal diseases. Curr Opin Gastroenterol. 2010 March; 26 (2): 95–101.

16. Christopher Duggan, Jennifer Gannon, and W Allan Walker. Protective nutrients and functional foods for the gastrointestinal tract 1,2,3.

4

Efficacy and Dose Determination

Daniel A. Abugri[1] and Melissa Johnson

[1]Department of Chemistry, Tuskegee University College of Arts and Science, Tuskegee, Alabama, USA; [2]Center for Plant Biotechnology Research, Tuskegee University, College of Agriculture, Environment and Nutrition Science, Tuskegee, Alabama 36088, USA

Introduction

Technology has enabled greater access to healthy food, yet chronic diet-related diseases continue to be the leading cause of morbidity and mortality in the developed world. Functional foods have thus become a major pillar in the campaign for health promotion and disease prevention. Bioactive compounds such as essential fatty acids, dietary fibers, antioxidants, vitamins, and minerals all perform in concert and are best consumed as whole foods. Although a consensus has not been reached regarding the exact dose-response of specific bioactive compounds to achieve a desired effect, the *in vivo*, *in vitro*, clinical, and epidemiological evidence suggests that there are upper limits of tolerance and tentative optimal intake levels. Furthermore, these recommendations are often for a population, rather than specific subpopulations. Those with certain diseases, metabolic disorders, and other conditions require specialized dosages. Analysis of functional food efficacy and dosage requires researchers to understand the specific class (e.g. carbohydrates, proteins, lipids, vitamins, minerals, etc.), metabolism (e.g. absorption, transport, metabolism and excretion), analysis (e.g. analytical, chromatographic, genetic, combination), laboratory and clinical evaluation (e.g. *in vivo*, *in vitro*, epidemiological) and assessment of intake levels (e.g. recommended, upper and lower levels, toxicity) (Figure 1). Thus, researchers draw upon the nutritional and food sciences, molecular biology, biochemistry, plant science, (epi)genetics, genomics, proteomics, metabolomics, and other disciplines to determine the subcellular, cellular, tissue and organismic outcomes of functional food and bioactive compound administration.

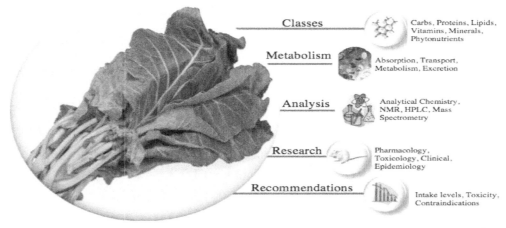

Figure 1. Components of determining the efficacy and dosage of bioactive compounds

Bioactive Compounds – Definition and Dietary Sources

According to Kris-Etherton et al., bioactive compounds are "*extranutritional constituents that typically occur in small quantities in foods,*" which are believed to exert salutary effect [8]. Bioactive compounds have also been defined as "*essential and non-essential compounds that occur in nature, are part of the food chain, and can be shown to have an effect on human health*" [2]. Dietary sources of bioactive compounds include fruits, vegetables, whole grains, nuts, and legumes [9]. Typically, more naturally-colorful and fragrant foods serve as more concentrated sources of bioactive compounds. The major classes of bioactive compounds and dietary sources are presented below.

Table 1. Common plant bioactive compounds classes, dietary source and bioactive component.

Class	Dietary Source	Bioactive Component
Anthocyanins Anthocyanidins	Berries (blueberries, cranberries, raspberries, strawberries)	Cyandin, malvidin
Caffeic acid	Extra virgin olive oil, sweet potato leaves	Caffeic acid
Dietary Fiber (soluble & insoluble)	Barley, oats, fruits, vegetables	β-glucan, pectin, psyllium
Flavonoids (Bioflavonoid), Flavonols, Flavones, Flavanones	Cocoa, green and black tea, citrus fruit, grapes, wine, berries, apples, plums, teas, herbs and spices	Catechin, epicatechin, kaempferol, myricetin, procyanidins, quercetin
Isoflavones	Legumes, soybeans, herbs	Daidzein, genistein
Isothiocyanates	Cruciferous vegetables	Benzyl isothiocyanates, phenethyl isothiocyanates, sulforaphanes
Lipids	Oily fish, nuts, vegetable oils	Omega-3 (α-linolenic acid, eicosapentaenoic acid)
Minerals	Green leafy vegetables	Selenium Zinc, magnesium, calcium, trace minerals
Omega-3 fatty acids	Oily fish; purslane	α-linolenic acid; eicosapentaenoic acid; docosahexaenoic acid
Organosulfur	Garlic, leek, onion	Allicin, diallyl disulfide, diallyl sulfide
Phenolic acid Polyphenol	Fruits, vegetables, tea, wine, coffee, chocolate, olives	Tannins
Phytochemicals	Blueberries, cranberries, strawberries, orange, grape, cocoa, broccoli, tomatoes, garlic, tea	Anthocyanins (cyaniding, malvidin), Carotenoid (α-carotene, β-carotene, β-cryptoxanthin, lutein, lycopene), organosulfides (allicin, isothiocyanates, sulforaphane), tocotrienols, tocopherols, xanthophylls, zeaxanthin

Class	Dietary Source	Bioactive Component
Phytoestrogen	Flaxseed, soybeans, legumes	Isoflavones, lycopene, resveratrol, lignans
Prebiotic compounds	Soybeans, Jerusalem artichoke, chicory root, raw oats, whaet, barley	Fruttooligosaccharide, galactooligosaccharide, oligofructose, inulin
(Plant) Sterols	Rice bran oil, soybean oil	Campesterol, sitostanol, stigmasterol
Vitamins	Fruits, vegetables, citrus fruits, sweet potatoes	B Vitamins, K Vitamins Vitamin C, Folate

Classes of Bioactive Compounds

Bioactive compounds are widely distributed in nature through different sources, with the highest compositions found in plants. They are classified into secondary metabolites, lipids, proteins, and carbohydrates. Each of these major classes is subcategorized by their chemical properties.

Bioactive compounds are often referred to as secondary metabolites, with their derivatives typically of low molecular weight and at low concentration. Bioactive compounds encompass flavonoids, capsaicinoids, lignin, terpenoids, carotenoids, chlorophylls, vitamins, stilbenes, phenolic acids, sterols, lipids, fatty acids, and polysaccharides (Figure 2). As Hippocrates once said, *"Let food be thy medicine and medicine be thy food."* Where total syntheses don't exist, bioactive compounds are derived from plants [1, 2]. Many early cultures hold herbs and functional foods aloft in their pharmacopeia. Many of these plants are antioxidants, anti-lipid peroxidation, anti-inflammatory and pro-inflammatory agents, antimalarial, anticancer agents, anti-ageing, cosmetics, dyes, antimicrobials. These claims have been supported in a variety of studies, including studies addressing the improvement of learning and memory in humans [3], downregulation of oncogenes at terminal stages of the disease during chemotherapy [4], inhibition of cell proliferation [5], effects on secretory processes of inflammatory cells, modulation of proinflammatory enzymatic activities [5], treatment of urinary tract infections [6], inhibition of seasonal allergic rhinoconjunctivitis in humans [7], and much more. [8]

Bioactive compounds are present in plants, algae, and some animals as secondary metabolites for defensive and other physiological purposes. Humans must obtain some via diet, as they cannot synthesize them. Examples include chlorophylls and essential fatty acids like linoleic and alpha linolenic acid. Many of these compounds have a short half-life upon being ingested. While some of these compounds are insoluble or slightly soluble in water (although readily soluble in most organic solvents), hot water can sometimes be used to extract or dissolve them.

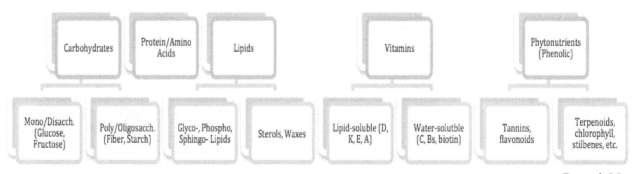

Figure 2. Bioactive compound classes from exogenous (dietary) sources

Metabolism of Bioactive Compounds

The metabolism of nutrients begins in the oral cavity or mouth, with α-amylase catalyzing the hydrolysis of α bonds within polysaccharides such as glycogen, to produce glucose and maltose. Following ingestion and degradation of major nutrient classes, cellular anabolic and catabolic pathways facilitate the transport and absorption to and excretion from various cellular components, depending upon the body's nutritional needs and physiological state. A brief synopsis of the ingestion, transport, absorption, metabolism, and excretion of nutrients and bioactive compounds is presented in Figure 2. Within the gastrointestinal tract, most nutrient absorption occurs in the small intestine. The presence of dietary fibers within the gastrointestinal tract facilitates the formation of a complex matrix, which "traps" nutrients and contributes to delayed gastric emptying (which can also act to attenuate blood glucose concentrations). Moreover, within the intestinal tract, prebiotics interact with polyunsaturated fatty acids and phytochemicals during their metabolism and transformation to secondary metabolites, which in turn influence bioavailability and health [35]. In contrast to bioavailability, which spotlights the rate of absorption and the extent to which active moieties of compounds are available at the target site, efficacy refers to the effectiveness of the bioactive compound in producing the desired effect(s) by interacting with relevant receptors. The bioavailability, transport, absorption, metabolism, and excretion of bioactive compounds (**pharmacokinetics**) ultimately influence the receptor affinity and efficacy (**pharmacodynamics**) of these compounds for different individuals.

Bioactive Compounds in Health Promotion and Disease Prevention

Evidence from many scientific disciplines emphasizes the influence of bioactive compounds on health promotion, in addition to disease prevention [10-12]. Phytochemicals are believed to function additively and synergistically as substrates and cofactors during metabolism. Administered compounds can interact to alter pharmacokinetics (ADME: absorption, distribution, metabolism, excretion) and pharmacodynamics (interactions with receptors). For example, lipid-soluble molecules are better absorbed when consumed with lipids, and minerals may be sequestered by nature chelators like phytic acid, reducing bioavailability [13-15]. These bioactive compounds also have the potential to influence pathways involved in inflammation, energy storage, and adipogenesis involved in conditions such as cancer and obesity [16, 17].

Further, anthocyanins are believed to exert their chemopreventive effects by targeting inflammatory and apoptotic pathways involved in anti-inflammatory, anti-carcinogenesis, and antitumor progression [18]. Plant sterols (**phytosterols**) (such as campesterol, sitosterol, and stigmasterol) promote anti-inflammatory, anti-oxidative, anti-atherogenic, and cardioprotective activities, in addition to facilitating decreases in total and LDL-C [19-21]. Flavonoids also demonstrate antioxidant and anti-inflammatory effects, which can be beneficial in preventing atherosclerosis [22].

Much scientific evidence is available supporting the role of medium-chain and omega-3 fatty acids (α-linolenic acid, eicosapentaenoic acid, docosahexaenoic acid) in reducing risk of diabetes, metabolic syndrome, stroke, cardiovascular disease, and other diseases [23-25]. More recently, the potential of **conjugated linoleic acids (CLAs),** found in animal products such as milk and meat and their products, as a functional food component with apparent health benefits, is being considered.

In a review highlighting the health benefits of CLAs, researchers emphasize the benefits of this nutrient class in terms of preventing diabetes, obesity, atherosclerosis, and carcinogenesis, in addition to modulating immune function [26]. The role of CLAs on lipid metabolism has been demonstrated by the suppression of triglyceride accumulation, inhibition of preadipocyte proliferation (induction of apoptosis) [27], increased palmitoyltransferase activity, and increased lipolysis and alteration of tissue fatty acid composition [28, 29]. Among obese individuals, CLAs supplemented into the diet reduced abdominal fat mass and increased adiponectin levels [30], as well as increased energy expenditure and fat oxidation [31]. Conversely, the excessive consumption of CLAs has supported the development of colon carcinogenesis, hyperinsulinemia, fatty liver, and fatty spleen [32]. However, others found that CLA supplemented into the diets of rats, as well as derived endogenously, was able to attenuate nonalcoholic fatty liver disease [33] and reduce the risk of cancer [34].

Although there is inadequate scientific evidence to make conclusive dietary recommendations for specific bioactive compounds, it is recommended that individuals consume diets abundant in whole grains, nuts, legumes, fruits, and vegetables, rich sources of bioactive compounds.

On the other hand, excessive intake of concentrated bioactive compounds (e.g. excessive dietary supplements) can cultivate an oxidative shift within the cellular environment, prompting these antioxidant molecules to act as pro-oxidants, contributing to oxidative stress, oxidative damage, and increased risk for disease [35]. Therefore, determining the efficacy of bioactive compounds and their potential role in pathways implicated in disease initiation, progression and/or termination is critical. It is suggested that an integrative approach, considering the dietary origins of bioactive compounds, metabolism, acute (short-term) and long term effects, subsequent biomarkers for disease, and ultimate health status be undertaken to demonstrate the efficacy of bioactive compounds (Figure 3).

Analysis of food bioactive compound content (extraction, identification, quantification)

Bioactive compounds are complexed with many other compounds bearing different functional groups and polarities, which makes their isolation and purification difficult [36]. It is therefore especially important to note that these properties of the compounds require careful and simple extraction techniques in order to release them from their bounded membranes into solution without contaminating or destroying their unique chemical and physical forms, which can render them biologically inactive.

Figure 3. An integrative approach in determining the efficacy of bioactive compounds

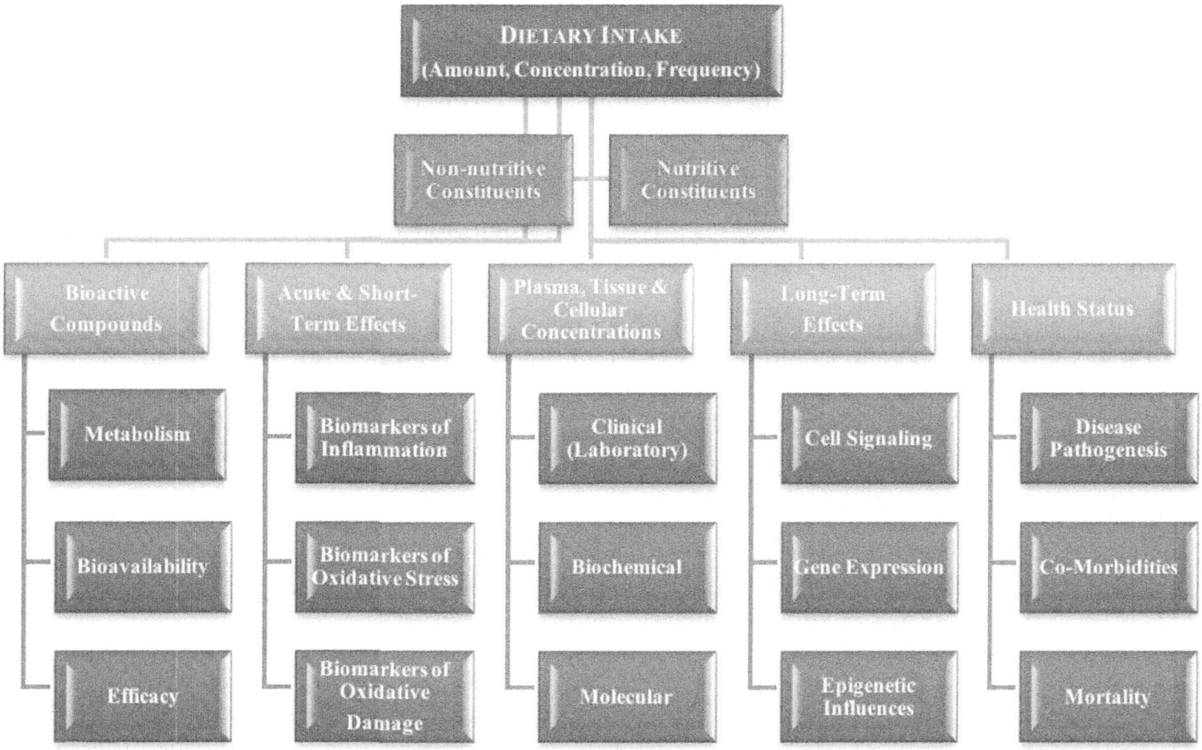

Extraction of bioactive compounds (using methanol, ethyl acetate)

Generally, there are several ways of extracting these bioactive compounds, depending on the bioactive compounds of interest. The techniques employed are maceration, infusion, percolation, digestion, decoction, and hot continuous extraction (Soxhlet). Other techniques also include aqueous-alcoholic extraction by fermentation, counter current extraction, microwave-assisted extraction, ultrasound extraction (sonication), supercritical fluid extraction, and phytonic extraction (with hydrofluorocarbon solvents) [37, 38]. Current techniques used in bioactive compound extraction include head space trapping, solid phase micro extraction, protoplast extraction, micro distillation, thermomicrodistillation, and molecular distillation [39]. All these methods of extraction are efficient. However, caution must be exercised, because some compounds do require long extraction time, low temperature, small particle size, more polar solvent type, and a proper solvent to solid ratio in order to release the bioactive compounds in maximum quantity in solution [38, 40]. Some solvents are toxic to the user and the environment, and as such it is recommended that alternative solvents of less or no toxicity should be adopted. For example, super critical fluid extraction using CO_2 as the solvent is preferable because it is cost effective, does not require the use of toxic chemicals and is less harmful to the environment (e.g. "green" methodology).

Analytical and Chromatographic Techniques

There are several analytical, chromatographic and molecular techniques for fingerprinting bioactive compounds. However, we will only focus on high performance liquid chromatography/high performance thin layer chromatography (HPLC/HPTLC), Fourier-transform infrared spectroscopy (FTIR), and immunoassay techniques.

Chromatographic Techniques

There is a requirement for comprehensive examination of the bioactive compounds in functional foods (nutraceuticals, dietary supplements, herbs, food colorants and additives). Also, market availability of bioactive compound supplements depends partly on their nutritional, nutraceutical, and pharmaceutical labels and proven uses, requiring a thorough analysis of isolated and identified compounds using modern analytical techniques.

Table 2. Common procedures employed to extract bioactive compounds

Extraction Procedure	Procedure Principles Solvent(s)	Strengths	Limitations	Reference
Homogenization	Samples ground with an organic solvent and homogenized in either a dry form or wet form Samples filtered with Whatman filter paper into clean amber bottles to avoid photolysis	Relatively simple and rapid (wet and dry) sample extraction. Reduced solvent requirement Ideal for lipid, phenolic, tannin and protein extraction	Electrical source Required. Time and labor intensive	[38]
Exhaustive Extraction	Samples are often prepared with one solvent, dried under a vacuum or using rotary evaporator. More polar solvents are used in re-extraction stages to produce optimum and wider classes of bioactive compounds.	It has the ability to release bioactive compounds that were not extracted by the initial solvent because of less polarity. Very fast.	Requires special rotary evaporators around bottles. Requires energy.	[41]
Maceration	The solvent of choice is often poured onto either a coarse grade or a fine grade sample and agitated frequently for anywhere between a few minutes to 24 hours in a Pyrex culture test tube until all the powder of the sample is completely dissolved. Sample (liquid extract) is carefully filtered and used for chromatographic or spectrophotometric analysis.	Excellent choice for thermolabile compounds, can be used for coarse or fine powdered samples, water bath can be used to assist in digestion of samples.	May require a long time to extract substantial amounts of bioactive compounds.	[38]
Decoction	Samples are boiled in the required solvent; the solvent used is usually water. The samples are then filtered and used for analysis.	Very good for thermolabile bioactive compounds; requires a short time (approximately 15 minutes); good for water soluble bioactive compounds.	Requires heat.	[38]

Sonication	Requires high voltage and energy, the frequency ranges from 20 kHz to 2000 kHz, the solvent could be water or any organic solvent.	Very fast, efficient in releasing bioactive compounds.	Results in free radical formation. Also requires high energy and non-economical for small sample extractions.	[39]

HPLC/HPTLC

High performance thin layer chromatography (HPTLC/HPLC) has been an essential tool for fingerprinting bioactive compounds in plants, fungi, and marine functional food sources. HPTLC is a new tool that replaces the previous TLC in that it has the ability to profile small molecules by comparing the sample fingerprints with that of the reference standards. It is a simpler, cheaper method in terms of solvent usage, and fast technique which is used in bioactive compound screening with the reference or selected constituents, which are then quantified using densitometry.

In the HPLTC process, a developing chamber is set up with a good solvent combination (for example, an ethyl acetate to hexane in a ratio of 1:1 is used if the original extraction solvents were hexane or ethyl acetate). Here the chamber is allowed to equilibrate or is saturated for about 5 to 20 minutes, depending on the protocol, with the mouth covered with a slit to prevent the organic solvents from evaporating. A 60 silica gel glass-backed layer is used for the samples to be spotted for analyses. This is done with nitrogen flow. For HPTLC, plates are measured from the bottom of about 5 mm where samples are spotted and allowed to dry for 20 seconds. Plates are then placed into the chamber, and compounds are allowed to migrate upward. Then, the plate is removed and a mark is made to indicate where the elution solvent front ends. Plates are typically allowed to sit for 20-30 minutes and then inspected under UV light of 254, 256, and 366 nm. Spots can also be viewed under white light on a CAMAG TLC visualizer [42, 43]. From the mark to the bottom where the sample was spotted becomes the solvent front (solvent distance) and from the bottom again as a reference point to where a visible spot is found becomes the compound distance. Retention times can be calculated and compare bands and retention factors (RF) values with standard and identification can then be confirmed.

HPLC identification of bioactive compounds

High performance liquid chromatography is a broadly used technique for the characterization of bioactive compounds [44]. For many years now, this technique has been popular among scientists for quality control purposes [45]. HPLC uses the principle of migration of the bioactive compounds according to their molecular size, polarity, charge-mass ratio, and UV visible absorption properties. The HPLC instrument is made up of a solvent delivery pump, a needle for sample injection into the column and an auto-sampler or a manual injection valve, an analytical column (e.g. 5μm with 250cm x 4.6cm), a guard column to pre filter any debris that might have escaped from initial filtration of bioactive compounds, detector (UV-Visible, photodiode array detector (PDAD), refractive index detector (RIFD), and a recorder or a printer connected to a computer.

Bioactive compounds are chemically separated and identified using HPLC by taking advantage of the fact that certain compounds have different migration rates (retention factors) due to their functional groups, size and polarity. This implies when a particular column and mobile phase is used, the individual compounds will elute differently. It is important to note that the level of separation of these compounds is greatly influenced by the type of stationary phase and mobile phase used [46]. The identification and separation of bioactive compounds are achieved by using an isocratic system (i.e. single unchanging mobile phase system). Solvent systems are either methanol or acetonitrile, or HPLC water at pH = 3.0.

It is also crucial that if many bioactive compounds are to be identified, gradient elution is the superior approach because the proportion of organic solvent to water is altered with time as a result of the differences in retention under the conditions selected. Purification done by HPLC is also based on the structural properties of each compound of interest, and therefore can be distinguished from contaminants. Each compound has a unique characteristic peak under certain chromatographic conditions, so if factors such as mobile phase, flow rate, and suitable columns and detectors are selected, identification and quantification is relatively straightforward.

For proper identification of bioactive compounds via HPLC, two things are of vital importance: first, a detector of functionality must be properly selected, and second, optimal detection settings and an assay of separation must be properly established. The actual set up should provide a clean peak chromatograph of the known sample. The peak identified should have a realistic retention time, along with well separated patterns from contaminants peaks when several runs are carried out under the set conditions. Caution needs to be exercised in sample preparation stages. For instance, the crude source material must be prepared in a suitable form for HPLC analysis. This means all solvents ideally should be of HPLC grade. Also, the choice of solvent for sample reformation must be carefully selected, since it has broader implications for the success of bioactive compound isolation and identification. The state of the sample must be considered as well. For example, dried samples need sufficient time for the bioactive compounds to dissolve into solution [46].

Fourier-transform infrared spectroscopy (FTIR)

FTIR is another popular analytical method [46-48]. This technique relies on the fact that FTIR spectra are often distinct, and as such look like a molecular "fingerprints" when the compound is in its pure state [46-48]. Identification of unknown compound spectra can be determined using an online database. Samples for FTIR can be prepared in a number of ways. One route is a liquid form: when liquid samples are tested, the analyst should place one drop of the bioactive compound extract between two plates of sodium chloride. Note that after the drop is made, the bioactive compounds will form a thin film between the plates, which can then be scanned using varying wavelengths to identify compounds. If the FTIR is coupled with a mass spectrometer (MS), mass-to-charge ratios of protons or fractions can be determined for structure. When testing with solid samples, the samples are first ground up with potassium bromide (KBr) and then compressed into a thin pellet form.

In order to double check with the analysis, solid samples can be dissolved in methylene chloride or another organic solvent and then placed onto a single salt plate. The solvent evaporates off, leaving the thin film of the original material on the plate for analysis with the FTIR [46-48].

Immunoassay

Immunoassays are a useful molecular tool for both qualitative and quantitative analyses of bioactive compounds using monoclonal antibodies. This technique is combined with chromatography and employs antigen-antibody binding properties, producing a rapid and sensitive detection of analytes. It is applied to drugs and bioactive compounds with smaller molecular weights (MW). For example, compounds such as peptides, some proteins, phenolic acids, flavonoids, and anthocyanidins can be detected and quantified. The advantages of immunoassay techniques are (1) high specificity and sensitivity for receptor binding analyses, (2) high specificity and sensitivity for enzyme assays, and (3) high specificity and sensitivity for qualitative and quantitative analysis of bioactive compounds [46, 49]. Enzyme-linked immunosorbent essay (ELISA) based on monoclonal antibodies is more efficient and sensitive than any conventional HPLC methods currently in use for extract mixture fingerprinting [46, 49]. The detection is often determined spectrophotometrically by using the intensity or level of absorbance as indicators. The more intense the color, the more binding affinity of the bioactive compound tested.

Evaluation of the Efficacy of Bioactive Compounds

A myriad of natural products have demonstrated efficacy and safety. Many act as antioxidants, neutralizing harmful free radical chain reactions. They perform these roles using their hydroxyls, methoxylated, carboxylic, and methyl functional groups as donating and accepting groups. Also, they create blockages of certain pathways of pathogens, resulting in a disruption of their glycolic pathways, DNA, RNA, and protein synthesis (antibiotics). The principle employed here is often by methylation, acetylation, sulfonation, or protein cleavage, among others. Other natural products inhibit COX-2, a mediator of inflammation. For example, naringin, tricin, genistein, and apigenin have been shown to inhibit COX-2 [5]. They have also been shown to inhibit phosphatase kinase C (PKC) and to modulate mitogen-activated protein kinase (MAPK). Modulation of NF-kB has also been studied using the compound morin in various cancer models, which has achieved markedly positive results [5].

Efficacy of bioactive compounds in vitro and in vivo

In vitro techniques, analysis

Cell culture

Fibroblast or **HeLa** cells are often cultured using 96 microwell plates. Depending on the type of medium that will enhance the cell growth, preparation involves ensuring the proper pH of the medium, as well as the addition of any necessary supplements or antibiotics. When cells are seeded, they are incubated at 37°C at 5% CO_2, monitoring of their growth is done by light microscope, or a fluorescence microscope if they are engineered to fluoresce. Another technique involves using a cell counter to validate their replication. However, this requires trypan blue and trypsin, as well as special slides for measuring the viability of the cells. Another technique is the spectrophotometer method, whereby a dye is added to the cultured cell lines to form chromophores, which can be read at an established wavelength as absorbance with a blank (without cells). Here, higher absorbance implies higher growth, and vice versa. The second step is to prepare the bioactive compounds in a concentration that can enable 50%, 90%, and 100% inhibition, or death of the cells. This concentration will enable one to determine the IC $_{50}$, IC $_{90}$, and LD$_{100}$ of such bioactive compounds.

The third step is the infection of a 96 plate well with grown cell lines with parasites or microbes of interest, and then introducing the sample bioactive compound in different concentrations to determine its efficacy on the same time of infection. In this technique, the cells plus the microorganisms can be monitored hourly or in 24 or 72-hour intervals, depending on the replication (growth) rate of the parasites/microorganisms. Using a light microscope or fluorescent microscope, the efficacy of bioactive compound inhibition properties can be measured by looking at the degree of florescence, and thus IC$_{50}$, LD$_{50}$, and LD$_{100}$ can be determined.

The first two techniques could be used in the presence of parasites. If the inhibition is positive, immunological assays, cloning, and PCR techniques may be employed to target the bioactive compound, and the pathway of disruption in such microorganisms can be investigated further. It is very important that attention is given to the extraction and purification stages of the bioactive compounds, as well as the cells and microorganism preparations for inoculation of the compounds. Also, these must be done in a sterile environment to reduce possible contamination and false positives.

Selected bioactive compounds and their efficacy in animals and humans

Plant flavonoids are present in most plants, fungi, and microalgae, and have been shown to have anti-inflammatory effects in many studies [50-53]. Table 5 summarizes the latest evidence of plant flavonoids derived bioactive compounds and their efficacy in animals and human subjects. It is also important to note that there are several bioactive compounds which still need to be thoroughly investigated because of their synergetic properties.

Table 5. Human Trials of Select Natural Products

Bioactive compound (quantity used)	Cohort /study design	Memory test	Results/ Activity (efficacy)	Reference
Galantamine (24 or 32 mg)	Patients with mild to moderate AD, R, DB, PC blind, parallel group, trial (6-months; n = 653)	ADAS-cog	Better scores on the disability assessment for dementia, slowed the decline of functional ability as well as cognition in subjects with mild to moderate AD as compared with placebo	[54]
Galantamine (24 mg/day)	Patients with Vascular dementia, M, DB (n = 592)	ADAS-cog and CIBIC-plus	Therapeutic on all key areas of cognitive and non-cognitive abilities, with improved activities of daily living; behavioral symptoms were also significantly improved in dementia patients	[55]
Galantamine (24 mg/day)	Patient with severe AD, R, DB, PC, blind (n = 207)	SIB and MDS-ADL	Improvement in memory, praxis, and visuospatial ability	[56]

Bioactive compound (quantity used)	Cohort /study design	Memory test	Results/ Activity (efficacy)	Reference
Huperzine A (0.2 mg twice daily)	R, DB, PC with AD (n = 80)	MQ test	Improved memory test scores over the individuals receiving the placebo	[57]
Huperzine A (200 and 400 µg; twice daily)	Patients with mild to moderate AD, M, R (N=16weeks; n=210)	ADL & ADS-Cog	Significant improvement in MQ test as compared to the control group	[58]
Huperzine A (400µg/day)	Subjects with diagnosis of possible or probable AD (n=100/12 weeks)	ADL & ADS-Cog	Remarkably improved cognition, behavior, ADL, and model of AD patients as assessed by ADAS-Cog.	[59]
Huperzine A (0.1 mg twice daily)	Patients with mild to moderate VaD, R, DB, PC (12 weeks; n =78)	CDR, MMSE, and ADL	Huperzine A 400 µg and not at 200ug had cognitive effect in patients with mild to moderate AD	[60]
Quercetin (500-1000 mg/day)	Healthy volunteers (human subjects)	Evaluate plasma quercetin concentration after 12 weeks of supplementation	6- to 10-fold increase of plasma quercetin concentration compared to the placebo	[61]
Quercetin (500 mg/day)	Healthy volunteers (human subjects)	Effects of quercetin on CYP2A6, CYP1A2, N-acetyl-transferase; xanthine-oxidase activities	Quercetin modulators CYP2A6, CYP1A2; N-acetyl-transferase and xanthine-oxidase enzyme activity in vivo	[62]
Quercetin (1000 mg/day with or without EGCG, Isoquercetin, eicosopentanoic acids	Healthy volunteers (human subjects)	Quercetin effects on mitochondrial biogenesis and immunity	Increase in plasma quercetin concentration. Quercetin increase granulocyte oxidative burst activity. Decrease of IL-10;IL-10;CRP	[63]
Quercetin (325µmol Q-3G, 331 µmol Q-4'G)	Healthy volunteers (Human subjects)	Bioavailability of Q-3G and Q-4'G	Plasmatic bioavailability; 5 µM Q-3G; 4.5 UM Q-4'G	[64]
Quercetin (150 mg/day)	High cardiovascular disease risk subjects (human subjects)	Serum lipid levels and blood pressure responses in overweight patients	Quercetin decreases systolic blood pressure, plasma oxidized LDL, and TNF-α in some subjects	[65]
Quercetin (150 mg/day	Overweight and obese subjects with metabolic syndrome traits (human subjects)	To evaluate the effects of quercetin supplementation on markers related to metabolic syndrome	Quercetin decrease plasma oxidized LDL and systolic blood pressure	[66]
Quercetin (4 x 500 mg/day)	Sarcoidosis (human subjects)	To evaluate effects of quercetin	Increased total plasma antioxidant capacity and reduced markers of	[67]

Bioactive compound (quantity used)	Cohort /study design	Memory test	Results/ Activity (efficacy)	Reference
		supplementation in sarcoidosis patients on markers of both oxidative stress and inflammation	oxidative stress and inflammation (TNF-α, IL-10, IL-8)	
Quercetin (500-1000 mg/day)	Upper respiratory tract infection (URT) (human subjects)	Quercetin supplementation and influences on upper respiratory tract infection	Reduction in URT in middle-aged and older subjects	[68]
Quercetin (166 mg plus 133 mg Vit- C)	Rheumatoid arthritis	Effects of quercetin on the level of plasma inflammatory biomarkers	No change in blood biomarkers of inflammation (TNF-α; IL-6;IL-β;CRP	[69]
Quercetin (Q) , vitamin C, Niacin (500 mg Q, 125 mg, Vit-C, 5 mg niacin/ 1000 mg Q, 250 mg Vit-C, and 10 mg niacin)	Healthy (humans subject) Supplement for 12 weeks in adults (n =1002; 60% women), difference in age & body mass index	Effects on body mass Cardiovascular risk factors	No major change existedCardiovascular risk factors, mean arterial blood pressure and inflammatory markers such as IL-6-interleukin-6 was observed to decrease moderately	[70]
Quercetin (730 mg/day)	Hypertensive patients, Trial used 28 days		Reduction of systolic, diastolic and mean arterial pressures	[71]
Quercetin (150 mg/day)	At risk overweight/obese (n = 93) 6 week trials	Metabolic syndrome traits, supplementation of 150 mg and its effect on patients	Decreased systolic blood pressure and plasma concentrations of atherogenic-oxidized LDL, no effect on TNF-α and C-Reactive protein (CRP)	[66,70]

TNF-α -tumor necrosis factor; CRP- C-Reactive protein; AD-Alzheimer's diseases; Q-quercetin; MMSE- mini-mental state examination; ADAS-cog- Alzheimer's disease assessment scale-cognitive; MDS-ADL-minimum data set activities of daily living; SIB- severe impairment battery; TNF- tumor necrosis factor-α and CRP- C-Reactive protein (CRP), URT- Upper respiratory tract infection (URT), CIBIC-Clinician's interview-based impression of change; SB-single blind; PC-Placebo controlled; R-randomized; DAT- Divided attention task; DB-double blind; VaD- vascular dementia; n- number of participants.

In vivo and clinical analyses

In vivo studies use live organisms, and the bioactive compound of interest is administered by injection or orally (syrup, tablet, gavage). Animal models or human subjects (clinical trials) are then tested with the concentration prepared. During the testing of the bioactive compounds in *in vivo* systems, the investigator usually screens subjects by taking physical and biochemical examinations. The study can be monitored, with samples collected hourly or every 24 hours, up to 30 days, as post-follow-up-treatment data to evaluate the efficacy and the safety of the bioactive compounds. Two arms are often chosen; one with the treated bioactive compound at different concentration based on body mass index, height, sex, and age, and the second arm without any bioactive compound administered. The latter arm is termed as the control arm of the study.

During clinical trials, three factors must be considered: (1) participants must give informed consent to the study, as well as potential benefits, adverse effects, outcomes, and handling of the information collected from participants; (2) participants are then screened for certain qualities and enrolled into the study; and (3) a physical examination is conducted, and physical data, biochemical and hematological samples such as blood, serum, plasma, urine, saliva, and sweat are collected for analysis. After the above steps are completed, bioactive compounds are then administered to each participant except the control group.

Studies of this nature vary from one clinical endpoint to another, depending on what one is trying to establish. Therefore, samples are taken at intervals varying from an hour to a few weeks, based on the protocol. Proteins, lipids, fatty acids, gene expression, and certain enzymes are carefully determined and compared to the untreated groups. Proteins, enzymes, and lipids can be determined by electrophoresis, high performance/thin layer chromatographic techniques, and gas-liquid chromatography or gas chromatography–mass spectrometer (GC-MS). Immunoassays are also used to test for antigen-antibody interaction, enzymes, and protein expression.

It is worth noting that *in vivo* studies rely heavily on proper informed consent, and the results of failing to acquire said consent could include legal and financial troubles for those conducting the study. Furthermore, given the fact that the studies are conducted on living beings, it is especially important that compounds be stored properly and administered safely.

Selected *In vivo* clinical evidence of bioactive compounds efficacy in some disease treatments
Urinary tract infection has been a significant health problem for women throughout the world [6]. It is estimated that over 50% of most women in the world will have at least one episode in their life time of a UTI [6]. Proanthocyanidin from cranberry (*Vaccinium macrocarpon*) powder has demonstrated to be effective in the treatment of urinary tract infections [6]. In a randomized study, 60 females ranging in age from 18 to 40 were recruited in India, where the study divided the participants into three groups: untreated, low dosage, and high dosage. The untreated group (n =16) were not given any of the PS-WCP; low dosage group (n =21) was given 500 mg daily; and the high dosage group (n =23) was given 1000 mg daily of PS-WCP. The authors assessed the biochemical and hematological compounds of all the groups on the 10th, 30th, 60th, and 90th days of the study and compared them to the baselines. The study concluded that those patients who were administered with 500 mg and 1000 mg daily had an effective curing of the UTI. This implies an intake of 500 mg or 1000 mg of PS-WCP could be an effective dosage to serve as antibiotic therapy against re-infection of UTIs in women [6].

Another study investigated osteoarthritis (OA), which is known in the USA as a major age-associated chronic disease and has contributed to significant mortality in the USA [72]. Furthermore, it has created practical loss as well as a significant financial burden upon its victims [72]. Levy et al. [72] stated that flavocoxid has been proven by screening and enzymatic testing to be effective in remedying OA. The flavonoid (catechin and baicailin) has been documented to manage both the cyclooxygenase and 5-lipoxygenase pathways of arachidonic acid metabolism identified to be the underlying route for the pathological processes of OA.

Curcumin and resveratrol have been used in traditional medicine for treatments of inflammatory disorders like hepatitis, arthritis, and colitis [73]. Resveratrol is a polyphenol compound commonly found in grapes and most berries. These bioactive compounds have demonstrated efficacy in a variety of ways, including acting as anti-inflammatories, anti-oxidants, anti-tumors, anti-platelet aggregators, anti-aging compounds, and anti-atherogenics [74-77].

One *in vivo* study on animals showed that resveratrol, curcumin, and simvastatin were effective in treating acute inflammation of the small intestine. According to the authors, these bioactive compounds were observed to increase the number of regulatory T cells and improved their intestinal epithelial cells, as well as reducing the neutrophilic granulocyte numbers in the treated mice. This implies that such compounds have the ability to up-regulate the immune system and help it act against infection by disease causative agents.

Furthermore, anti-inflammatory cytokine IL-10 in ileum and mesenteric lymph nodes were observed to increase, whereas that of the pro-inflammatory cytokine expression (IL-23p19, IFN-γ, TNF-α, IL-6, MCP-1) were significantly lower in the ileum of the treated animals as compared to the placebo controls [77]. This was attributed to their ability to down-regulate the Th1-type immune responses. In conclusion, there is sufficient evidence that these three bioactive compounds can be used to treat acute small intestinal inflammation. These findings indicate new treatment options for patients suffering from inflammatory bowel disease [77]. Table 5 summarizes the efficacy and the desired intake of bioactive compounds that can bring about a desired outcome. Table 1 presents a summary of different bioactive compounds used to study their efficacy in improving learning and memory.

Assessment of lower and upper intake levels of bioactive compounds

Determining safe dosages of bioactive compounds is crucial. There are few dietary reference intakes estimated for some of the bioactive compounds proven to be effective in providing a desired outcome (Tables 7, 8, and 9). It is difficult to specifically give an estimated dietary intake of most of these bioactive compounds, because of the difference in structure, sources, and their variations in the food source ingested [78], and even geographical area, age, height, body mass index and sex of consumers. Erdman et al. [79] stated that in measuring the optimal intake of some of these bioactive compounds in humans, especially flavonoids, there are two approaches that could be considered. The first is **absolute intake**, while the second is **relative intake**.

The absolute intake of a bioactive compound is often determined by gathering data on the flavonoid content of foods and then calculating of the amount ingested by humans. In order to determine the absolute intake levels of bioactive compounds, accurate and comprehensive food composition tables are necessary. Determining the relative intake level of a bioactive compound requires the use of biomarkers of flavonoids consumed in biological framework. In the US alone it is estimated that the dietary intake of polyphenols is 1g/d, which goes beyond the intake levels for other common bioactive compounds, such as vitamin C (90 mg/d), carotenoids (5 mg/d), and vitamin E (12 mg/d) [79]. A summary of selected bioactive compound intakes in mg/d in different countries is presented in Table 6.

Table 6. Dietary reference intakes (DRIs): Recommended Dietary Allowances and Adequate Intakes of Vitamins*.

Life stage	Vit A (µg/)	Vit C (mg/d)	Vit D (mg/d)	Vit E (mg/d)	Vit K (µg/d)	Thiamin (mg/d)	Riboflavin (mg/d)	Niacin (mg/d)	Vit B6 (mg/d)	Folate (µg/d)	Choline (g/d)	Vit B12 (ug/d)	Pantothenic acid (mg/d)	Biotin (ug/d)
Infants														
0-6 mo	400*	40*	10	4*	2.0*	2*	0.3*	2*	0.1*	65*	125*	0.4*	1.7*	5*
6-12 mo	500*	50*	10	5*	2.5*	.3*	0.4*	4*	0.3*	80*	150*	0.5*	1.8*	6*
Children														
1-3y	300	15	15	6	30*	0.5	0.5	6	0.5	50	200*	0.9	2*	8*
4-8 y	400	25	15	7	35*	0.6	0.6	8	0.6	200	250*	1.2	3*	12*
Males														
9-13y	600	45	15	11	60*	0.9	0.9	12	1.0	300	375*	1.8	4*	20*
14-18y	900	75	15	15	75*	1.2	1.3	16	1.3	400	550*	2.4	5*	25*
19-30y	900	90	15	15	120*	1.2	1.3	16	1.3	400	550*	2.4	5*	30*
31-50y	900	90	15	15	120*	1.2	1.3	16	1.3	400	550*	2.4	5*	30*
51-70y	900	90	15	15	120*	1.2	1.3	16	1.7	400	550*	2.4	5*	30*
>70 y	900	90	20	15	120*	1.2	1.3	16	1.7	400	550*	2.4	5*	30*
Females														
9-13y	600	45	15	11	60*	0.9	0.9	12	1.0	300	375*	1.8	4*	20*
14-18y	700	65	15	15	75*	1.0	1.0	14	1.2	400	400*	2.4	5*	25*
19-30y	700	75	15	15	90*	1.1	1.1	14	1.3	400	425*	2.4	5*	30*
31-50y	700	75	15	15	90*	1.1	1.1	14	1.3	400	425*	2.4	5*	30*
51-70y	700	75	15	15	90*	1.1	1.1	14	1.5	400	425*	2.4	5*	30*
>70 y	700	75	20	15	90*	1.1	1.1	14	1.5	400	425*	2.4	5*	30*
Pregnancy														
14-18y	750	80	15	15	75*	1.4	1.4	18	1.9	600	450*	2.6	6*	30*
19-30y	770	85	15	15	90*	1.4	1.4	18	1.9	600	450*	2.6	6*	30*
31-50y	770	85	15	15	90*	1.4	1.4	18	1.9	600	450*	2.6	6*	30*
Lactation														
14-18y	1,200	115	15	19	75*	1.4	1.6	17	2.0	500	550	2.8	7*	35*
19-30y	1,300	120	15	19	90*	1.4	1.6	17	2.0	500	550	2.8	7*	35*
31-50y	1,300	120	15	19	90*	1.4	1.6	17	2.0	500	550	2.8	7*	35*

Adapted from Dietary reference intakes for thiamin, riboflavin, niacin, vitamin B6, Folate, vitamin B12, Pantothenic acid, biotin, and choline [83]; dietary reference intakes for vitamin C, Vitamin E, selenium, and carotenoids [84]. Accessed 06/05/2013 via www.nap.deu.*- means adequate intakes (AIs) levels, bold type is for recommended dietary allowances (RDAs), mo - months.

Recommended intake and adequate intake

Most bioactive compounds have been labeled with the recommended dosage needed by the manufacturers, that can bring an effective outcome, while higher dosages might have a toxic effect on the body [80]. For instance, it is recommended that isoflavone consumption should be 50 mg/d, or 100-300 mg/d of grape seeds, which are rich in proanthocyanidins [80]. These ranges conformed to the intake levels which are closer to those consumed typically from soy products, grapes, and wine in Japan and European countries [81, 82].

Lower and upper intake levels

The lower and upper intake levels of bioactive compounds vary depending on the type of bioactive compounds ingested as well as the subclass of bioactive compounds under study. Table 7 below summarizes bioactive compounds as vitamin subclasses of those compounds.

Table 7. Dietary reference intakes (DRIs): Tolerable Upper Levels, Vitamins*.

Life stage	Vit A (ug/d)	Vit C (mg/d)	Vit D (mg/d)	Vit E (mg/d)	Niacin (mg/d)	Vit B6 (mg/d)	Folate (ug/d)	Choline (g/d)
Infants								
0-6 mo	600	ND	25	ND	ND	ND	ND	ND
6-12 mo	600	ND	38	ND	ND	ND	ND	ND
Children								
1-3y	600	400	63	200	10	30	300	1.0
4-8 y	600	650	75	300	5	40	400	1.0
Males								
9-13y	1,700	1,200	100	600	20	60	600	2.0
14-18y	2,800	1,800	100	800	30	80	800	3.0
19-30y	3,000	2,000	100	1,000	35	100	1,000	3.5
31-50y	3,000	2,000	100	1,000	35	100	1,000	3.5
51-70y	3,000	2,000	100	1,000	35	100	1,000	3.5
>70 y	3,000	2,000	100	1,000	35	100	1,000	3.5
Females								
9-13y	1,700	1,200	100	600	20	60	600	2.0
14-18y	2,800	1,800	100	800	30	80	800	3.0
19-30y	3,000	2,000	100	1,000	35	100	1,000	3.5
31-50y	3,000	2,000	100	1,000	35	100	1,000	3.5
51-70y	3,000	2,000	100	1,000	35	100	1,000	3.5
>70 y	3,000	2,000	100	1,000	35	100	1,000	3.5
Pregnancy								
14-18y	2,800	1,800	100	800	30	80	800	3.0
19-30y	3,000	2,000	100	1,000	35	100	1,000	3.5
31-50y	3,000	2,000	100	1,000	35	100	1,000	3.5
Lactation								
14-18y	2,800	1,800	100	800	30	80	800	3.0
19-30y	3,000	2,000	100	1,000	35	100	1,000	3.5
31-50y	3,000	2,000	100	1,000	35	100	1,000	3.5

*Adapted from Dietary reference intakes for thiamin, riboflavin, niacin, vitamin B6, Folate, vitamin B12, Pantothenic acid, biotin, and choline [83]; dietary reference intakes for vitamin C, Vitamin E, selenium, and carotenoids [84]. Accessed via www.nap.deu. ND- not determined, mo -months.

Table 8 below summarizes global consumption of bioactive compounds by adults.

Table 8. Global consumption of select bioactive (phenolic) compounds by adults

Bioactive compounds	Country/Region	Intake, mg/d	Reference
Flavonols	Netherlands	21-29	[85-87]
	Germany	13.1-22.6	[88; 89]
	Japan	15.3-15.6	[90; 91]
	Korea	24.6	[92]
	UK	26	[93]
	US	9.4	[94]
Flavones	Netherlands	1.6	[95]
	Japan	1.0-1.1	[96]
	Korea	2.1	[92]
	US	1.3	[94]
Flavonones	Germany	21-29.4	[88]
	Finland	20	[89]
	Greece	31-78	[96]
	Italy	31	[97-99]
	Australia	23	[100]
	US	2.7	[94; 101]
Isoflavones	Netherlands	0.9	[102]
	Ireland	‹ 1	[103]
	Italy	1‹ 1.0-3	[104-105]
	Netherlands UK	0.8	[106]
	UK	0.5-25	[94]
	Finland	31.7-63.9	[107]
	US	24.6-38	[108-112]
	Japan	4-6	[113; 96]
	Korea	N/A	[114; 90]
	Finland	N/A	[115-116; 92]
Flavan-3-ols (monomeric)	Germany	11	[88]
	Netherlands	50	[117]
	US	4-25	[118; 119]

Anthocyanidins	US	6.5	[88
	Germany	1.3	[94]
Proanthocyanidins	US	58	[118]

Toxicity

Toxicity of bioactive compounds comes from high doses. It is been reported that overconsumption of some bioactive compounds can cause negative effects on the body's vital organs, cells, and tissues [120]. Studies using octyl gallate or dodecyl gallate as the bioactive compound have shown such compounds to be toxic when ingested above a certain level. For instance, a concentration of 25,000-50,000 mg/kg or higher has been shown to cause growth retardation, anemia, patchy hyperplasia in the tubuli of the outer kidney medulla, and increased activity of several microsomal and cytoplasmic hepatic drug-metabolite enzymes [120]. In other studies, concentrations of 11,700 -23,400 mg/kg resulted in reduced food intake, growth inhibition, low blood hemoglobin, and kidney damage [121]. Dacre et al. [122] observed that bioactive compounds (gallates) with ingestion ranges of 0-10,000 mg/kg resulted in spleen reduction in the mice. Table 9 below summarizes toxicity and chemoprevention doses of some bioactive compounds.

Table 9. Systematic toxicity and chemoprevention doses of some bioactive compounds in single *in vivo* studies in animals.

Bioactive compounds	Dose	Effect	Reference
Isoflavone	140 mg/kg (mice)	No effect	[123]
Genistein	250 mg/kg (rats)	No effect	[124]
Daidzein			[125]
Phenoxodiol			
Flavonoids of *Vitex negundo*	15 mg/l (amphibian)	Male reproductive toxicity	[126]
Naringenin	10 mg/l (amphibian)	teratogenic	[127; 128]
Epigallo catechin gallate (EGCG)	100 mg/kg (mice)	hepatoxicity	[119; 120]
Pyrogallol	100 mg/kg (rats)	hepatoxicity	[121]
Propyl gallate	5 g/kg oral (rats)	hepatoxicity	[122]
Tannic acid	10 mg/kg (fish, carp), 120 mg/kg (mice)	hepatoxicity	[119;121;122, 126,127]

Proposed Mechanisms of Bioactive Compounds in Health Promotion and Disease Prevention

Some bioactive compounds act as modulators of pro-inflammatory enzymes, anti-inflammatory agents, modulators of inflammatory cells and **cytokines**, or free radical scavengers. Flavonoids, phenolic acids, certain omega 3 and omega 6 polyunsaturated fatty acids (PUFAs), and chlorophylls and carotenoids have demonstrated these properties in both *in vitro* and *in vivo* studies. For example, studies have shown that abdominal or visceral fat depots (which result in high TH, low HDL, high LDL dyslipemia, and insulin resistance) has a metabolic linkage. These result in metabolic impaired regulation of the production of free fatty acids in most adipose tissue [129]. Huang et al. [130] observed that cyaniding-3-glucoside found in mulberry caused a decrease in fatty acid synthesis by down regulating TG and TC, and also decrease lipid accumulation, which results in a decrease in LDL, up regulation of HDL, and an increase in fatty acid oxidation, which protects the liver from cardiovascular diseases. The positive benefit in this type of mechanism is that it stimulates the adenosine monophosphate activated–protein kinase (AMPK) [131].

Waltner-Law et al [132] found epigallocatechin gallate (EGCG) to decrease glucose production in H4IIE rat hepatoma cells. The mechanism used by EGCG is associated with its ability to mimic the insulin structure. This mock-insulin structure can cause an increase in tyrosine phosphorylation of the receptors responsible for the production of insulin. This causes a reduction of the gluconeogenic enzyme phosphoenolpyruvate carboxykinase [132].

Another promising group is polysaccharides. Studies using polysaccharides found in mushrooms have been carried out in Asia, and satisfactory outcomes have been achieved. These compounds are capable of stimulating the non-specific immune system, which then triggers their antitumor activity using the stimulation of host defense mechanisms [133-136]. Polysaccharides and their protein complexes first activate effectors such as macrophages, T lymphocytes, and natural killer (NK) cells to produce certain cytokines (for instance, TNF-alpha, IFN-gamma, and IL-1beta, among others) which then exert anti-proliferation properties as well as induce the apoptosis and differentiation in the turmor cells [137]. In addition, β-D glucans have been reported to have biological responses, such as binding to membrane complement (CR3, alphaMb2 integrin or CD11b/CD18) receptor type 3 on immune effector cells. The good thing is that the ligand receptor complex has the ability to be internalized [137]. Although the above evidence is known, the intercellular events that occur after glucan-receptor binding properties is still hidden to scientists [138]. A recent experiment has shown that schizophyllan (produced by a type of mushroom known as *S. commune Fr.: Fr*) has the ability to bind the mRNA poly (A) tail [139]. These capabilities of the polysaccharides have been observed because of their molecular weight, degree of branching, number of substituents, and ultrastructure, including the presence of single and triple helices, which greatly influence their biological activities, especially β-glucans [137,140]. In agreement with these observations, several studies have found higher antitumor activities were correlated with the degree of molecular weight (higher), lower level of branching, and greater water solubility of β-glucans [137; 141].

Bioactive compounds therefore utilize their varying chemical and physical properties (such as acidic, basic, chelating, hydrophobic and hydrophilic properties) as well as their amphipathic properties to either bind tightly to proteins, enzymes, free radicals, glycolipids, and membranes of most microbial organisms or infected cells to stop metastasis of further pathogenic infection. As a result, such binding ability could disrupt the replication cycle leading to the inhibition of disease pathogen growth. Other bioactive compounds also affect certain vital enzyme expressions, which consequently lead to the death of such pathogens internally. The body has a mechanism that eventually flushes out such dead pathogens through the excretory pathways in the body. In another school of thought, some polysaccharides may have the ability to disrupt the transcription process.

SUMMARY

➢ Researchers draw upon many different disciplines including nutritional and food sciences, molecular biology, biochemistry, plant science, epigenetics, genomics, and many other areas in order to determine specific outcomes of functional food and bioactive compound administration.

➢ Bioactive compounds are defined as essential and non-essential compounds that occur in nature, are part of a food chain, and can be shown to have an effect on human health.

➢ The consumption of diets rich in bioactive compounds is preferred to thwart excessively active inflammatory and oxidative pathways involved in disease.

➢ The metabolism of nutrients begins in the oral cavity (mouth), with alpha-amylase catalyzing the hydrolysis of alpha-bonds within polysaccharides such as glycogen, to produce glucose and maltose.

➢ Conjugated linoleic acids (CLAs) are found in animal products and may prevent many diseases including diabetes, obesity, and may also improve immune function.

➢ There are several techniques used to extract bioactive compounds: maceration, infusion, percolation, digestion, decoction, hot continuous extraction, and many others.

➢ Overconsumption of some bioactive compounds can cause negative effects on the vital organs, cells, and tissues within the body.

➢ Although extensive research has been carried out *in vitro*, the need for further research into the subclasses of bioactive compounds is needed *in vivo*.

REVIEW QUESTIONS

1. Bioactive compounds can be classified into major classes, including:
   a. Lipids
   b. Sugar
   c. Salt
   d. All of the above

2. _____ has been an essential tool for fingerprinting bioactive compounds in plants, fungi, and marine functional food sources.
   a. HPLC
   b. PDAD
   c. HPTLC
   d. FTIR

3. Why is it difficult to specifically give an estimated dietary intake of most bioactive compounds?
   a. The difference in structure, sources, and their variations in the food source ingested
   b. Geographical area, age, height, body mass index
   c. A and B
   d. None of the above

4. The ____, such as bioavailability, transport, absorption, metabolism, and excretion of bioactive compounds ultimately influence the ____, such as receptor affinity and efficacy, of these compounds for different individuals.

   a. Biokinetics; biodynamics
   b. Pharmacodynamics; pharmacokinetics
   c. Biodynamics; biokinetics
   d. Pharmacokinetics; pharmacodynamics

5. Isolating and purifying bioactive compounds is difficult because.
   a. They are usually found with other compounds bearing different polarities
   b. The isolation and purification of bioactive compounds from their sources will ultimately deprive them of their effect
   c. Chemical separation of bioactive compounds requires a long period of time
   d. Solating bioactive compounds is not difficult due to the vast amount of instrumentation available to use
6. Where does the metabolism of nutrients begin?
   a. Mouth
   b. Esophagus
   c. Stomach
   d. As soon as it comes into contact with the body
7. What is not a factor that must be considered when conducting a clinical trial?
   a. Informed consent must be given to participants
   b. A physical analysis is conducted where collected data is analyzed
   c. Participants must be screened for certain traits
   d. None of the above
8. HPLC separates compounds through the usage of
   a. Molecular "fingerprints" that are recorded for each compound run
   b. The compounds' different retention rates in certain solvents
   c. Antigen-antibody binding properties
   d. The compounds' boiling points with a ramping of temperature
9. What is not true about bioactive compounds?
   a. Overconsumption can cause negative effects to the body
   b. Can be difficult to separate due to various chemical factors
   c. When taken at appropriate amounts, can have a beneficial effect to the body
   d. Must be paired with subscribed supplements to take effect
10. In measuring the optimal intake of bioactive compounds in humans, what is an approach that can be considered?
    a. Absolute intake
    b. Relative intake
    c. Suggested intake
    d. A and B

Answers: 1. **(A)** 2. **(C)** 3. **(C)** 4. **(D)** 5. **(A)** 6. **(A)** 7. **(D)** 8. **(B)** 9. **(D)** 10. **(D)**

REFERENCES:

1. Abugri DA, Tiimob BJ, Apalangya VA, Pritchett G, McElhenney WH. (2013). Bioactive and Nutritive Compounds in *Sorghum bicolor* (Guinea corn) Red Leaves and Their Health Implication. Food Chemistry, 718-723.

2. Johnson M and Pace RD. Sweet potato leaves: properties and synergistic interactions that Promotes health and prevent disease. 2010. Nutrition Reviews, Special Article. 68(10): 604-615.

3. Kumar H, More SV, Han S-D, Choi J-Y, Choi C-K (2012). Promising therapeutics with natural bioactive compounds for improving learning and memory- A review of randomized trials. Molecules, 17: 10503-10539.

4. Finley (2005). Proposed Criteria for Assessing the Efficacy of Cancer Reduction by Plant Foods Enriched in Carotenoids, Glucosinolates, Polyphenols and Selenocompounds. Annals of Botany 95: 1075–1096.

5. Ana Garcı́a-Lafuente, Eva Guillamo'n, Ana Villares, Mauricio A. Rostagno, Jose' Alfredo Martı́nez (2009). Flavonoids as anti-inflammatory agents: implications in cancer and cardiovascular disease. Inflammation Research, 58: 537–552.

6. Sengupta, K..; V. Alluri, K.; Golakoti, T.; V. Gottumukkala, G.; Raavi, J.; Kotchrlakota, L.; C. Sigalan, S.; Dey, D.; Ghosh, S.; Chatterjee, A. (2011). A Randomized, Double Blind, Controlled, Dose Dependent Clinical Trial to Evaluate the Efficacy of a Proanthocyanidin Standardized Whole Cranberry (Vaccinium macrocarpon) Powder on Infections of the Urinary Tract. Current Bioactive Compounds, 7(1): 39-46(8).

7. Takano H, Osakabe N, Sanbongi C, Yanagisawa R, Inoue K, Yasuda A, Natsume M, Baba S, Ichiishi E, Yoshikawa T (2004). Extract of Perilla frutescens enriched for rosmarinic acid, a polyphenolic phytochemical, inhibits seasonal allergic rhinoconjunctivitis in humans. Experimental Biology Medicine (Maywood). 229(3): 247-54.

8. Kris-Etherton PM, Hecker KD, Bonanome A, Coval SM, Binkoski AE, Hilpert KF, Griel AE, Etherton TD. Bioactive compounds in foods: their role in the prevention of cardiovascular disease and cancer. Am J Med 2002; 113: 71-88.

9. Biesalski HK, Dragsted LO, Elmadfa I, Grossklaus R, Müller M, Schrenk D, Walter P, Weber PC. Bioactive compounds: Definition and assessment of activity. Nutrition 2009; 25:1202-1205.

10. Martin KR. Targeting Apoptosis with Dietary Bioactive Agents. Exp Biol Med 2006; 231:117-129.

11. Milner JA. Molecular Targets for Bioactive Food Components. J Nutr 2004; 134:2492S-2498S.

12. Siddiqui IA, Mukhtar H. Nanochemoprevention by Bioactive Food Components: A Perspective. Pharm Res 2010; 27:1054-1060.

13. Dillard CJ, German JB. Phytochemicals: nutraceuticals and human health. J Sci Food Agr 2000; 80:1744-1756.

14. Liu RH. Health benefits of fruit and vegetables are from additive and synergistic combinations of phytochemicals. Am J Clin Nutr 2003; 78:517S-520S.

15. Wallig MA, Heinz-Taheny KM, Epps DL, Gossman T. Synergy among Phytochemicals within Crucifers: Does It Translate into Chemoprotection? J Nutr 2005; 135:2972S-2977S.

16. González-Castejón M, Rodriguez-Casado A. Dietary phytochemicals and their potential effects on obesity: A review. Pharmacol Res 2011; 64:438-455.

17. Liu RH. Potential Synergy of Phytochemicals in Cancer Prevention: Mechanism of Action. J Nutr 2004; 134:3479S-3485S.

18. Hou D-X, Fujii M, Terahara N, Yoshimoto M. Molecular Mechanisms Behind the Chemopreventive Effects of Anthocyanidins. J Biomed Biotechnol 2004; 2004:321-325.

19. Berger A, Jones PJH, Abumweis SS. Plant sterols: factors affecting their efficacy and safety as functional food ingredients. Lipids Health Dis 2004; 3:5.

20. Marangoni F, Poli A. Phytosterols and cardiovascular health. Pharmacol Res 2010; 61:193-199.

21. Marinangeli C, Jones P. Plant sterols, marine-derived omega-3 fatty acids and other functional ingredients: a new frontier for treating hyperlipidemia. Nutr Metab 2010; 7:76.

22. Kris-Etherton PM, Lefevre M, Beecher GR, Gross MD, Keen CL, Etherton TD. Bioactive compounds in nutrition and health-research methodologies for establishing biological function: the antioxidant and anti-inflammatory effects of flavonoids on atherosclerosis. Annu rev Nutr 2004; 24:511-538.

23. Lopez-Huertas E. Health effects of oleic acid and long chain omega-3 fatty acids (EPA and DHA) enriched milks. A review of intervention studies. Pharmacol Res 2010; 61:200-207.

24. Nagao K, Yanagita T. Medium-chain fatty acids: Functional lipids for the prevention and treatment of the metabolic syndrome. Pharmacol Res 2010; 61:208-212.

25. Nguemeni C, Delplanque B, Rovère C, Simon-Rousseau N, Gandin C, Agnani G, Nahon JL, Heurteaux C, Blondeau N. Dietary supplementation of alpha-linolenic acid in an enriched rapeseed oil diet protects from stroke. Pharmacol Res 2010; 61:226-233.

26. Benjamin S, Spener F. Conjugated linoleic acids as functional food: an insight into their health benefits. Nutr Metab 2009; 6:1-13.

27. Evans M, Geigerman C, Cook J, Curtis L, Kuebler B, McIntosh M. Conjugated linoleic acid suppresses triglyceride accumulation and induces apoptosis in 3T3-L1 preadipocytes. Lipids 2000; 35:899-910.

28. Ostrowska E, Suster D, Muralitharan M, Cross RF, Leury BJ, Bauman DE, R DF. Conjugated linoleic acid decreases fat accretion in pigs: evaluation by dual-energy X-ray absorptiometry. Brit J Nutr 2003; 89:219-229.

29. Ostrowska E, Cross RF, Muralitharan M, Bauman DE, Dunshea FR. Dietary conjugated linoleic acid differentially alters fatty acid composition and increases conjugated linoleic acid content in porcine adipose tissue. Brit J Nutr 2003; 90:915-928

30. Sneddon AA, Tsofliou F, Fyfe CL, Matheson I, Jackson DM, Horgan G, Winzell MS, Wahle KWJ, Ahren B, Williams LM. Effect of a Conjugated Linoleic Acid and ω-3 Fatty Acid Mixture on Body Composition and Adiponectin. Obesity 2008; 16:1019-1024.

31. Close RN, Schoeller DA, Watras AC, Nora EH. Conjugated linoleic acid supplementation alters the 6-mo change in fat oxidation during sleep. Am J Clin Nutr 2007; 86:797-804.

32. Clément L, Poirier H, Niot I, Bocher V, Guerre-Millo M, Krief S, Staels B, Besnard P. Dietary trans-10,cis-12 conjugated linoleic acid induces hyperinsulinemia and fatty liver in the mouse. J Lipid Res 2002; 43:1400-1409.

33. Nagao K, Inoue N, Wang Y-M, Shirouchi B, Yanagita T. Dietary Conjugated Linoleic Acid Alleviates Nonalcoholic Fatty Liver Disease in Zucker (fa/fa) Rats. J Nutr 2005; 135:9-13.

34. Corl BA, Barbano DM, Bauman DE, Ip C. cis-9, trans-11 CLA Derived Endogenously from trans-11 18:1 Reduces Cancer Risk in Rats. J Nutr 2003; 133:2893-2900.

35. Laparra JM, Sanz Y. Interactions of gut microbiota with functional food components and nutraceuticals. Pharmacol Res 2010; 61:219-225.

36. Crowe KM, Francis C. Position of the Academy of Nutrition and Dietetics: Functional Foods. J Acad Nutr Diet 2013; 113:1096-1103.

37. Sarker S D, Latif Z and Gray AI. Natural products isolation. Second edition, 2006, Humana press pg 29.

38. Tiwari P, Kumar B, Kaur M, Kaur G, Kaur H. 2011. Phytochemical screening and extraction:Areview. *International pharmaceuticaSciencia,* 1(1): 98-106.

39. Handa SS, Khanuja SPS, Longo G, Rakesh DD. Extraction technologies for medicinal and aromatic plants. International centre for science and high technology, Trieste, 2008, 21-25.

40. Abugri DA· McElhenney WH. (2013). Extraction of Total Phenolic and Flavonoids from Edible Wild and Cultivated Medicinal Mushrooms as Affected by Different Solvents. Journal of Natural Products and Plant Resources, 3 (3):37-42.

41. Das K, Tiwari RKS, Shrivastava DK. Techniques for evaluation of medicinal plant Products as antimicrobial agent: current methods and future trends. Journal of medicinal plants research. 2010.4(2):104-111.

42. Piccin A, Toniolo C, Nicoletti M. Analytical tools for digestive plants extracts: application of HPTLC fingerprint. Nutrafoods (2012) 11:29-35.

43. Nicoletti M, Toniolo C (2012) HPTLC Fingerprint Analysis of Plant Staminal Cells Products. J. Chromatography Separation Techniques 3:148. doi.

44. Canell RJP. (1998). Natural products isolation. Human Press Inc. New Jersey, pp.165-208.

45. Fan XH, Cheng YY, Ye ZL, Lin RC, Qian ZZ (2006). Multiple chromatographic fingerprinting and its application to the quality control of herbal medicines. Anal. Chim. Acta 555:217-224.

46. Sasidharan S, Chen Y, Saravanan D, Sundram KM, Latha Yoga L. (2011). Extraction, isolation and characterization of bioactive compounds from plants extracts. African Journal of complement Alternative Medicine, 8(1) 1:10.

47. Eberhardt TL, Li X, Shupe TF, Hse CY. (2007). Chinese tallow tree (sapium Sebiferum) utilization: characterization of extractives and cell-wall chemistry. Wood Fiber Sci. 39:319-324.

48. Hazra KM, Roy RN, Sen SK, Laska S. (2007). Isolation of antibacterial pentahydroxy flavones from the seeds of Mimusops elengi Linn. Afri.J.Biotechnology. 6(12):1446-1449.

49. Imsungnoen N., Phrompittayarat W., Ingkaninan, Tanaka H, and Putalum W. 2009. Immunochromatographic assay for the detection of pseudojujubogenin glycosides. Phytochemicals Analysis. 20:64-67.

50. Habtemariam S. Natural inhibitors of turmor necrosis factor-alpha production, secretion and function. PlantaMedica 2000; 66:303-13.

51. Gerritsen ME, Carley WW, Ranges GE, Shen CP, Phan SA, Ligon GF, Perry CA. Flavonoids inhibit cytokines- induced endothelial cell adhesion protein gene expression. American Journal of Pathology 1995; 147:278-92

52. Middleton E Jr. Effect of plant flavonoids on immune and inflammatory cell function. Advance Experimental Medicine and Biology 1998; 439:175-82.

53. Di Carlo G, Mascolo N, Izzo AA, Capasso F. Flavonoids: old and new aspects of a class of natural therapeutic drugs. Life Sciences 1999; 65:337-53.

54. Wilcock, GK.; Lilienfeld, S,; Gaens, E. (2000). Efficacy and safety of galantamine in patients with mild to moderate Alzheimer's disease: multicenter randomized controlled trial. Galantamine International-1 study Group. BMJ 2000, 321, 2261-228.

55. Erkinjuntti T, Kurz A, Gauthier S, Bullock R, Lilienfeld S, Damaraju CV. (2002). Efficacy of galantamine in probable vascular dementia and Alzheimers disease combined with cerebrovascular disease: a randomized trial. Lancet 2002, 359, 1283-1290.

56. Burns A, Bernabei R, Bullock R, Cruz Jentoft AJ, Frolich L, Hock C; Raivio M, Triau E, Vandewoude M, Wimo A et al. (2009). Safety and efficacy of galantamine (Reminyl) in severe Alzheimer's disease (the SERAD study): A randomized, placebo-controlled, double-blind trial. Lancet neurol.2009, 8, 39-47.

57. Liu, F.G.; Fang, Y.S.; Gao, Z.X.; Zuo, J.D.; Sou, M.L.(1995). Double-blind control treatment of huperzine-A and placebo in 28 patients with Alzheimer disease. Chin. J. Pharmacoepidemiol. 4, 196–198.

58. Ma, Y.X.; Zhu, Y.; Gu, Y.D.; Yu, Z.Y.; Yu, S.M.; Ye, Y.Z. (1998). Double-blind trial of huperzine-A (HUP) on cognitive deterioration in 314 cases of benign senescent forgetfulness, vascular dementia, and Alzheimer's disease. *Ann. NY Acad. Sci.*, *854*, 506–507.

59. Zhang, Z.; Wang, X.; Chen, Q.; Shu, L.; Wang, J.; Shan, G. (2002). Clinical efficacy and safety of huperzine Alpha in treatment of mild to moderate Alzheimer disease, a placebo-controlled, double-blind, randomized trial. *Zhonghua Yi Xue Za Zhi*, *82*, 941–944.

60. Rafii, M.S.; Walsh, S.; Little, J.T.; Behan, K.; Reynolds, B.; Ward, C.; Jin, S.; Thomas, R.;Aisen, P.S. (2011). A phase II trial of huperzine A in mild to moderate Alzheimer disease. *Neurology; 76*, 1389–1394.

61. Jin F; Nieman DC; Shanely RA; Knab AM; Austin MD; Sha W. (2010). The variable plasma quercetin response to 12- week quercetin supplementation in humans. Eur J Clin Nutr 64:692-7.

62. Chen Y; Xiao P; Ou-Yang DS; Fan L; Guo D; Wang YN; et al. (2009). Simultaneous action of the flavonoid quercetin oncytochrome P450 (CYP) 1A2, CYP2A6, N-acetyltransferase and xanthine oxidase activity in healthy volunteers. Clin Exp. Pharmacol Physio. 36:828-33.

63. Nieman DC; Henson DA; Maxwell KR; Williams AS; McAnulty SR; Jin F; et al. (2009). Effects of quercetin and EGCG on mitochondrial biogenesis and immunity. Med Sci Sports Exerc; 41:1467-75.

64. Olthof MR; Hollman PC; Vree TB; Katan MB. (2000). Bioavailabilities of quercetin-3-glucoside and quercetin-4'-glucoside do not differ in humans. J Nutrition, 130:1200-3.

65. Egert S; Boesch-Saadatmandi C; Wolffram S; Rimbach G; Muller MJ. (2009). Serum lipid and blood pressure responses to quercetin vary in overweight patients by apolipoprotein E genotype. J Nutrition, 140:278-84.

66. Egert S; Bosy- Westphal A; Seiberl J; Kurbitz C; Settler U; Plachta-Danielzik S; et al. (2009). Quercetin reduces systolic blood pressure and plasma oxidized low density lipoprotein concentrations in overweight subjects with a high –cardiovascular disease risk phenotype: a double- blinded, placebo- controlled cross-over study. Br J Nutr; 102:1065-74.

67. Boots AW; Drent M; de Boer VC; Bast A; Haenen GR. (2011). Quercetin reduces markers of oxidative stress and inflammation in sarcoidosis. Clinical Nutrition, 30:506-12.

68. Heinz SA; Henson DA; Austin MD; Jin F; Nieman DC. (2010). Quercetin supplementation and upper respiratory tract infection: a randomized community clinical trial. Pharmacol Res 62:2337-42.

69. Bae SC; Jung WJ; Lee EJ; Yu R; Sung MK. (2009). Effects of antioxidant supplements intervention on the level of plasma inflammatory molecules and disease severity of rheumatoid arthritis patients. J American Coll Nutrition, 28:56-62.

70. Russo M; Spagnuolo C; Tedesco I; Bilotto S; Russo GL. (2012). The flavonoid quercetin in disease prevention and therapy: Facts and fancies; *Biochemical pharmacology,* 83:6-15.

71. Edwards RL; Lyon T; Litwin SE; Rabovsky A; Symons JD; Jalilli T. (2007). Quercetin reduces blood pressure in hypertensive subjects. J Nutrition, 137:2405-11.

72. Levy RM, Pillai L, Burnett BP. (2010). Nutritional benefits of flavocovid in patients with osteoarthritis: efficacy and safety. Nutrition and Dietary Supplements, 2:27-38.

73. Baur JA, Pearson KJ, Price NL, Jamieson HA, Lerin C, et al. (2006). Resveratrol improves health and survival of mice on a high-calorie diet. Nature, 444:337–342.

74. Elmali N, Baysal O, Harma A, Esenkaya I, Mizrak B. (2007). Effects of resveratrol in inflammatory arthritis. Inflammation, 30:1–6.

75. Ma ZH, Ma QY, Wang LC, Sha HC, Wu SL, et al. (2005). Effect of resveratrol on peritoneal macrophages in rats with severe acute pancreatitis. Inflammation Research, 54:522–527.

76. Bereswill S, Mun˜oz M, Fischer A, Rita Plickert R, Lea-Maxie Haag L, Otto B, Ku¨hl, AA, Loddenkemper C, Go bel UB, Heimesaat MM, (2010). Anti-Inflammatory Effects of Resveratrol, Curcumin and Simvastatin in Acute Small Intestinal Inflammation PLos one 5(12/e), 15099.

77. Scalbert A, Williamson G. (2000). Dietary intake and bioavailability of polyphenols. Journal of Nutrition, 130:8 Suppl: S2073–85.

78. Erdman JW, Balentine Jr. D, Arab L, Beecher G, Dwyer JT, Folts J, Harnly J, Hollman P, Keen CL, Mazza G, Messina M, Scalbert A,Vita J, Williamson G, and Burrowes J. (2005). Flavonoids and Heart Health: Proceedings of the ILSI North America Flavonoids Workshop, May 31–June 1, 2005, Washington, DC.

79. Mennen L I, Walker R, Bennetau-Pelissero C, Scalbert A. (2005). Risks and safety of polyphenol consumption. Am J Clin Nutr: 81(suppl):326S-9S.

80. Scalbert A, Williamson G. (2000). Dietary intake and bioavailability of polyphenols. Journal Nutrition, 130:2073S-85S.

81. Manach C, Scalbert A, Morand C, Remesy C, Jimenez L. (2004). Polyphenols: food sources and bioavailability. Am J Clin Nutr 79:727-47.

82. Dietary reference intakes for thiamin, riboflavin, niacin, vitamin B6, Folate, vitamin B12, Pantothenic acid, biotin, and choline (1998).

83. Dietary reference intakes for vitamin C, Vitamin E, selenium, and carotenoids (2000). Accessed 06/ 05/2013 via www.nap.deu

84. Hertog MG, Feskens EJ, Hollman PC, Katan MB, Kromhout D. (1993). Dietary antioxidant flavonoids and risk of coronary heart disease: the Zutphen Elderly Study. Lancet, 342:1007–11.

85. Hertog MG, Hollman PC, Katan MB, Kromhout D. (1993). Intake of potentially anticarcinogenic flavonoids and their determinants in adults in the Netherlands. Nu ional Cancer, 20:21–9.

86. Geleijnse JM, Launer LJ, Van der Kuip DA, Hofman A, Witteman JC. (2002). Inverse association of tea and flavonoid intakes with incident myocardial infarction: the Rotterdam Study. American Journal of Clinical Nutrition, 75:880–6.

87. Linseisen J, Radtke J, Wolfram G. (1997). Flavonoid intake of adults in a Bavarian subgroup of the national food consumption survey. Z Ernahrungswiss, 36:403–12.

88. Radtke J, Linseisen J, Wolfram G. (2002). Fasting plasma concentrations of selected flavonoids as markers of their ordinary dietary intake. European Journal of Nutrition, 41:203–9.

89. Arai Y, Uehara M, Sato Y, Kimira M, Eboshida A, Adlercreutz H, Watanabe S. (2000). Comparison of isoflavones among dietary intake, Plasma concentration and urinary excretion for accurate estimation of phytoestrogen intake. Journal of Epidemiology, 10:127–35.

90. Hertog MG, Kromhout D, Aravanis C, Blackburn H, Buzina R, Fidanza F, Giampaoli S, Jansen A, Menotti A, et al. (1995). Flavonoid intakeand long-term risk of coronary heart disease and cancer in the seven countries study. Arch Internal Medicine, 155:381–6.

91. Park YK, Kim Y, Park E, Kim JS, Kang M-H. (2002). Estimated flavonoids intake in Korean adults using semiquantitative food frequency questionnaire. Korean J Nutrition, 35:1081–8.

92. Hertog MG, Sweetnam PM, Fehily AM, Elwood PC, Kromhout D. (1997). Antioxidant flavonols and ischemic heart disease in a Welshpopulation of men: the Caerphilly Study. American Journal Clinical Nutrition. 65:1489–94.

93. Chun OK, Chung S, Kerver JM, Obayashi S, Song WO. (2005). Estimated dietary intakes and major food sources of flavonoids among the U.S. population and within socioeconomic subgroups. FASEB J, 19: Abstract 75.1.

94. Kimira M, Arai Y, Shimoi K, Watanabe S. (1998). Japanese intake of flavonoidsand isoflavonoids from foods. Journal of Epidemiology, 8:168–75

95. Kirk P, Patterson RE, Lampe J. (1999). Development of a soy food frequencyquestionnaire to estimate isoflavone consumption in U.S. adults. Journal American Diet Assoc, 99:558–63.

96. Lagiou P, Samoli E, Lagiou A, Katsouyanni K, Peterson J, Dwyer J, Trichopoulos D. (2004). Flavonoid intake in relation to lung cancer risk: case-control study among women in Greece. Nutritional Cancer, 49:139–43.

97. Lagiou P, Samoli E, Lagiou A, Peterson J, Tzonou A, Dwyer J, Trichopoulos D. (2004). Flavonoids, vitamin C and adenocarcinoma of the stomach. Cancer Causes Control, 15:67–72.

98. Bosetti C, Spertini L, Parpinel M, Gnagnarella P, Lagiou P, Negri E, Franceschi S, Montella M, Peterson J, et al. (2005). Flavonoids and breast cancer risk in Italy. Cancer Epidemiological Biomarkers Prevention, 14:805–8.

99. Lyons-Wall P, Autenzio P, Lee E, Moss R, Gie S, Samman S. (2004). Catechins are the major source of flavonoids in a group of Australian women. Asia Pacific Journal of Clinical Nutrition, 13: Suppl: S72.

100. Boker LK, Van der Schouw YT, de Kleijn MJ, Jacques PF, Grobbee DE, Peeters PH. (2002). Intake of dietary phytoestrogens by Dutch women. Journal of Nutrition, 132:1319–28.

101. van Erp-Baart MA, Brants HA, Kiely M, Mulligan A, Turrini A, Sermoneta C, Kilkkinen A, Valsta LM. (2003). Isoflavone intake in four different European countries: the VENUS approach. Britain Journal of Nutrition, 89:1 Suppl: S25–30.

102. Jones AE, Price KE, Fenwick GR. (1989). Development and application of a high performance liquid Chromatographic method for the analysis of phytoestrogens. Journal of Science and Food Agriculture, 46:357-64.

103. Clarke DB, Lloyd AS. (2004). Dietary exposure estimates of isoflavones from the 1998 UK total diet study. Food additives and contaminants, 21:305-16.

104. Valsta L, Kilkkinen A, Mazur W, Nurmi T, Lampi AM, Ovaskainen M, Korhonen T, Adlercreutz H, Pietinen P. (2003). Phyto-estrogen database of foods and average intake in Finland. Britian Journal of Nutrition, 89:1 Suppl: S31-8.

105. de Kleijn MJ, van der Schouw YT, Wilson PW, Adlercreutz H, Mazur W, Grobbee DE, Jacques PF. (2001). Intake of dietary phytoestrogens is low in postmenopausal women in the United States: the Framingham Study (1–4). Journal of Nutrition, 131:1826–32.

106. Horn-Ross PL, Lee M, John EM, Koo J. (2000). Sources of phytoestrogen exposure among non-Asian women in California, USA. Cancer Causes Control, 11:299–302.

107. Kirk P, Patterson RE, Lampe J. (1999). Development of a soy food frequency questionnaire to estimate isoflavone consumption in U.S. adults. Journal of American Diet Association, 99:558–63.

108. Rimm EB, Katan MB, Ascherio A, Stampfer MJ, Willett WC. (1996). Relation between intake of flavonoids and risk for coronary heart disease in male health professionals. Ann Internal Medicine, 125:384–9.

109. Yochum L, Kushi LH, Meyer K, Folsom AR. (1999). Dietary flavonoid intake and risk of cardiovascular disease in postmenopausal women. American Journal of Epidemiolology, 149:943–9.

110. Sesso HD, Gaziano JM, Liu S, Buring JE. (2003). Flavonoid intake and the risk of cardiovascular disease in women. American Journal of Clinical Nutrition, 77:1400–8.

111. Wakai K, Egami I, Kato K, Kawamura T, Tamakoshi A, Lin Y, Nakayama T, Wada M, Ohno (1999). Dietary intake and sources of isoflavones among Japanese. Nutritional Cancer, 3:139–45.

112. Arts IC, Jacobs DR, Harnack LJ, Gross M, Folsom AR. (2001). Dietarycatechins in relation to coronary heart disease among postmenopausal women. Journal of Epidemiology, 12:668–75.

113. Arts IC, Hollman PC, Feskens EJ, Bueno de Mesquita HB, Kromhout D. (2001). Catechin intake and associated dietary and lifestyle factors in a representative sample of Dutch men and women. Europena Journal of Clinical Nutrition, 55:76–81.

114. Gu L, Kelm MA, Hammerstone JF, Beecher G, Holden J, Haytowitz D Gebhardt S, Prior RL. (2004). Concentrations of proanthocyanidins in common foods and estimations of normal consumption. Journal of Nutrition, 134:613–7.

115. Van der Heijden CA; Janssen PJ; Strik JJ. (1986). Toxicology of gallates: a review and evaluation. Food Chemical Toxicolology, 24:1067-1070.

116. Orten JM; Kuyper AC; Smith AH. (1948). Studies on the toxicity of propyl gallate and of antioxidant mixtures containing propyl gallate. Food Technolology, 2:308.

117. Dacre JC. (1974). Long-term toxicity study of n- propyl gallate in mice. Food Cosmetic Toxicology, 12:125

118. Uckun FM; Narla RK; Zeren T; Yanishevski Y; Myers DE; Waurzyniak B; Ke O; Schneider E; Messinger Y; Chelstrom LM; Gunther R; Evans W. (1998). In vivo toxicity, pharmacokinetics, and anticancer activity of genistein linked to recombinant human epidermal growth factor. Clinical Cancer Research, 4:1125-1134

119. Lamartiniere CA; Wang J; Smith-Johnson M; Eltoum I-E. (2002). Daidzein: bioavailability, potential for reproductive toxicity, and breast cancer chemoprevention in female rats. Toxicological. Science, 65:228-238

120. Constantinou AI; Mehta R; Husband A. (2003). Phenoxodiol, a novel isoflavone derivative, inhibits dimethylbenz(a)anthracene (DMBA)-induced mammary carcinogenesis in female Sprague-Dawley rats. European Journal of Cancer, 39:1012-1018.

121. Das S; Parveen S; Kundra CP; Pereria BMJ. (2004). Reproduction in male rats in vulnerable to treatment with the flavonoid-rich seed extracts of Vitex negundo. Phytotherapy Research, 18:8-13.

122. Perez-Coll CS; Herkovits J. (2004). Lethal and teragenic effects of naringenin evaluated by means of an amphibian embryo toxicity test (AMPHITOX). Food Chemical Toxicology, 42:299-306.

123. Menon LG; Kuttan R; Kuttan G. (1995). Inhibition of lung metastasis in mice induced by BI6F10 melanoma cells by polyphenolic compounds. Cancer Letters, 95:221-225.

124. Galati G. (2004). Dietary flavonoid/polyphenolic reactive metabolites and their biological properties. Toronto: University of Toronto: Ph.D. thesis.

125. Li ZG; Shimada Y; Sato F; Maeda M; Itami A; Kaganoi J; Komoto I; Kawabe A; Imamura M. (2002). Inhibitory effects of epigallocatechin-3-gallate on N-nitrosomethyl benzylamine induced esophageal tumorigenesis in F344 rats. International Journal of Oncology, 21:1275-1283.

126. Gupta YK; Sharma M; Chaudhary G. (2002). Pyrogallo-induced hepatotoxicity in rats: a model to evaluate antioxidant hepatoprotective agents. Methods Find. Experimental Clinical Pharmacology, 24:497-500.

127. Varanka Z; Rojik I; Varanka I; Nemcsok J; Abraham M. (2001). Biochemical and morphological changes in carp (Cyprinus carpio L.) liver following exposure to copper sulfate and tannic acid. Comprehensive Biochemistry and Physiolology, 128:467-477.

128. Gali-Muhtasib HU; Yamount SZ; Sidani MM. (2000). Tannins protect against skin tumor promotion induced by ultraviolet–B radiation in hairless mice. Nutritional Cancer, 37:73-77.

129. Desperes JP. (2006). Is visceral obesity the cause of the metabolic syndrome? Ann medicine, 38:52-63.

130. Huang H-P, Ou T-T, Wang C-J (2013). Mulberry (Sang Shèn Zǐ) and its Bioactive Compounds, the Chemoprevention Effects and Molecular Mechanisms *In Vitro and In Vivo*. Journal of Traditional and Complementary Medicine 3: 7-15.

131. Ou TT, Hsu MJ, Chan KC, Huang CN, Ho HH, Wang CJ. (2011). Mulberry extract inhibits oleic acid-induced lipid accumulation via reduction of lipogenesis and promotion of hepatic lipid clearance. Journal of Science and Food Agriculture, 91:2740-8.

132. Waltner-Law ME, Wang XL, Law BK, Hall RK, Nawano M, and Granner DK. (2002). Epigallocatechin Gallate, a Constituent of Green Tea, Represses Hepatic Glucose Production. Journal of Biological Chemistry, 277, 34933-34940.

133. Chihara G, Maeda Y, Sasaki T, Fukuoka F. (1969). Inhibition of mouse sarcoma 180 by polysaccharides from Lentinusedodes (Berk.). Nature, 222:687–8.

134. Mizuno T. (1999). The extraction and development of antitumor-active polysaccharides from medicinal mushrooms in Japan (review). International Journal of Medicinal Mushrooms, 1:9–30.

135. Wasser SP, Weis AL. (1999). Medicinal properties of substances occurring in higher Basidiomycetes mushrooms: current perspectives (review). Intertional Journal of Medicinal Mushrooms; 1:31–62.

136. Reshetnikov SV, Wasser SP, Tan KK. (2001). Higher basidiomycetes as a source of antitumor and immunostimulating polysaccharides (review). International Journal of Medicinal Mushrooms; 3:361–94.

137. Lindequist U, Niedermeyer THJ, Jülich W-D. (2005). The Pharmacological Potential of Mushrooms Review. eCAM, 2(3)285–299.

138. Zhou S, Gao Y. (2002). The immunomodulating effects of *Ganoderma lucidum* (Curt.:Fr.) P.Karst (LingZhi, Reishi Mushroom) (Aphylloromycetidae).International Journal of Medicinal Mushrooms, 4:1–11.

139. Karinaga R, Mizu M, Koumoto K, Anada T, Shinkai S, Kimura T, et al. (2004). First observation by fluorescence polarization of complexation between mRNA and the natural polysaccharide schizophyllan. Chemical Biodiversity, 1:634–945.

140. Adachi Y, Suzuki Y, Jinushi T, Yadomae T, Ohno N. (2002). Th 1 orientedimmunomodulating activity of geforming fungal (1-3) beta-glucans. International Journal of Medicinal Mushrooms, 4:95-109.

141. Zjawiony J. (2004). Biologically active compounds from Aphyllophorales (polypore) fungi. Journal of Natural Product, 67:300-10.

5

Healthy, Functional, and Medical Foods: Similarities and Differences

Cara J. Westmark

Department of Neurology, University of Wisconsin Madison, Madison, WI, 53705, USA

Introduction

Food is a material consisting essentially of protein, carbohydrates, and fat, together with supplementary substances (minerals, vitamins, and condiments) that are used in the body of an organism to sustain growth, repair, and vital processes, as well as to furnish energy [1]. Food serves both as a fuel (providing calories for energy expenditures), and as a medicine (for the prevention and treatment of disease). Harvesting energy from food begins with mechanical digestion in the mouth, where amylase in the saliva starts to digest the starch. The food **bolus** then moves by peristalsis through the esophagus to the stomach and is further digested by gastric juice consisting of hydrochloric acid and pepsin. The resulting **chyme** enters the small intestine, where it is fully digested and absorbed into the bloodstream through villi lining the wall of the small intestine [2]. Once in the bloodstream, nutrients are distributed throughout the body. Daily energy requirements for males in their twenties range from 2,400-3,000 calories; females 1,800-2,400 calories [3].

In addition to serving as the body's fuel source, food contains chemicals that can protect against or increase the likelihood of developing chronic diseases. There is a growing interest on the part of consumers and medical professionals to identify health-promoting chemicals in foods and thus provide dietary means to promote wellness. The food industry has accommodated this trend by marketing numerous nutritional and dietary supplements, as well as medical foods for specific disorders. However, the package labeling and government regulation of these products is varied and often confusing. It is imperative to understand how chemicals in our food affect the body at the molecular and genetic levels. In the words of Ann Wigmore [4], "The food you eat can either be the safest and most powerful form of medicine or the slowest form of poison."

Definition of Functional Food

In the United States, the term "functional food" is a marketing expression with no legal meaning or regulation by the Food and Drug Administration (FDA). The Functional Food Center defines a functional food as "a natural or processed food that contains known or unknown biologically-active compounds; which in defined amounts, provide a clinically proven and documented health benefit, and thus are important sources in the prevention, management and treatment of chronic diseases in the modern age [5]." The American Dietetic Association (ADA), the largest organization of food and nutrition professionals in the United States, classifies all foods as functional at some physiological level [6]. Furthermore, the ADA subdivides food into conventional foods, modified foods, foods for special dietary use, and medical foods. Conventional foods are unmodified whole foods such as fruits (e.g. apples) and vegetables (e.g. broccoli). These foods are in their natural state and have not been modified by enrichment or fortification. Modified foods are foods that have been fortified, enriched or enhanced. For instance, orange juice can be fortified with calcium to promote bone health, cereal products can be enriched with folic acid to reduce birth defects, and margarine can be enhanced with plant esters to reduce cholesterol. Modified foods have been a staple in the American diet since 1924, when the essential trace mineral iodine was added to table salt to prevent goiter [7]. Special dietary foods are commercially available foods formulated for persons with specific dietary requirements, but don't require supervision by a health care provider. For example, infant formula for babies, gluten-free products for individuals with Celiac disease and dairy-free foods for those who are lactose-intolerant. Medical foods are specially formulated, regulated products for the dietary management of specific diseases. In 1988, the FDA, through the Orphan Drug Amendment, defined medical food as, "food which is formulated to be consumed or administered internally under the supervision of a physician and is intended for the specific dietary management of a disease or condition for which distinctive nutritional requirements, based on recognized scientific principles, are established by medical evaluation [8]. The 5 criteria that clarify the characteristics of medical food include:

1. It is a specifically formulated and processed product for the partial or exclusive feeding of a patient by means of oral intake or enteral feeding by tube
2. It is intended for the dietary management of a patient who, because of therapeutic or chronic medical needs, has limited or impaired capacity to ingest, digest, absorb, or metabolize ordinary foodstuffs or certain nutrients, or who has other special medically determined nutrient requirements, in which the dietary management cannot be achieved by the modification of the normal diet alone
3. It provides nutritional support that is specifically modified for the management of the unique nutrient needs resulting from the specific disease or condition, as determined by medical evaluation
4. It is intended to be used under medical supervision
5. It is intended only for a patient receiving active and ongoing medical supervision, wherein the patient requires medical care on a recurring basis for, among other things, instructions on the use of the medical food.

Medical foods cannot prevent or cure illness, but are used to manage the course of a disease. A medical food can also be defined by what it is not. A medical food is not a change in diet, a vitamin-rich health food, a dietary supplement, or sold over the counter.

Other food-related terminology that one encounters includes "dietary supplement," "nutritional supplement," "nutraceutical," "organic food," "free-range food," "hormone-free food," "natural food," and "essential nutrient." Dietary and nutritional supplements are nutrients derived from food products and intended to provide extra health benefits in addition to the basic nutritional value found in foods. They include vitamins, minerals, herbs or other botanicals, amino acids, and enzymes. They can be extracts or concentrates, as well as in liquid, capsule, tablet, softgel, gelcap or powder form. "**Nutraceutical**" is a combination of the words "nutrition" and "pharmaceutical", coined in 1989 by Dr. Stephen DeFelice, founder and chairman of the Foundation for Innovation in Medicine [9]. He defined nutraceutical as "a food (or part of a food) that provides medical or health benefits, including the prevention and/or treatment of a disease [10]." Thus, Dr. DeFelice's definition of a nutraceutical and the Functional Food Center's definition of a functional food are very similar. The term nutraceutical has no regulatory definition and is commonly used interchangeably with dietary or nutritional supplement. Organic food refers to food that is produced without using the conventional inputs of modern industrial agriculture, including pesticides, synthetic fertilizers, sewage sludge, genetically modified organisms (GMOs), irradiation or food additives [11]. Animal-based organic food, such as meat, eggs and dairy, come from animals that are not given any antibiotics or hormones and are fed 100% organic feed. The free-range label on food denotes the method of farming husbandry. Free-range animals roam freely for food with extensive locomotion and sunlight rather than being confined in an enclosure. Free-range applies to meat, egg and dairy farming, but the current United States Department of Agriculture (USDA) regulations only apply to poultry and indicate that the animals have been allowed access to the outside (although the size of the outdoor range and the duration are not specified) [12]. Hormone-free food also refers to farming husbandry methods. Farmers often fatten cattle by giving them sex hormones that increase the amount of meat produced without requiring extra feed, or they treat the cattle with genetically engineered growth hormones to increase milk output. Hormone-free meat and dairy products come from animals that are not treated with hormones [12]. Natural foods generally imply that foods are minimally processed and do not contain artificial ingredients. However, there is no legal meaning for natural foods in the United States. Essentially all foodstuffs are derived from natural components of plants and animals and are processed in some manner, making them all "natural" in the broadest definition of the term. Just because a food is labeled free-range, hormone-free or natural does not guarantee that it is organic; nonetheless, USDA-certified organic foods cannot contain any artificial hormones. An essential nutrient is a nutrient that is required for normal body function and must be obtained from a dietary source, because it is not synthesized by the body or is not synthesized in adequate amounts. The interrelationship between functional foods, medical foods, and dietary supplements is depicted in Figure 1.

Examples of Healthy, Functional and Medical Foods

Main food groups include fruits, vegetables, grains, dairy and proteins. A healthy diet is a combination of these food groups in amounts that provide a balance of dietary fats, carbohydrates, proteins, vitamins and minerals. Dietary fats include trans fats, saturated fats, cholesterol, polyunsaturated fats and monounsaturated fats. Carbohydrates include complex carbohydrates (dietary fiber) and simple carbohydrates (sugars). Proteins can be a complete protein source that provides all of the essential amino acids, or an incomplete protein source that is low in one or more of the essential amino acids. Vitamins are organic substances made by plants or animals whereas minerals are inorganic elements that come from the earth. Animals, including humans, absorb minerals from the plants that they eat. Next we will briefly describe the health benefits of a functional food from each of the main food groups: apples (fruit), broccoli (vegetable), oatmeal (grains), tuna (protein) and yogurt (dairy), all excellent examples of nutrient-rich foods that contribute to a healthy diet.

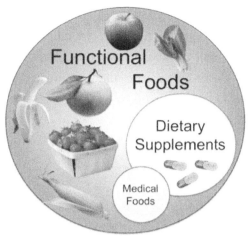

Figure 1: The interrelationship between functional foods, medical foods and dietary supplements.

"A functional food is a natural or processed food that contains known or unknown biologically-active compounds; which in defined amounts, provide a clinically proven and documented health benefit, and thus are important sources in the prevention, management and treatment of chronic diseases in the modern age"- the functional food definition by Functional Food Center Inc. at Dallas, TX, USA. Both medical foods and dietary supplements fall under the umbrella of functional foods, but each has unique definitions and regulatory guidelines. Medical foods are specially formulated and regulated products for the dietary management of specific diseases. They may contain dietary supplements, but are more than dietary supplements. Dietary and nutritional supplements are nutrients derived from food products and are intended to provide extra health benefits in addition to the basic nutritional value found in foods. They include vitamins, minerals, herbs or other botanicals, amino acids, and enzymes.

The old adage, "An apple a day keeps the doctor away," likely stems from the high nutritional value of this popular fruit. Apple skins contain pectin, which is a form of soluble fiber that humans cannot digest. Fiber helps maintain gastrointestinal health by slowing food transit time, resulting in lower glucose and low-density lipoprotein (LDL) "bad" cholesterol levels. The flesh of the apple is rich in vitamins including A, B_1 (thiamine), B_2 (riboflavin), B_6, C, E, and K, as well as niacin, folic acid, pantothenic acid and the minerals (potassium, phosphorus, calcium, manganese, magnesium, iron and zinc). Vitamin C is thought to boost immunity. Apples are also rich in phytonutrients such as quercetin, a flavonoid that may reduce free radical damage and the risk of cancer [13]. In addition, apples have a low caloric density and cleanse the teeth, thus killing bacteria in the mouth. Broccoli is another "super" functional food that is rich in phytonutrients, including glucosinolates, kaempferol, quercetin, vitamins (E, C and K) and dietary minerals (iron, zinc, selenium), which potentially promote cardiovascular health and have anti-cancer activity [14]. Oatmeal contains the most soluble fiber of any grain in the form of beta-glucan and decreases

LDL levels [15]. In addition to fiber, oatmeal contains vitamin B complex, vitamins E and K, thiamine, niacin, folic acid, selenium, iron, phosphorus, magnesium, manganese, calcium, and zinc. Tuna and salmon are good sources of lean protein rich in omega-3 fatty acids, which may benefit cardiovascular health [16]. These cold-water fish also contain vitamins E and K, potassium, iron and iodine. Vitamin E is an antioxidant, vitamin K promotes blood clotting, potassium supports heart contractions, iron carries oxygen in the bloodstream, and iodine is an essential component of thyroid hormones. Yogurt is a dairy product rich in probiotics, which modulate the microflora ("good bacteria") content of the intestines. Yogurt contains numerous vitamins; A, B_1, B_2, B_6, B_{12}, and E, as well as calcium, potassium, magnesium and zinc. Several additional nutrient-rich functional foods are depicted in Figure 2, along with some other examples, with the health benefits of their bioactive compounds.

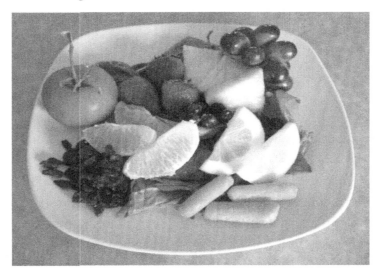

Figure 2: Color your plate with a variety of colors for a healthy diet.

Nutrient-rich foods derive their bright colors from the phytochemicals they contain. Strawberries, blueberries, cranberries and grapes derive their colors from anthocyanins. Anthocyanins are powerful antioxidants that support healthy blood pressure, improved memory, and lower risks of cancer and heart disease. These flavonoid pigments can be used as pH indicators because they change color dependent on acid levels: pink (acidic), purple (neutral), greenish-yellow (alkaline) and colorless (very alkaline). Pineapple, lemons, oranges, carrots and tomatoes derive their colors from carotenoids. Some carotenoids such as beta-carotene can be converted into vitamin A in the body. Vitamin A aids vision and immune system function. Other carotenoids such as lycopene, which is prevalent in tomatoes, and lutein found in spinach, have no vitamin A activity. However, lycopene is the most potent antioxidant of the estimated 600 naturally occurring carotenoids and reduces the risk of prostate cancer. Lutein lowers the risk of developing cataracts. The green of leafy vegetables derives from chlorophyll, which allows plants to absorb light from the sun and convert that light into energy. Chlorophyll has anti-oxidant, anti-inflammatory, and wound-healing properties.

Medical Foods

Medical foods are used to treat inborn metabolism errors, such as phenylketonuria, commonly called PKU. In the 1960s, PKU was the first condition targeted for newborn screening. About 1 in every 15,000 babies in the United States is born with this rare, autosomal recessive disorder caused by a mutation in a protein called phenylalanine hydroxylate (PAH). PAH is an enzyme in the liver that metabolizes the essential amino acid phenylalanine. If PKU is not treated with a low phenylalanine diet soon after birth, the build-up of phenylalanine in the body damages nerve cells and causes mental retardation. There are significant levels of phenylalanine in milk, eggs and other common foods. Babies with PKU are fed special infant formula that is extremely low in phenylalanine and balanced for the remaining essential amino acids. Recently, scientists at the University of Wisconsin, Madison, discovered a special protein known as glycomacropeptide (GMP), derived from cheese whey that contains only trace amounts of phenylalanine, and they are developing GMP medical foods as safe and more palatable protein sources for individuals with PKU [17]. Other examples of medical foods include Axona, a formulation of medium-chain triglycerides that can provide an alternative energy source for the brains of Alzheimer's disease patients [18]; Banatrol Plus, consisting of banana flakes and a prebiotic for the treatment of diarrhea [19]; Deplin or L-methylfolate, for the dietary management of suboptimal folic acid levels in depressed patients [20]; Fosteum, a blend of the soybean isoflavone genistein with chelazome (a form of zinc) and vitamin D3 which is a medical food for osteopenia and osteoporosis [21].

The Similarities and Differences between Functional and Medical Foods

Functional and medical foods are similar in that both contain nutrients that promote health, and both are regulated by the FDA under the provisions of the Federal Food, Drug and Cosmetic Act and the Fair Packaging and Labeling Act [22-23]. For the purposes of package labeling, medical foods are considered food products and require a statement of identity and a declaration of net quantity of content on the Principal Display Panel (PDP). The Information Panel (immediately to the right of the PDP) must contain a designation of ingredients, name and place of business of manufacturer, packer or distributor, country of origin, nutrition labeling, nutrient content claims, material facts (adverse effects), warning and caution statements and allergy labeling. Medical foods differ from other functional foods in that they are specially formulated and regulated for the dietary management of a specific disease (such as PKU), and while a prescription is not required, they are consumed under medical supervision. Other functional foods including dietary supplements are generally used by otherwise healthy individuals, and do not require the guidance of a medical practitioner.

Functional and medical foods also share connections with medications. All of these products are intended to promote health. Unlike prescription drugs and medical foods (which must be proven safe and effective for their intended use by scientific and clinical studies), dietary and nutritional supplements require no pre-market efficacy testing by the FDA. Pharmaceutical labels have directions informing consumers exactly what dose to take, how often and for how long to take it, and who should not take it, as well as possible adverse reactions. Conversely, dietary supplements do not have to undergo testing to see if they cause cancer, birth defects, liver toxicity, allergies, drug interactions, drowsiness, adverse side effects or other serious problems.

However, dietary supplements are included under the general umbrella of foods, not drugs, and do not have to be approved by the FDA prior to marketing; companies must register their manufacturing facilities with the FDA and products must be labeled as dietary supplements. They may not claim to treat a specific disease or condition, but their labels may include ambiguous claims stating that they prevent chronic disease, improve health, delay the aging process, increase life expectancy, or support the structure or function of the body. These claims are often not supported by scientific scrutiny. In contrast to the lack of regulation with dietary supplements, organic food production is heavily controlled in the United States and farms and companies that produce or handle organic food must be certified to meet United States Department of Agriculture (USDA) organic standards [24].

Table 1: An Alphabet of Functional Foods

Food	Bioactive Compound
Apples	Quercetin
Blueberries	Anthocyanins
Cranberries	Proanthocyanidins
Dark chocolate	Epicatechin
Eggs	Lutein
Fatty fish	Omega-3 fatty acids
Grape juice	Resveratrol
Horseradish	Sulforaphane
Iodized salt	Iodine
Jalapeno	Antioxidants
Kale	Iron
Lamb	Conjugated linoleic acid
Milk	Calcium
Nuts	Vitamin E
Oats	Fiber
Pumpkin	Beta-carotene
Quinoa	Phytosterols
Rye	Beta glucan
Sage	Monoterpenes
Tomatoes	Lycopene
Uube (purple yams)	Potassium
Vegetables (leafy)	Folate
Walnuts	Alpha-linolenic acid
Watermelon	Vitamin C
Yogurt	Active bacterial cultures
Zucchini	Magnesium

Strict labeling requirements ensure that consumers know the exact organic content of products. A USDA organic seal signifies that a product is at minimum 95% organic. However, current labeling requirements do not guarantee that organic food is free of genetically modified organisms (GMOs); i.e. plants genetically engineered with gene(s) from a different species than the host, resulting in the expression of a trait such as pesticide resistance. Even though GMOs are prohibited in the production of organic food, cross-pollination between neighboring farms can result in GMO-contamination of organically grown crops.

Bioactive Food Compounds

Bioactive food compounds are the essential and non-essential compounds (for example, vitamins and polyphenols) that occur in nature. They are part of the food chain and can be shown to have an effect on human health [25]. Several conventional foods are listed in Table 1, alongside an example of a prevalent bioactive compound that they contain. Bioactive compounds include essential amino acids, vitamins, and minerals that are not synthesized in adequate amounts by the human body and therefore must be obtained from the diet. Essential amino acids include isoleucine, lysine, leucine, methionine, phenylalanine, threonine, tryptophan, valine and histidine. Essential vitamins include vitamin A (retinol), B_1 (thiamin), B_2 (riboflavin), B_3 (niacin), B_5 (pantothenic acid), B_6 (pyridoxine), B_7 (biotin), B_9 (folic acid), B_{12} (cobalamin), C (ascorbic acid), D (cholecalciferol), E (tocopherol, tocotrienols), and K (naphthoquinones). The essential dietary minerals include calcium, chloride, chromium, cobalt, copper, fluoride, iodine, iron, magnesium, manganese, molybdenum, phosphorus, potassium, selenium, sodium, sulfur, and zinc. Perhaps the most well-recognized bioactive compound is vitamin C, which was extensively promoted as a cancer therapeutic by the famous chemist and Nobel laureate Dr. Linus Pauling [26]. Inadequate consumption of vitamin C can cause the nutritional deficiency of scurvy, commonly associated with sailors in the 16th-18th centuries. Bioactive food compounds also include nonessential biomolecules such as phytochemicals, which are predominantly found in plant foods (whole grains, fruits and vegetables). A summary of the major classification of groups is given in Table 2.

Table 2: Classification of Phytochemicals

Phenolic Compounds
Monophenols
Flavonoids / Polyphenols
Phenolic Acids
Lignans
Tyrosol Esters
Stilbenoids
Terpenes / Isoprenoids
Carotenoids
Monoterpenes
Saponins
Lipids
Betalains
Organosulfur Compounds
Protease Inhibitors
Other Organic Acids

Phenolic compounds are chemical compounds consisting of a hydroxyl group bonded to a phenyl ring. The monophenols have a single phenyl ring and are found in parsley, rosemary, dill weed, oregano and thyme. Polyphenols (or flavonoids), contain multiple phenyl rings and a varying number of hydroxyl groups. Flavonoids are the most plentiful bioactive compounds, numbering in the thousands. These plant pigments function in UV filtration, symbiotic nitrogen fixation and floral pigmentation. Flavonoids are further subdivided into flavonols, flavanones, flavones, flavan-3-ols, anthocyanins and anthocyanidins, isoflavones, dihydroflavonols, chalconoids, coumestans and prenylflavonoids, dependening on the location of the phenolic ring and modifications. Common examples of flavonoids include quercetin, a flavonol found in apples, and epigallocatechin gallate (EGCG), a flavan-3-ol prevalent in green tea. Phenolic acids are non-flavonoid polyphenolic compounds, subdivided into benzoic acid and cinnamic acid derivatives based on their carbon backbone structure [27]. Examples of benzoic acids include salicyclic acid (aspirin), which is found in peppermint and licorice, and capsaicin, which is found in chili peppers. Examples of cinnamic acids include caffeic acid found in artichokes and cinnamic acid found in cinnamon and aloe. Lignans are a major class of phytoestrogens along with isoflavones and coumestans. Plant lignans are derived from the amino acid phenylalanine by dimerization of substituted cinnamic alcohols to a dibenzylbutane skeleton. Lignans are found in seeds, whole grains, bran, fruits, and vegetables. Tyrosol esters are phenylethanoids with powerful antioxidant activity that are found in olive oil. The stilbenoids are hydroxylated derivatives of stilbene (1,2 diphenylethene). The best-known member of this family of phenolic compounds is resveratrol, which is found in red grapes and wine. Resveratrol is under study for potential anti-cancer, anti-inflammatory, blood sugar-lowering and neuroprotective properties.

In addition to phenolic compounds, phytochemicals contain terpenes, betalains, organosulfur compounds, protein inhibitors and other organic acids. Terpenes are composed of two or more structural units derived from isoprene (a five-carbon hydrocarbon with a branched-chain structure), two double bonds, and the molecular formula C_5H_8. These can be further sub-divided into carotenoids, monoterpenes, saponins and lipids. Carotenoids are lipid-soluble plant pigments consisting of oxygenated or non-oxygenated hydrocarbon chains with a minimum of 40 carbons and an extensive conjugated double bond system. Examples are beta-carotene, lutein and lycopene. Lycopene, a red pigment found in tomatoes, watermelon, pink grapefruit and papaya, is the most potent antioxidant of the estimated 600 naturally occurring carotenoids. Limonene is a monoterpine found in the rinds of lemons and other citrus fruits. Saponins contain one or more hydrophilic glycoside moieties combined with a lipophilic triterpene derivative, and are prevalent in soybeans. Lipids include phytosterols, tocopherols and omega-fatty acids. Phytosterols are the plant equivalent of mammalian cholesterol and are found in nuts, seeds and legumes. The tocopherols and tocotrienols of the vitamin E family contain a phenolic-chromanol ring linked to an isoprenoid side chain that is either saturated (tocopherols) or unsaturated (tocotrienols). Vitamin E is an antioxidant found in vegetable oils, nuts and the germ portion of grains. Omega-3 fatty acids are polyunsaturated fatty acids with a double bond at the 3rd carbon atom from the end of the carbon chain. Omega-3 fatty acids are an example of an essential nutrient that is not synthesized by humans and must be acquired through diet. Plant sources include dark-green leafy vegetables, grains, legumes and nuts. This bioactive food compound is also found in cold-water fish. Betalains are red and yellow indole-derived pigments that have powerful antioxidant activity. They were first extracted from beets, where their name is derived. Organosulfur compounds contain sulfur atoms bound to a cyanate group or a carbon atom in a cyclic or noncyclic configuration, and are found in cruciferous vegetables such as broccoli, cauliflower and brussel sprouts. Protein inhibitors are found in soy, seeds, legumes, potatoes, eggs and cereals. In addition to the phenolic acids, other organic acid bioactive compounds include oxalic, phytic, tartaric and anacardic acids which are found in spinach, cereals, avocados, and cashews, respectively.

The mechanism of action of these bioactive compounds largely remains to be determined. Many are purported to have antioxidant, anti-cancer, anti-aging, and cholesterol-reducing properties. For example, higher intake of carotenoids (vitamin A) is associated with a lower risk of age-related macular degeneration [28], and a high fiber diet is associated with lower cholesterol [15]. Some bioactive compounds may function to bind toxins or carcinogens and expedite their removal from the body. Adversely, the bioactive compounds in foods can potentially augment or interfere with the activity of over-the-counter and prescription drugs. For example, the bioactive compound bergamottin, found in grapefruit, inhibits cytochrome P-450, which is involved in the metabolism of statin drugs [29]. Thus, consuming grapefruit juice with statin prescriptions causes the drug to accumulate in high amounts in the body, potentially resulting in an overdose. It is rare for a plant food to contain a single bioactive component. For example, strawberries are rich in numerous phenolic compounds, such as quercetin, kaempferol and ellagic acid as well as fiber, vitamin C, manganese, calcium, iron, potassium and folic acid [30]. Extensive scientific and clinical research is required to determine which bioactive compounds are responsible for beneficial health effects and how those components synergistically interact with each other and with pharmaceuticals. A major issue confronting the use of bioactive compounds to promote health and treat chronic disease is the lack of controlled clinical trials that demonstrate compound efficacy and safety. Clinical trials are expensive, and natural compounds don't offer the prospect of large monetary returns on patents for the pharmaceutical industry. Another issue is that functional foods may benefit certain individuals, while being toxic to others depending on genetic makeup. The term "nutrigenomics" surfaces in the discussion of the health benefits of bioactive compounds. **Nutrigenomics** is the understanding of the effects of nutrients in molecular level processes in the body, as well as the variable effects nutrients and non-nutritive dietary phytochemicals have on individual persons [31]. As the medical field moves forward in patient-based whole genome sequencing and personalized medicine, it will be important to develop personalized nutrition based on an individual's genetic makeup [32].

The term "bioactive compound" connotes a health benefit, but we would be remiss if we did not mention that biological compounds that have deleterious health effects also exist; for example, mushroom toxins such as amatoxins and phallotoxins. Over two thousand years ago, Hippocrates said, "Let food be thy medicine and medicine be thy food," and all medicine at some dose is a poison. Similarly, phytoestrogens are heavily marketed as dietary supplements, and are thought to have health benefits in terms of hormone-dependent breast and prostate cancers, osteoporosis, cognitive function, cardiovascular disease, immunity, inflammation, reproduction and fertility. However, there is often scarce or conflicting scientific data to support these claims [33]. Phytoestrogens can exert biological activity by mimicking the effects of mammalian estrogens, and thus disrupt the endocrine cycle. They were originally discovered in clover after cattle and sheep eating the plants exhibited decreased fertility [34]. Approximately 20 percent of infants are fed soy-based infant formulas, which are rich in phytoestrogens [35]. Emerging evidence suggests that a soy-based diet is associated with increased seizure incidence [36], which could have important implications for babies genetically predisposed to seizure-related disorders, such as epilepsy, autism, Down syndrome and Fragile X syndrome.

SUMMARY

- A functional food is a natural or processed food that contains known or unknown biologically-active compounds; which in defined amounts, provide a clinically proven and documented health benefit, and thus are important sources in the prevention, management and treatment of chronic diseases in the modern age.

- Bioactive food compounds are essential and non-essential compounds (for example, vitamins and polyphenols) that occur in nature, are part of the food chain, and can be shown to have an effect on human health.

- There are well established roles for dietary components in disease, including sugar (diabetes), cholesterol (heart disease), calcium and vitamin D (bone density), phenylalanine (PKU) and gluten (Celiac disease).

- Scientific data regarding bioactive compounds for preventing chronic diseases is scarce and requires more research to be able to support such information. The mission of the next generation of scientists and health care professionals is to understand the mechanisms of the action of functional foods and bioactive compounds on health.

- Many bioactive compounds, although largely undetermined, may have antioxidant, anti-cancer, anti-aging, and cholesterol-reducing properties.

- Non-physiological, high concentrations of bioactive compounds are tested *in vitro* studies, but these may not correlate with *in vivo* activity.

- Special dietary foods are commercially available foods formulated for persons with specific dietary requirements, but don't require supervision by a health care provider. Examples include infant formula for babies, gluten-free products for individuals with Celiac disease and dairy-free foods for those who are lactose-intolerant. Medical foods are specially formulated, regulated products for the dietary management of specific diseases and must only be used under the supervision of a physician.

REVIEW QUESTIONS

1. A medical food can be defined by all of the following EXCEPT:
   a. A food intended to be used under the supervision of a physician
   b. A change in a person's diet to control chronic diseases
   c. Is not able to prevent or cure any illness
   d. Not a vitamin-rich health food

2. The American Dietetic Association (ADA) subdivides functional foods into four groups:
   a. Vitamins, enzymes, botanicals, amino acids
   b. Medical foods, modified foods, standardized foods, conventional foods
   c. Vitamins, minerals, botanicals, amino acids
   d. Medical foods, modified foods, special diets, conventional foods

3. Food that is produced without using the conventional inputs of modern industrial agriculture, including pesticides, synthetic fertilizers, sewage sludge, genetically modified organisms (GMOs), irradiation or food additives
    a. Functional Food
    b. Free-ranged food
    c. Medical Food
    d. Organic food

4. A lack of consumption of vitamin C is associated with which health effect?
    a. Scurvy
    b. Arthritis
    c. Low blood glucose
    d. Insomnia

5. Which of the following is not an essential amino acid?
    a. Tryptophan
    b. Isoleucine
    c. Glycine
    d. Histidine

6. What is not true about bioactive compounds?
    a. There are a lack of controlled clinical compounds to support the effects of bioactive compounds
    b. Much of their mechanism of action has yet to be determined
    c. Can possibly interfere with other prescription drugs
    d. Promote health proportional to the amount consumed

7. Dietary supplements
    a. Must undergo testing to see if they cause cancer
    b. Have to be approved by the FDA prior to marketing
    c. May not claim to treat a specific disease or condition
    d. Can't have ambiguous labels claiming to prevent diseases

8. What is a similarity between medical foods and dietary supplements?
    a. Both are regulated products to treat specific diseases
    b. Both are considered functional foods
    c. Both are taken without prescription
    d. Both are said to treat diseases

9. _____ are organic substances made by plants or animals whereas _____ are inorganic elements that come from the earth.
    a. Amino acids; peptides
    b. Vitamins; minerals
    c. Bioactive compounds; metallic compounds
    d. Functional food; Medical food

10. Which of the following statements is true?
    a. A high fiber diet is associated with a lower risk of cholesterol
    b. Consuming grapefruit juice with certain prescriptions may lead to an overdose
    c. A and B

d. None of the above

Answers: 1. **(B)** 2. **(D)** 3. **(D)** 4. **(A)** 5. **(C)** 6. **(D)** 7. **(C)** 8. **(B)** 9. **(B)** 10. **(C)**

REFERENCES:
1. Merriam-Webster.com [http://www.merriam-webster.com] (25 April 2013).
2. National Digestive Diseases Information Clearinghouse. "Your Digestive System and How It Works." [http://www.digestive.niddk.nih.gov/ddiseases/pubs/yrdd/] (25 April 2013).
3. Gerrior, S., WenYen, J., Basiotis, P.: An Easy Approach to Calculating Estimated Energy Requirements. Preventing Chronic Disease Public Health Research, Practice, and Policy 2006, 3(4):1-4.
4. Ann Wigmore National Health Institute [http://www.annwigmore.org/] (25 April 2013).
5. Functional Food Center [http://www.functionalfoodscenter.net] {25 April 2013).
6. Hasler, C.M., Brown, A.C., American Dietetic Association.: Position of the American Dietetic Association: Functional Foods. Journal of the American Dietetic Association 2009, 109 (4): 435-46.
7. Markel, H.: When it Rains it Pours: Endemic Goiter, Iodized Salt, and David Murray Cowie, MD. American Journal of Public Health 1987, 77(2): 219-29.
8. U.S. Food and Drug Administration
9. [http://www.fda.gov/regulatoryinformation/legislation/federalfooddrugandcosmeticact fdcact/significantamendmentstothefdcact/orphandrugact/default.htm] (25 April 2013).
10. The Foundation for Innovation in Medicine [http://www.fimdefelice.org/] (25 April 2013).
11. Kalra, E.K.: Nutraceutical – Definition and Introduction. American Association of Pharmaceutical Scientists 2003, 5(3): 1-2.
12. Allen, G.J., Albala, K: The Business of Food: Encyclopedia of the Food and Drink Industries. Greenwood Press; Westport, CT, 2007.
13. United States Department of Agriculture
14. [http://www.fsis.usda.gov/factsheets/meat_&_poultry_labeling_terms/#4] (25 April 2013).
15. Eberhardt, M.V., Lee, C.Y., Liu, R.H.: Nutrition: Antioxidant Activity of Fresh Apples 2000, 405(6789): 903-4.
16. Vasanthi, H.R., Mukherjee, S., Das, D.K.: Potential Health Benefits of Broccoli- a Chemico-Biological Overview 2009, 9(6): 749-59.
17. Brown, L., Rosner, B., Willett, W.W., Sacks, F.M.: Cholesterol-lowering Effects of Dietary Fiber: a Meta Analysis 1999, 69(1):30-42.
18. Covington, M.B. Omega-3 Fatty Acids: American Family Physician 2004 70(1):133-40.
19. Van Calcar, S.C., Ney, D. M.: Food Products Made with Glycomacropeptide, a Low-Phenylalanine Whey Protein, Provide a New Alternative to Amino Acid-Based Medical Foods for Nutrition Management of Phenylketonuria 2012, 112(8):1201-10.
20. Accera [http://www.accerapharma.com/axona.html] (25 April 2013).

21. Medtrition [http://www.medtrition.com/banatrol-diarrhea-relief/] (25 April 2013).

22. Deplin [http://www.deplin.com/] (25 April 2013).

23. Primus Pharmaceuticals [http://www.primusrx.com/prescription_discounts.php] (25 April 2013).

24. U.S. Food and Drug Administration

25. [http://www.fda.gov/RegulatoryInformation/Legislation/FederalFoodDrugandCosmeti cActFDCAct/FDCActChapterIVFood/default.htm] (26 April 2013).

26. U.S. Food and Drug Administration

27. [http://www.fda.gov/RegulatoryInformation/Legislation/ucm148722.htm] (26 April 2013).

28. United States Department of Agriculture

29. [http://www.usda.gov/wps/portal/usda/usdahome?navid=ORGANIC_CERTIFICATIO] (26 April 213).

30. Biesalski, H-K., Dragsted, L.O., Elmadfa, I., Grossklaus, R., Muller, M., Shrenk, D., Walter, P., Weber, P.: Bioactive Compounds: Definition and Assessment of Activity 2009, 25(11-12):1202-5.

31. Linus Pauling Institute [http://lpi.oregonstate.edu/infocenter/vitamins.html] (26 April 2013).

32. Tsao, R.: Chemistry and Biochemistry of Dietary Polyphenols Nutrients 2010, 2(12):1231-1246.

33. Seddon, J.M., Ajani, U.A., Sperduto, R.D., Hiller, R., Blair N., Burton, T.C., Farber, M.D., Gragoudas, E.S., Haller, J., Miller, D.T., Lawrence, A., Yannuzzi, M.D., Willett, W.: Dietary Carotenoids, Vitamins A, C, and E, and Advanced Age-Related Macular Degeneration. Journal of the American Medical Association 1994, 272(18):1413-20.

34. He, K., Iyer, K.R., Hayes, R.N., Sinz, M.W., Woolf, T.F., Hollenberg, P.F.: Inactivation of Cytochrome P450 3A4 by Bergamottin, a Component of Grapefruit Juice 1998, 11(4):252-9.

35. Giampieri, F., Tulipani, S., Alvarez-Suarez, J.M., Quiles, J.L, Mezzetti, B., Battino, M.: The Strawberry: Composition, Nutritional Quality, and Impact on Human Health. Nutrition 2012, 28(1):9-19.

36. Peregrin, T.: The New Frontier of Nutrition Science: Nutrigenomics 2001, 101(11):1306.

37. Green, M.R., van der Ouderaa, F.: Nutrigenetics: Where Next for the Foods Industry. Pharmacogenomics Journal 2003, 3(4):191-3.

38. Daniel, K.T.: The Whole Soy Story: The Dark Side of America's Favorite Health Food. New Trends Publishing, Inc.; Washington, DC, 2005.

39. Dixon, R.A.: Phytoestrogens. Annual Review of Plant Biology 2004, 55:225-61.

40. Setchell, K.D., Zimmer-Nechemias, L., Cai, J., Heubi, J.E.: Exposure of Infants to Phyto-oestrogens from Soy-Based Infant Formula. Lancet 1997, 350(9070):23-7.

41. Westmark, C.J., Westmark, P.R., Malter J.S.: Soy-Based Diet Exacerbates Seizures in Mouse Models of Neurological Disease. Journal of Alzheimer's Disease 2013, 33(3):797-805.

6

Vitamin C: optimal dosages, supplementation and use in disease prevention

Callen Pacier and Danik M. Martirosyan

Functional Food Center/Functional Food Institute, Dallas, TX 75252, USA

Introduction

Vitamin C was first identified in fruits (citrus), vegetables and adrenal glands as hexuronic acid in the 1920s by Albert Szent-Györgyi, a Hungarian biochemist. With the help of an American physician named Joseph Svibely, Szent-Györgyi was able to identify that hexuronic acid was vitamin C through scurvy research on guinea pigs. It was later named ascorbic acid (meaning "without scurvy" from Latin) by Szent-Györgyi and Norman Haworth, a scientist who also studied vitamin C [1].

Vitamin C is a crucial component to human health. This particular vitamin is water soluble (causing quick elimination and preventing storage) and cannot be synthesized by humans; therefore, it is essential that vitamin C be incorporated into our diet [2]. The particular mechanism that prevents synthesis is the absence of gulonolactone oxidase (GLO) [3], which is necessary to catalyze the enzyme L-gulono-1,4-lactone oxidase, the final step in the biosynthetic pathway of vitamin C [4]. There are numerous reasons why vitamin C is important to our health, but many relate to how it is essential for the synthesis of collagen, carnitine and norepinephrine [5].

The two main components of vitamin C are ascorbate and dehydroascorbic acid (DHA) [3]. The transport of ascorbate through the human body involves two sodium-dependent vitamin C transporters (SVCT): SVCT1 and SVCT2 [6]. The majority of ascorbate is transported by SVCT1 in epithelial cells (e.g. intestine, kidney and liver), and the remaining is transported by SVCT2 in specialized cells (e.g. brain and eye) [7]. DHA (the oxidized form of ascorbate) is transported in the human body through 2 glucose transporters (GLUT): GLUT1 and GLUT3 [6] (a third transporter, GLUT 4, is used only for insulin-sensitive tissues [8]). Once DHA has been transported inside the cell by a GLUT, it is reduced back to ascorbate [6]. The distribution and homeostasis of vitamin C in the human body is regulated by the SVCTs, GLUTs, facilitated diffusion through channels and exocytosis in secretory vesicles [9]. The main concentrations of vitamin C are located in brain and adrenal cells.

Vitamin C as an Antioxidant

The importance of vitamin C stems from its powerful antioxidant capacity. The term antioxidant has been defined as, "any substance that, when present at low concentrations compared to those of an oxidisable substrate, significantly delays or prevents oxidation of that substrate" [10]. Out of the three different antioxidant defense systems, vitamin C is classified as a chain breaking antioxidant; specifically, an aqueous phase chain breaking antioxidant [11]. As an antioxidant, vitamin C protects low-density lipoproteins (LDLs) from being oxidized, decreases damaging oxidation in the stomach, and facilitates the absorption of iron [8].

In one study examining the chemical composition of broccoli and cauliflower, vitamin C was shown to have the highest positive correlation of phytochemicals (phenol, flavonoid and glucosinolate), and the second highest antioxidant activity (only 9.5% lower than total phenol) [12]. In another study highlighting the antioxidant capacity of jujube fruits, vitamin C had the highest correlation coefficient in the 2,2'-azinobis (3-ethylbenzothiazoline-6) sulfonic acid (ABTS) scavenging method (which establishes antioxidant activity) [13].

Why Vitamin C is So Important to Health

Vitamin C is crucial to our overall health and wellbeing. It should be considered a functional food ingredient, as it is an important bioactive compound with antioxidant properties. A functional food is defined as "natural or processed foods that contain known or unknown biologically active compounds; which, in defined amounts, provide a clinically proven and documented health benefit for the prevention, management, or treatment of chronic disease" [14]. Those health benefits are numerous, and will be discussed further in a later section. One of its most important aspects involves its role in cognitive functions, due to its high concentration in the brain [15]. This affects us in different ways throughout our life. Concerning our early years, there is animal-model data that suggests vitamin C deficiency in newborns could result in impaired spatial memory, due to decreased neurons (~30% loss) in the hippocampus [16]. As we get older, the importance of an adequate amount of daily vitamin C over a lifetime could help prevent certain degenerative diseases. For example, vitamin C is a main defense against dopamine auto toxicity, a major component of Parkinson's disease [17].

Physiological Role of Vitamin C

In a general sense, vitamin C acts as a cofactor and reduces certain enzymes by providing them with electrons, due to its chemical structure [8]. Those enzymes can react with biomolecules known as lipids, proteins and DNA, and cause harm. In order to help prevent this, vitamin C reduces oxygen species when lipid peroxidation is formed, reduces radical inhibitors in protein oxidation, and prevents nitrosamine formation to reduce DNA damage [18].

The role of vitamin C in health could be related to its recycling ability in the presence of microorganisms [19]. When microorganisms are present, the amount of vitamin C in neutrophils is 30 times higher than in neutrophils that do not have microorganisms [19]. This is important due to the ability of vitamin C to provide oxidant protection by scavenging excessive reactive oxygen species (ROS), which causes oxidant damage [19-20]. When more vitamin C is produced due to recycling, the ability to protect the body against damage is increased.

Another reason why vitamin C is important is due to its ability to facilitate proper iron levels. In one comparison study, individuals who consumed 247 mg of vitamin C daily had 35% higher iron absorption levels than those who consumed 51 mg of vitamin C daily [21].

Vitamin C Deficiency

Individuals at risk: One reason for this review is the high prevalence of vitamin C deficient individuals. There is a strong correlation that individuals who smoke tobacco are at risk to be deficient in vitamin C [22]. This has been demonstrated by the United States Department of Agriculture (USDA), which specifies on their Recommended Dietary Allowances (RDA) that smokers require an additional 35 mg of vitamin C daily to maintain adequate levels [23]. One reason for this association is that smokers tend to consume a less healthy diet (specifically less fruits and vegetables) [24], leading to a 16% decrease in vitamin C intake [25]. Another reason is that cigarette smoke causes vitamin C to be depleted at a much faster rate, in order to compensate for the oxidative stress [25]. In one study conducted, ascorbate was completely depleted from human plasma after six puffs of cigarette smoke [26].

There is also an association between lower-income households and vitamin C deficiency. In the United Kingdom, a study was conducted on the 15% lowest income households to determine plasma vitamin C levels [27]. The results indicated that 26% of men and 16% of women were vitamin C deficient (<11 μmol), and 21% of men and 18% of women had depleted vitamin C levels (11–28 μmol) [27]. A main reason for this is that households with lower socioeconomic status tend to consume less fruits and vegetables, which are essential sources of vitamin C. In one study, it was shown that 53% of low-income households spend less than $1.00 a week on fresh fruit and vegetables [28].

Individuals who have more stressful lives (thereby creating more oxidative damage) are at risk for low vitamin C levels. Vitamin C decreases more quickly with increased oxidative stress, so higher intakes can help to better manage the increased emotional/physical pressure. It has been shown that helicopter pilots have a more stressful job compared to non-flight staff, based on serum levels of stress indicators, with 21.1% higher malondialdehyde (MDA), 21.7% higher superoxide dismutase (SOD), and 25.1% higher total antioxidant capacity (TAC) [29]. There are also issues of oxidative stress which result from a worker's environment, and not necessarily the job itself. Workers who have been exposed to lead (73 μg of lead/dl of blood) compared to those who haven't (6.7 μg of lead/dl) show a 46.2% higher thiobarbituric acid reactive species concentration (TBARS (nmol MDA/ml PG)), 60.9% higher SOD, 70.3% higher chloramphenicol acetyltransferase (CAT) activity, and a 40% higher TAC [30]. When these lead-exposed workers were given daily oral 1 g vitamin C supplements (in addition to 400 IU vitamin E) for one year, their TBARS decreased by 46.2%, TAC decreased by 36.4%, CAT decreased by 59.5%, and SOD decreased by 48.5%, bringing them back down to levels of their non-lead exposed workers [30].

Elderly individuals are at risk for malnutrition from multiple factors, including disease, medications, diminished senses (taste/smell), physical limitations (reaching/bending), depression, oral issues (difficulty chewing/swallowing, mouth pain, tooth loss, poorly fit dentures), financial issues, and stress (death of a loved one) [31]. An insufficient amount of calories also leads to diminished nutrients, such as vitamin C. In one study of over 400 community-dwelling elders (mean age of 76.8) with varying diets, the average intake of vitamin C was 55.57 mg [32], which is 25.9% lower than the RDA for women and 38.3% lower than the RDA for men.

Another group of individuals who are at risk include those who suffer from certain addictions. It has been shown that increased alcohol consumption leads to a decrease in plasma vitamin C due to the action of ethanol and/or poor diet: low drinkers (~10.6 g/d) have 41.4 µmol/L, moderate drinkers (~59 g/d) have 32.4 µmol/L, and alcoholics (~194.3 g/d) have 24.2 µmol/L [33]. This relationship has also been demonstrated in heroin addicts, where increased use led to a further decrease in vitamin C levels [34]. In another study, various drug addicts were shown to have a 43.6% lower vitamin C level than control subjects [35].

Women who are pregnant are also at risk for vitamin C deficiency, due to increased oxidative stress [36]. Pregnant women who are obese (BMI >30 kg m−2) have a greater risk of low vitamin C levels than pregnant women of a healthy weight (BMI 18–25 kg m−2), because their oxidative stress has been shown to be greater [37]. Low vitamin C levels during pregnancy can lead to various health issues to the fetus, such as low birth weight [36]. Many women take iron supplements during pregnancy, which have been shown to decrease vitamin C levels. In one study, pregnant women who were taking iron supplements had a 24% decrease in vitamin C levels from the 1st to the 3rd trimester, while women who were not taking iron supplements only had a 3.7% loss [38].

Individuals who are being treated in hospitals may also suffer from vitamin C deficiency. This is especially true for maintenance haemodialysis (MHD) patients. One study determined that 44.1% of MHD patients are vitamin C deficient with <2 µg/mL (or <11 µmol/L) [39]. This is due to multiple factors, one being that MHD patients need to avoid foods that are high in potassium in order to help prevent hyperkalemia. Potassium-rich foods tend to be high in vitamin C; therefore, a decrease in potassium also causes a decrease in vitamin C [39]. Another reason these patients are at risk is that each dialysis treatment they receive can remove an average of 66 mg of vitamin C from their plasma levels [40].

Symptoms: A person who has a normal intake of vitamin C will have plasma levels of >28 µmol/L or 0.4-0.99 mg/dl [41-42]. An individual with depleted vitamin C will have plasma levels between 11–28 µmol/L or 0.2-0.39 mg/dl [41-42]. In order for an individual to be deficient, their vitamin C plasma levels must be <11 µmol/L or <0.2 mg/dl [41-42]. Though the human body is resilient, vitamin C is an essential and water-soluble nutrient that is quickly excreted. Vitamin C has a half-life of 16 days in our bloodstream; if ingestion of it stops completely, it will be eliminated within 35-40 days [43]. While blood plasma levels drop fairly quickly, the symptoms of deficiency take much longer to develop [44]. In order to prevent deficiency, humans must ingest 10 mg of vitamin C daily (this prevents deficiency, but does not provide enough to reach normal plasma levels) [45]. Unfortunately, one of the earliest symptoms is very non-specific: fatigue. This is because vitamin C is involved in the biosynthesis of carnitine, a compound essential for producing energy by transporting long-chain fatty acids into the mitochondria [46]. A plethora of symptoms in vitamin C deficiency are related to collagen, an essential element in tendon, cartilage, bone and skin function [47]. Vitamin C is required by proline hydroxylase and lysine hydroxylase (enzymes in procollagen biosynthesis), and a deficiency leads to unstable collagenous structures [46, 48]. This causes tooth loss, joint pain, bone and connective tissue disorders, poor wound healing and more specifically: bleeding, bruising, edema, hemorrhage, gingivitis, and corkscrew hairs [48-50].

Vitamin C Overdose

The side effects of normal vitamin C intake are very minor, if non-existent, because it is water soluble and quickly excreted [51]. There have been some reports of negative effects in larger doses; to help prevent negative side effects and overdose, the USDA set the upper tolerable limit (UL) for vitamin C at 2 g [23]. Gastrointestinal distress and diarrhea are the most common side effects, which have been shown in single oral doses of 5-10 g or greater than 2 g daily, with symptoms disappearing within 1-2 weeks [51-52]. However, there has been evidence to suggest there are a few more severe side effects with high-dose vitamin C. The most note-worthy is the production of calcium oxalate stones in patients with renal issues (though some healthy individuals can also produce excessive oxalate at doses greater than 1 g daily [53]). This is because vitamin C converts to oxalate during the elimination process, which can cause formation of stones at high doses. In a fairly recent study there was evidence to support limited, but still statistically significant, oxalate formation with high dose vitamin C. Both groups took an oral 1 g vitamin C supplement twice daily for 6 days (2 trials were completed); the healthy group reported a 20% increase in oxalate, while the group with renal issues had a 33% increase [54]. This study helps explain the controversy of whether high dose vitamin C is dangerous or not. There are documented cases of oxalate stone formation in subjects with renal issues, but the incidence rate is low. While a majority of the data surrounding oxalate formation provides statistically significant findings, there are no clinically significant ones [55]. An additional concern deals with an overproduction of iron. Vitamin C increases iron absorption by helping to transport iron across the epithelium in the small intestine [15]. Though this is a beneficial effect in most cases, there is potential for an iron overload in some individuals with diseases such as hemochromatosis, sideroblastic anemia, beta-thalassemia major and sickle cell anemia [56-57].

Optimal Daily Intake

As with most nutrients, there are always questions about optimal intake. This can vary dramatically when considering different factors of age, health, lifestyle and gender. In regards to determining a daily amount best suited for the general population, the most recent RDA has been calculated at 90 mg for men and 75 mg for women, daily [23]. Many researchers believe this amount is too low, and have conducted experiments and reviews to explain why a higher daily intake would better benefit our health (Table 1).

Table 1: Comparison of optimal vitamin C intake

Study/Organization	Recommended Intake (Healthy Adults)	Reasoning
USDA RDA (IOM, FNB, 2000 [23])	90 mg oral (men), 75 mg oral (women)	Meets nutrient requirements for 97-98% of the population; calculated from an EAR

Vitamin C depletion-repletion pharmacokinetic studies in 7 healthy inpatient volunteers by using 7 doses from 30-2500mg (Levine et al., 1996 [59])	200 mg oral	Bioavailability was complete at 200 mg
The combined evidence from human metabolic, pharmacokinetic, and observational studies and Phase II RCTs. (Frei, Birlouez-Aragon, & Lykkesfeldt, 2012 [60])	200 mg oral	Maximizes the vitamin's potential health benefits with the least risk of inadequacy or adverse health effects.
15 healthy female inpatientsreceived in succession daily vitamin C doses of 30, 60, 100, 200, 400, 1,000, and 2,500 mg. (Levine, Wang, Padayatty, & Morrow, 2001 [58])	90 mg oral (women)	Using FNB guidelines and on the basis of determination of an EAR; produces a median of ≈80% vitamin C saturation of neutrophils; minimal urine excretion
Review of past findings, and analysis of recent findings, on optimal vitamin C dosage. (Ordman, 2010 [61])	500 mg oral twice daily	500 mg of vitamin C taken every 12 hrs may reduce many major causes of chronic disease, aging decline, and colds

In terms of gender, there is evidence to suggest that both men and women should have a RDA of 90 mg [58]. The RDA of 90 mg for men was calculated from depletion-repletion study data [59], and the RDA for women was calculated from the men's dose by accounting for weight differences (depletion-repletion study data was not available for women) [23]. Levine, Wang, Padayatty, and Morrow (2001) conducted their own depletion-repletion study specifically for women and determined that both sexes should have the same 90 mg daily intake, based off neutrophil saturation and urinary excretion [58]. Some studies and reviews have determined that 200 mg daily is the optimal intake [59-60], with others claiming that 1,000 mg (500 mg twice daily) provides the best health effects [61]. In terms of bioavailability, the absorption efficiency of vitamin C is 89% for 15 mg/day, 87% for 30 mg/day, 85% for 50 mg/day, 80% for 100 mg/day, 72% for 200 mg/day, 63% for 500 mg/day, and 46% for 1250 mg/day [62]. Although the higher intake is tolerated and absorbed to a certain extent, the maximum bioavailability seems to peak at 500 mg [51].

Though vitamin C tends to be well tolerated, even with high doses, maximum limits have been established. While the USDA has determined the UL for vitamin C at 2 g daily, the maximum tolerated *single* dose is 3 g [63], and the maximum tolerated *daily* dose is 18 g [64]. Those doses cannot be reached from food and beverage consumption; they must be administered through either oral supplementation or intravenous (IV) injection.

IV and Oral Supplementation

Though vitamin C intake should primarily come from whole foods (to be discussed later), there are reasons to take either IV or oral supplements. Many individuals do not have access to foods high in vitamin C due to financial (e.g. high cost of produce) or physical (e.g. no local grocery store) limitations. Others may require more vitamin C due to a genetic predisposition, disease, or diet restriction [65]. Outside of trying to ensure a proper daily intake, another reason for taking supplements is for a pharmacologic effect in the treatment of diseases [65].

For individuals looking to ensure a proper daily intake of vitamin C, oral supplementation is efficient. In the clinical setting, however, IV dosing is more regularly used. This is because IV dosing of vitamin C produces a much higher plasma concentration than an oral dose. It has been shown that a 3 g oral dose produces a peak plasma concentration of 220 µmol/L, whereas a 3 g IV dose produces a peak plasma concentration of 1760 µmol/L [63]. IV dosing also has the potential to increase peak plasma concentrations with an increased dose, whereas oral dosing eventually reaches a plateau in peak plasma concentration [63].

Incorporating Vitamin C in the Diet

Vitamin C is a crucial element to a healthy diet, and there are a number of ways to make sure we are ingesting an adequate daily amount. Though the chemical components of vitamin C supplements (oral/IV) and vitamin C in food are identical, the benefit of ingesting natural food-based vitamin C allows for the consumption of other important nutrients simultaneously [66]. This is important for both a balanced diet and for the increased health effects of certain nutrients. As mentioned earlier, vitamin C is able to help facilitate iron absorption [15, 21], so consuming foods rich in those nutrients together (i.e. a spinach salad topped with strawberries), would improve nutritional benefits. Another healthy combination is vitamin C and vitamin E, as they work together to inhibit oxidation [67]. Furthermore, vitamin C can help restore vitamin E levels by reducing α-tocopheroxyl (vitamin E radical) back to vitamin E [67]. Multiple studies have also shown that there is either little difference (in terms of plasma levels and urinary excretion) between supplemental and food-based vitamin C, or that food-based vitamin C provides better absorption than supplements [68-70]. With the benefit of symbiotic nutrient relationships and similar/better reactions to that of supplements, food-based vitamin C may be the best choice for healthy individuals to obtain their daily requirement.

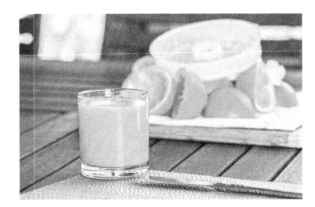

Figure 1. Orange Juice is a popular food-based source of vitamin C.

In order to ensure that individuals are getting the most vitamin C in their diet, there are a few items to consider. One concerns the area in which individuals live, and the availability of produce. In areas with limited produce due to the climate, individuals can attain vitamin C from herbs and organ meats [15]. If people live in an area without a fresh or even frozen produce section in their local market, they will be limited to canned fruits and vegetables, which have a much lower vitamin

C content [5]. Even orange juice (the most frequently purchased vitamin C rich food [71]) tends to be an inadequate source. At 4 weeks before expiration, orange juice may only have ~75% of the vitamin C claimed on the nutrition label, and it degrades by ~2% every day after it is opened, leading to ~25% at expiration [72]. In these situations, the best method would be to purchase canned fruits and vegetables that have the highest vitamin C content, and to choose the latest expiration date on juices rich in vitamin C, consuming them promptly after purchasing.

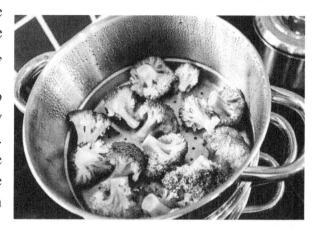

Even when individuals do have access to fresh fruits and vegetables, there are many factors which can degrade vitamin C content. Preparation of foods is one factor that can make a huge difference. Boiling tends to degrade the vitamin C content of vegetables, with an average of 50.9% loss in common vegetables (table 2) [73-77]. This evidence is further shown in a recent randomized double-blind placebo control study. The 2 test groups both

Figure 2. Steaming is the preferred method of cooking for preventing vitamin C loss.

consumed 350 g of vegetables daily. Group A cooked the food using specialized cookware that did not require the use of excess water, while group B cooked the food using standard methods (i.e. boiling). In just 2 weeks, the blood vitamin C levels in group A increased by ~17%, whereas group B only increased by ~9% [78]. As shown by that study, cooking vegetables without the use of excess water can help to preserve vitamin C content. Stir frying is one method, which shows a fairly minimal 29.9% average vitamin C loss (table 2) [73, 75-77]. Steaming foods (in a microwave or stovetop) can be a good compromise to boiling. The vitamin C content is preserved fairly well in steaming, with only an average 14.3% loss (Table 2) [73, 75-77, 79].

Table 2: Vitamin C loss in vegetables with different cooking methods

Reference	Vegetable	Boiling	Stir Frying	Steaming
Hwang, Shin, Lee S, Lee J, & Yoo, 2012 [73]	Red Pepper	66.5% loss	14% loss	34.2% loss
Gil, Ferreres, &Tomás-Barberán, 1999 (boiling) [74]; Zeng, 2013 (steaming) [79]	Spinach	60% loss	(no data)	11.1% loss
Ahmed, & Ali, 2013 [75]	Cauliflower	50% loss	15% loss	15% loss
Xu et al., 2014 [76]	Red Cabbage	40% loss	62.5 % loss	6% loss
Yuan G, Sun, Yuan J, & Wang, 2009 [77]	Broccoli	38% loss	28% loss	5% loss
Average Loss:		**50.9 %**	**29.9%**	**14.3 %**

Food storage is also a major factor for maintaining adequate vitamin C levels, and it has been established that high temperature and/or long storage periods degrade the vitamin C concentration of foods [80-82]. If food will not be eaten immediately after purchasing, the best method of storage (to maintain the highest level of vitamin C) would be freezing. For example, baby corn loses 11.6% after 3 months (0°C) [83], and broccoli and peas lose 10% after 12 months (-20°C) [84].

For individuals who have access to fresh produce, the necessary amount needed to achieve the RDA of 75 mg (women) and 90 mg (men) [23] is not difficult to attain. As shown in table 3, some common foods (such as kiwi and red pepper) can provide more than double the RDA of vitamin C for men and women with just 1 cup. This is even more exaggerated in Rose hips, providing an incredible 473.3% RDA for men and 568% RDA for women (Table 3). If individuals abide by the recommendation to eat 5 servings of fruits and vegetables daily (or 400-500g as determined by the World Health Organization (WHO) and the Food and Agricultural Organization of the United Nations (FAO) [85]) then their vitamin C intake would be between 210-280 mg [53]. In summary, some of the best ways to ensure proper intake are: consume fruits, vegetables and juices high in vitamin C; choose fresh and/or frozen products over canned when available; consume fresh produce/juice within a week of purchasing; eat foods raw or cook by steaming; and store produce not intended for immediate use in freezer.

Table 3: Amount of vitamin C in fruits and vegetables

Food	Measurement		Vitamin C (mg)	% RDA	
	Serving	Weight (g)		Men	Women
Rose hips (raw)	½ cup	100	426	473.3%	568%
Gold kiwifruit (raw)	1 cup, sliced	186	196	217.8%	261.3%
Sweet red pepper (raw)	1 cup, chopped	149	190.4	211.6%	253.9%
Broccoli (boiled)	1 cup, chopped	156	101.2	112.4%	134.9%
Orange (raw)	1 cup, sections	180	95.8	106.4%	127.7%
Strawberries (raw)	1 cup, halves	152	89.4	99.3%	119.2%
Orange juice	1 cup	249	83.7	93%	111.6%
Grapefruit (raw)	1 cup, sections	230	79.1	87.9%	105.5%
Cherry tomatoes (raw)	1 cup	149	20.4	22.7%	27.2%
Spinach (boiled)	1 cup	180	17.6	19.6%	23.5%
Potato (baked)	1 potato w/ skin	148	14.2	15.8%	18.9%

(Modified from U.S. Department of Agriculture, Agricultural Research Service. USDA National Nutrient Database for Standard Reference Release 27 [86], & National Nutrient Database for Standard Reference [87])

Even with the high vitamin C content of some foods, many individuals are still not reaching an adequate intake. One way to facilitate an increase of vitamin C in the diet is to supplement foods with additional vitamin C. A review of the pros and cons of vitamin C enhancement in plants has been completed, including methods using biosynthesis improvement and vitamin C recycling [2]. This type of genetic engineering could help communities with a limited variety of produce. For example, potatoes are a heavily consumed vegetable in both whole and processed varieties, and individuals usually have access to them in one form or another. Studies have shown 2-3 fold increases in typical vitamin C levels of potatoes using the overexpression of genes [88-89]. With that improvement, potatoes could compete with the vitamin C amounts in fresh produce not available to some communities, such as grapefruit and cherry tomatoes.

Management and Prevention of Chronic Diseases with Vitamin C

Though proper vitamin C intake can improve our diets and health, there is also evidence to suggest successful clinical applications in disease prevention and management.

There are many studies which demonstrate the disease management benefits of vitamin C on certain diseases, with a few shown in table 4. One study has shown that vitamin C can help treat diseases that current medicines cannot, such as Epstein-Barr virus (EBV). After high dose (7.5-50 g) IV vitamin C treatments, subjects with EBV showed a 40% decrease in early antibody (EA) immunoglobulin G (IgG) levels and a positive effect on disease duration (table 4) [90]. In a review on the effect of vitamin C on non-alcoholic fatty liver disease (NAFLD) and non-alcoholic steatohepatitis (NASH), human trials have shown that individuals afflicted with those diseases tend to have low vitamin C plasma concentrations and/or a low dietary intake of vitamin C [91]. This review also highlighted that treating those diseases with vitamin C (300-1000 mg daily) can facilitate improvement with disease symptoms (i.e. steatosis) [91]. One of those review studies by Kawanaka et.al., (2013) is highlighted in table 4 [92]. Another major health issue is hypertension, and vitamin C has been shown to lower blood pressure. After an initial vitamin C dose of 2 g, and subsequent daily doses of 500 mg for one month, the participants' mean blood pressure dropped 9.1%, providing evidence that long-term vitamin C treatment can reduce blood pressure in patients with hypertension (table 4) [93]. The use of vitamin C can also aid patients who are undergoing treatment. One study on breast cancer patients undergoing chemotherapy/radiotherapy showed that a once weekly IV dose of 7.5 g vitamin C decreased their overall side-effects (such as nausea, loss of appetite, and fatigue) by 37.5%, showcasing its benefits in conjunction with standard therapies (Table 4) [94]. Another study on the use of supplemental oxygen revealed that hyperoxia can cause negative side effects, including reduced coronary blood velocity (CBV) by 28%, increased relative coronary resistance by 34%, and decreased left ventricular (LV) systolic velocity by 11%, all of which were eliminated with an IV dose of 3 g vitamin C [95].

In addition to disease management, vitamin C is also a good indicator of certain diseases. Low plasma levels of vitamin C are associated with oxidative stress, a good marker for certain diseases. As mentioned earlier, vitamin C helps to reduce oxidative stress in the body, such as malonyldialdehyde (MDA), which leads to an inverse correlation. Patients with chronic obstructive pulmonary disease (COPD) can have a 55.3% higher level of MDA and a 69.4% lower level of vitamin C than healthy controls [96]. Patients with chronic hepatitis C virus (CHC) can have a 41.5% higher level of MDA and a 27.5% lower level of vitamin C than healthy controls [97]. Patients with chronic kidney disease (CKD) also show an inverse correlation between MDA and vitamin C, with a correlation coefficient of -0.36 [98]. Vitamin C plasma levels have also an inverse correlation with the incidence of heart disease, with every 20 µmol/L increase in plasma yielding a 17% decrease in risk for heart failure [99].

Table 4: Disease management with vitamin C

Study/EBM*	Analysts	N	Patients	Duration	Intervention	Outcome
A clinical study of EBV infected patients at the Riordan Clinic treated with IV vitamin C between 1997-2006, compared to a systematic review of current vitamin C/viral infection evidence. (Mikirova & Hunninghake, 2014 [90])	IV vitamin C	218 total; 35 with full data	Patients with elevated levels of EBV EA IgG (range 25 to 211 AU)	Varying durations.	IV vitamin C ranging from 7.5 g-50 g, administered 1-20 times.	Average improvement of 40% in EBV EA IgG levels; a 2.7% improvement was seen with each additional IV vitamin C treatment. Positive effect on disease duration and reducing viral antibodies.
A nonrandomized pilot study evaluating the effects of antioxidant therapy on patients with liver disease. (Kawanaka et al., 2013 [92])	Oral vitamin C and E	23	Patients with nonalcoholic steatohepatitis (NASH)	12 months	300 mg/day of both vitamin C and E	Decrease of 58.2% serum alanine aminotransferase and 49.4% of high-sensitivity C-reactive protein Combination therapy of vitamins C and E minimize damage and slow disease progression.
A randomized, double-blind, placebo-controlled study evaluating the effects of ascorbic acid on blood pressure. (Duffy et al., 1999 [93])	Oral vitamin C	45 initial; 39 final	Patients with hypertension	1 month	One initial 2 g dose, then 500 mg/day for 30 days	Decrease in systolic blood pressure (8.4%) and mean blood pressure (9.1%) Long-term vitamin C treatment reduces blood pressure in patients with hypertension.
An epidemiological, retrospective cohort study with parallel groups evaluating the safety and efficacy of vitamin C for breast cancer patients. (Vollbracht et al., 2011 [94])	IV vitamin C-Injektopas®/Pascorbin®	125	Patients with breast cancer in their first postoperative year	12 months	7.5 g once a week for 4 weeks during adjuvant therapies (not administered on the days of chemo- and radiotherapy).	37.5% reduction in complaints from side-effects during therapy and 52.5% reduction during aftercare compared to control IV vitamin C optimizes standard tumor-destructive therapies and reduces quality of life-related side-effects.

*Evidence-based medicine

There are many ways in which vitamin C can be used as a preventative measure, rather than a treatment. Though most research focuses on oral or IV routes, there is evidence to suggest the effectiveness of topical applications as well. A solution containing 10% l-ascorbic acid in a hydroglycolic base (water, butylene glcycol, dipropylene glycol, and ethanol), 0.5% ferulic acid and 2% phloretin has been shown to decrease the incidence of sunburned cells by ~90.2%, and

DNA damage (thymine dimers) by ~92.7% [100]. Topical vitamin C solutions can have protective effects against UV radiation, which can act as a potential prevention against certain skin cancers. Preventative effects have also been seen in diabetes, and individuals diagnosed with that disease are at risk for many complications. One of those complications involves high glucose concentrations, which activates the receptor for advanced glycation end products (RAGE) that can lead to pericyte apoptosis [101]. In a cell-culture study, ascorbate loading of 100 μM was shown to completely prevent apoptosis due to RAGE activation, presenting the importance for diabetes patients to ingest enough vitamin C to maintain plasma concentrations of 50–100 μM [101]. Outside of the lab, evaluations of vitamin C consumption and its preventative effects on certain populations have shown some promising results. Through the third National Health and Nutrition Examination Survey, women were shown to have a 13% lower prevalence of clinical gallbladder disease with each 27 μmol/L increase in their serum ascorbic acid level [102]. In an 11 year cohort study on the association of vitamin supplementation and upper gastrointestinal cancers, it was shown that multivitamin use did not help to lower risk, but specific vitamin C supplementation revealed a 21% lower risk of gastric noncardia adenocarcinoma (GNCA) [103]. Higher plasma levels of vitamin C have also been linked with a decrease in overall mortality, the greatest preventative measure. In a prospective population study, it was found that "a 20 μmol/L increase in plasma ascorbic acid was associated with about a 20% decline in death due to all cause, cardiovascular disease, and ischaemic heart disease" [104].

SUMMARY

- Vitamin C is a powerful functional food ingredient with numerous health applications. Proper intake over a lifetime helps maintain our current health and prevents future ailments.

- At least 10 mg daily of vitamin C will prevent clinical deficiency and scurvy, although current research suggests 90-500 mg daily for optimal benefits. Much higher doses (many beyond the 2 g UL) are used in the clinical setting, with the greatest blood plasma levels achieved through IV injection.

- The risks of high-dose vitamin C supplementation are almost negligible when compared to some current treatments. However, extremely high-doses should be administered with caution and treated as a pharmaceutical agent.

- Continued clinical and epidemiological research will help to further understand and confirm the positive health effects from vitamin C in the prevention and treatment of numerous conditions. tudies on the long-term effects of over-the-counter oral supplementation should be focused on, due to increasing awareness of vitamin C benefits. Future studies should also focus on how to safely and effectively implement vitamin C into diets of populations at risk for deficiency.

List of Abbreviations: 2,2′-azinobis (3-ethylbenzothiazoline-6) sulfonic acid, ABTS; chloramphenicol acetyltransferase, CAT; chronic hepatitis C virus, CHC; chronic kidney disease, CKD; chronic obstructive pulmonary disease, COPD; coronary blood velocity, CBV; dehydroascorbic acid, DHA; early antibody, EA; Epstein-Barr virus, EBV; estimated average requirement, EAR; Food and Agricultural Organization of the United Nations, FAO; food and nutrition board, FNB; gastric noncardia adenocarcinoma, GNCA; glucose transporter, GLUT; gulonolactone oxidase, GLO; immunoglobulin G, IgG; institute of medicine, IOM; intravenous, IV; left ventricular, LV; low-density lipoprotein, LDL; maintenance haemodialysis, MHD; malondialdehyde, MDA; malonyldialdehyde, MDA; non-alcoholic fatty liver disease, NAFLD; non-alcoholic steatohepatitis, NASH; reactive oxygen species, ROS; receptor for advanced glycation end products, RAGE; recommended dietary allowances, RDA; sodium-dependent vitamin C transporter, SVCT; superoxide dismutase, SOD; thiobarbituric acid reactive species, TBARS; total antioxidant capacity, TAC; United States department of agriculture, USDA; upper tolerable limit, UL; World Health Organization, WHO;

REVIEW QUESTIONS

1. Ascorbate is transported to epithelial cells in the body by a transporter called
    a. SVCT1
    b. SVCT2
    c. GLUT1
    d. GLUT3

2. Which of the following is not a function of vitamin C in the body?
    a. prevent oxidation of low-density lipoproteins (LDLs)
    b. facilitate absorption of iron
    c. scavenge excessive reactive oxygen species
    d. support bone growth

3. Which of the following is not a population that is likely to be at risk of vitamin C deficiency?
    a. smokers
    b. low-income households
    c. vegetarian
    d. pregnant women

4. The minimum amount of vitamin C required daily to prevent deficiency is
    a. 10mg
    b. 90mg
    c. 25mg
    d. 50mg

5. The cooking method with the least amount of vitamin C loss is
    a. boiling
    b. stir frying
    c. steaming
    d. stewing

Answers: 1. **(A)** 2. **(D)** 3. **(C)** 4. **(A)** 5. **(C)**

REFERENCES:

1. Grzybowski A, Pietrzak K: Albert Szent-Györgyi (1893-1986): the scientist who discovered vitamin C. Clinics in Dermatology 2013, 31(3):327-331.

2. Gallie DR: Increasing vitamin C content in plant foods to improve their nutritional value-successes and challenges. Nutrients 2013, 5:3424-3446.

3. Mandl J, Szarka A, Bánhegyi G: Vitamin C: update on physiology and pharmacology. British Journal of Pharmacology 2009, 157:1097-1110.

4. Chatterjee IB: Evolution and the biosynthesis of ascorbic acid. Science 1973, 182:1271-1272.

5. Doll S, Ricou B: Severe vitamin C deficiency in a critically ill adult: a case report. European Journal of Clinical Nutrition 2013, 67:881-882.

6. Li Y, Schellhorn HE: New developments and novel therapeutic perspectives for vitamin C. J Nutr 2007, 137(10):2171-2184.

7. Tsukaguchi H, Tokui T, Mackenzie B, Berger UV, Chen XZ, Wang YX, Brubaker RF, Hediger MA: A family of mammalian Na+-dependent L-ascorbic acid transporters. Nature 1999, 399:70-5.

8. Padayatty SJ, Levine M: New insights into the physiology and pharmacology of vitamin C. CMAJ 2001, 164(3):353-355.

9. Wilson JX: Regulation of vitamin C transport. Annu Rev Nutr 2005, 25:105-125.

10. Halliwell B, Gutteridge JMC: The definition and measurement of antioxidants in biological systems. Free Radical Biology & Medicine 1995, 18(1):125-126.

11. Young IS, Woodside JV: Antioxidants in heath and disease. J Clin Pathol 2001, 54:176-186.

12. Bhandari SR, Kwak JH: Chemical composition and antioxidant activity in different tissues of brassica vegetables. Molecules 2015, 20(1):1228-1243.

13. Kou X, Chen Q, Li X, Li M, Kan C, Chen B, Zhang Y, Xue Z: Quantitative assessment of bioactive compounds and the antioxidant activity of 15 jujube cultivars. Food Chem 2015, 173:1037-1044.

14. Martirosyan DM: Definition of functional food. Introduction to Functional Food Science. Volume 1. 2nd edition. Dallas, TX: Food Science Publisher; 2013:26.

15. Lykkesfeldt J, Michels AJ, Frei B: Vitamin C. Adv Nutr 2014, 5:16-18.

16. Tveden-Nyborg P, Johansen LK, Raida Z, Villumsen CK, Larsen JO, Lykkesfeldt J: Vitamin C deficiency in early postnatal life impairs spatial memory and reduces the number of hippocampal neurons in guinea pigs. Am J Clin Nutr 2009, 90(3):540-546.

17. Smythies JR: The role of ascorbate in brain: therapeutic implications. J R Soc Med 1996, 89(5):241.

18. Padayatty SJ, Katz A, Wang Y, Eck P, Kwon O, Lee JH, Chen S, Corpe C, Dutta A, Dutta SK, Levine M: Vitamin C as an antioxidant: evaluation of its role in disease prevention. J Am Coll Nutr 2003, 22(1):18-35.

19. Wang Y, Russo TA, Kwon O, Chanock S, Rumsey SC, Levine M: Ascorbate recycling in human neutrophils: induction by bacteria. Proc Natl Acad Sci USA 1997, 94(25):13816-13819.

20. Traber MG, Stevens JF: Vitamins C and E: beneficial effects from a mechanistic perspective. Free Radic Biol Med 2011, 51(5):1000-1013.

21. Cook JD, Reddy MB: Effect of ascorbic acid intake on nonheme-iron absorption from a complete diet. Am J Clin Nutr 2001, 73(1):93-98.

22. Ravindran RD, Vashist P, Gupta SK, Young IS, Maraini G, Camparini M, Jayanthi R, John N, Fitzpatrick KE, Chakravarthy U, Ravilla TD, Fletcher AE: Prevalence and risk factors for vitamin C deficiency in North and South India: a two centre population based study in people aged 60 years and over. PLoS ONE 2011, 6(12):1-8

23. Institute of Medicine. Food and Nutrition Board. Dietary Reference Intakes for Vitamin C, Vitamin E, Selenium, and Carotenoids. Washington, DC: National Academy Press; 2000.

24. Morabia A, Wynder EL: Dietary habits of smokers, people who never smoked, and exsmokers. Am J Clin Nutr 1990, 52:933-937.

25. Alberg AJ: The influence of cigarette smoking on circulating concentrations of antioxidant micronutrients. Toxicology 2002, 180(2):121-137.

26. Eiserich JP, tan der Vliet A, Handelman GJ, Halliwell B, Cross CE: Dietary antioxidants and cigarette smoke-induced biomolecular damage: a complex interaction. Am J Clin Nutr 1995, 62(6):1490S-1500S.

27. Mosdøl A, Erens B, Brunner EJ: Estimated prevalence and predictors of vitamin C deficiency within UK's low-income population. J Public Health 2008, 30(4):456-460.

28. Phipps EJ, Stites SD, Wallace SL, Braitman LE: Fresh fruit and vegetable purchases in an urban supermarket by low-income households. J Nutr Educ Behav 2013, 45(2):165-170.

29. Taleghani EA, Sotoudeh G, Amini K, Araghi MH, Mohammadi B, Yeganeh HS: Comparison of antioxidant status between pilots and non-flight staff of the Army Force: pilots may need more vitamin C. Biomed Environ Sci 2014, 27(5):371-377.

30. Rendón-Ramírez AL, Maldonado-Vega M, Quintanar-Escorza MA, Hernández G, Arévalo-Rivas BI, Zentella-Dehesa A, Calderón-Salinas JV: Effect of vitamin E and C supplementation on oxidative damage and total antioxidant capacity in lead-exposed workers. Environ Toxicol Pharmacol 2014, 37(1):45-54.

31. Sharkey JR, Branch LG, Zohoori N, Giuliani C, Busby-Whitehead J, Haines PS: Inadequate nutrient intakes among homebound elderly and their correlation with individual characteristics and health-related factors. Am J Clin Nutr 2002, 76(6):1435-1445.

32. Hsiao PY, Mitchell DC, Coffman DL, Allman RM, Locher JL, Sawyer P, Jensen GL, Hartman TJ: Dietary patterns and diet quality among diverse older adults: the University of Alabama at Birmingham Study of Aging. J Nutr Health Aging 2013, 17(1):19-25.

33. Lecomte E, Herbeth B, Pirollet P, Chancerelle Y, Arnaud J, Musse N, Paille F, Siest G, Artur Y: Effect of alcohol consumption on blood antioxidant nutrients and oxidative stress indicators. Am J Clin Nutr 1994, 60(2):255-261.

34. Zhou JF, Yan XF, Ruan ZR, Peng FY, Cai D, Yuan H, Sun L, Ding DY, Xu SS: Heroin abuse and nitric oxide, oxidation, peroxidation, lipoperoxidation. Biomed Environ Sci 2000, 13(2):131-139.

35. Nazrul Islam SK, Jahangir Hossain K, Ahsan M: Serum vitamin E, C and A status of the drug addicts undergoing detoxification: influence of drug habit, sexual practice and lifestyle factors. Eur J Clin Nutr 2001, 55(11):1022-1027.

36. Saker M, Soulimane Mokhtari N, Merzouk SA, Merzouk H, Belarbi B, Narce M: Oxidant and antioxidant status in mothers and their newborns according to birthweight. Eur J Obstet Gynecol Reprod Biol 2008, 141(2):95-99.

37. Sen S, Iyer C, Meydani SN: Obesity during pregnancy alters maternal oxidant balance and micronutrient status. Journal of Perinatology 2014, 34:105-111.

38. Anetor JI, Ajose OA, Adeleke FN, Olaniyan-Taylor GO, Fasola FA: Depressed antioxidant status in pregnant women on iron supplements: pathologic and clinical correlates. Biol Trace Elem Res 2010, 136(2):157-170.

39. Zhang K, Dong J, Cheng X, Bai W, Guo W, Wu L, Zuo L: Association between vitamin C deficiency and dialysis modalities. Nephrology (Carlton) 2012, 17(5):452-457.

40. Morena M, Cristol J-P, Bosc J-Y, Tetta C, Forret G, Leger C-L, Delcourt C, Papoz L, Descomps B, Canaud B: Convective and diffusive losses of vitamin C during haemodiafiltration session: a contributive factor to oxidative stress in haemodialysis patients. Nephrol Dial Transplant 2002, 17(3):422-427.

41. Jacob RA: Assessment of human vitamin C status. J Nutr 1990, 120(11):1480-1485.

42. Loria CM, Whelton PK, Caulfield LE, Szklo M, Klag MJ: Agreement among indicators of vitamin C status. Am J Epidemiol 1998, 147(6):587-596.

43. Noble M, Healey CS, McDougal-Chukwumah LD, Brown TM: Old disease, new look? A first report of Parkinsonism due to scurvy, and of refeeding-induced worsening of scurvy. Psychosomatics 2013, 54(3):277-283.

44. Delanghe JR, Langlois MR, De Buyzere ML, Na N, Ouyang J, Speeckaert MM, Torck MA: Vitamin C deficiency: more than just a nutritional disorder. Genes Nutr 2011, 6(4):341-346.

45. Lindblad M, Tveden-Nyborg P, Lykkesfeldt J: Regulation of vitamin C homeostasis during deficiency. Nutrients 2013, 5:2860-2879.

46. Carr AC, Frei B: Toward a new recommended dietary allowance for vitamin C based on antioxidant and health effects in humans. Am J Clin Nutr 1999, 69:1086-1107.

47. Kadler KE, Baldock C, Bella J, Boot-Handford RP: Collagens at a glance. J Cell Sci 2007, 120:1955-1958.

48. Phillips CL, Yeowell HN: Vitamin C, collagen biosynthesis, and aging. In Vitamin C in Health and Disease. Edited by Packer L, Fuchs J. New York: Marcel Dekker Inc; 1997:205-230.

49. Zammit P: Vitamin C deficiency in an elderly adult. JAGS 2013, 61(4):657-658.

50. Al-Dabagh A, Milliron B-J, Strowd L, Feldman SR: A disease of the present: scurvy in "well-nourished" patients. J Am Acad Dermatol 2013, 69(5):e246-e247.

51. Fukushima R, Yamazaki E: Vitamin C requirement in surgical patients. Current Opinion in Clinical Nutrition and Metabolic Care 2010, 13(6):669-676.

52. Deruelle F, Baron B: Vitamin C: is supplementation necessary for optimal health? The Journal of Alternative and Complementary Medicine 2008, 14(10):1291-1298.

53. Levine M, Rumsey SC, Daruwala R, Park JB, Wang Y: Criteria and recommendations for vitamin C intake. JAMA 1999, 281(15):1415-1423.

54. Traxer O, Huet B, Poindexter J, Pak CY, Pearle MS: Effect of ascorbic acid consumption on urinary stone risk factors. J Urol 2003, 170(2 Pt 1):397-401.

55. Auer BL, Auer D, Rodgers AL: The effect of ascorbic acid ingestion on the biochemical and physicochemical risk factors associated with calcium oxalate kidney stone formation. Clin Chem Lab Med 1998, 36:143-148.

56. Nienhuis AW: Vitamin C and iron. N Engl J Med 1981, 304:170-171.

57. Gerster H: High-dose vitamin C: a risk for persons with high iron stores? Int J Vitam Nutr Res 1999, 69(2):67-82.

58. Levine M, Wang Y, Padayatty SJ, Morrow J: A new recommended dietary allowance of vitamin C for healthy young women. Proc Natl Acad Sci USA 2001, 98:9842-9846.

59. Levine M, Conry-Cantilena C, Wang Y, Welch RW, Washko PW, Dhariwal KR, Park JB, Lazarev A, Graumlich JF, King J, Cantilena LR: Vitamin C pharmacokinetics in healthy volunteers: evidence for a recommended dietary allowance. Proc Natl Acad Sci USA 1996, 93(8):3704-3709.

60. Frei B, Birlouez-Aragon I, Lykkesfeldt J: Authors' perspective: what is the optimum intake of vitamin C in humans? Crit Rev Food Sci Nutr 2012, 52:815-829.

61. Ordman AR: Vitamin C twice a day enhances health. Health 2010, 2(8):819-823.

62. Graumlich JF, Ludden TM, Conry-Cantilena C, Cantilena Jr LR, Wang Y, Levine M: Pharmacokinetic model of ascorbic acid in healthy male volunteers during depletion and repletion. Pharmaceutical Research 1997, 14(9):1133-1139.

63. Padayatty SJ, Sun H, Wang Y, Riordan HD, Hewitt SM, Katz A, Wesley RA, Levine M: Vitamin C pharmacokinetics: implications for oral and intravenous use. Annals of Internal Medicine 2004, 140(7):533-538.

64. Padayatty SJ, Riordan HD, Hewitt SM, Katz A, Hoffer LJ, Levine M: Intravenously administered vitamin C as cancer therapy: three cases. CMAJ 2006, 174(7):937-942.

65. Zeisel SH: Is there a metabolic basis for dietary supplementation? Am J Clin Nutr 2000, 72:507S-5011S.

66. Carr AC, Vissers MCM: Synthetic or food-derived vitamin C—are they equally bioavailable? Nutrients 2013, 5(11):4284-4304.

67. Niki E, Noguchi N, Tsuchihashi H, Gotoh N: Interaction among vitamin C, vitamin E, and beta-carotene. The American Journal of Clinical Nutrition 1995, 62(6):1322S-1326S.

68. Carr AC, Bozonet SM, Vissers MC: A randomised cross-over pharmacokinetic bioavailability study of synthetic versus kiwifruit-derived vitamin C. Nutrients 2013, 5(11):4451-4461.

69. Nelson EW, Streiff RR, Cerda JJ: Comparative bioavailability of folate and vitamin C from a synthetic and a natural source. Am J Clin Nutr 1975, 28(9):1014-1019.

70. Vinson JA, Bose P: Comparative bioavailability to humans of ascorbic acid alone or in a citrus extract. Am J Clin Nutr 1988, 48(3):601-604.

71. Johnston CS, Taylor CA, Hampl JS: More Americans are eating "5 a day" but intakes of dark green and cruciferous vegetables remain low. J Nutr 2000, 130(12):3063-3067.

72. Johnston CS, Bowling DL: Stability of ascorbic acid in commercially available orange juices. Journal of the American Dietetic Association 2002, 102(4):525-529.

73. Hwang IG, Shin YJ, Lee S, Lee J, Yoo SM: Effects of different cooking methods on the antioxidant properties of red pepper (Capsicum annuum L.). Prev Nutr Food Sci 2012, 17(4):286-292.

74. Gil MI, Ferreres F, Tomás-Barberán FA: Effect of postharvest storage and processing on the antioxidant constituents (flavonoids and vitamin C) of fresh-cut spinach. J Agric Food Chem 1999, 47(6):2213-2217.

75. Ahmed FA, Ali RFM: Bioactive compounds and antioxidant activity of fresh and processed white cauliflower. Biomed Res Int 2013, 2013:1-9.

76. Xu F, Zheng Y, Yang Z, Cao S, Shao X, Wang H: Domestic cooking methods affect the nutritional quality of red cabbage. Food Chemistry 2014, 161:162-167.

77. Yuan G, Sun B, Yuan J, Wang Q: Effects of different cooking methods on health-promoting compounds of broccoli. J Zhejiang Univ Sci B 2009, 10(8):580-588.

78. Mori M, Hamada A, Mori H, Yamori Y, Tsuda K: Effects of cooking using multi-ply cookware on absorption of potassium and vitamins: a randomized double-blind placebo control study. Int J Food Sci Nutr 2012, 63(5):530-536.

79. Zeng C: Effects of different cooking methods on the vitamin C content of selected vegetables. Nutrition & Food Science 2013, 43(5):438-443.

80. Chaudhary PR, Jayaprakasha GK, Porat R, Patil BS: Low temperature conditioning reduces chilling injury while maintaining quality and certain bioactive compounds of 'Star Ruby' grapefruit. Food Chem 2014, 153:243-249.

81. Fan X, Sokorai KJ: Changes in quality, liking, and purchase intent of irradiated fresh-cut spinach during storage. J Food Sci 2011, 76(6):S363-S368.

82. Robles-Sánchez RM, Islas-Osuna MA, Astiazarán-García H, Vázquez-Ortiz FA, Martín-Belloso O, Gorinstein S, González-Aguilar GA: Quality index, consumer acceptability, bioactive compounds, and antioxidant activity of fresh-cut "ataulfo" mangoes (mangifera indica L.) as affected by low-temperature storage. J Food Sci 2009, 74(3):S126-S134.

83. Hooda S, Kawatra A: Effect of frozen storage on nutritional composition of baby corn. Nutrition & Food Science 2012, 42(1):5-11.

84. Favell DJ: A comparison of the vitamin C content of fresh and frozen vegetables. Food Chemistry 1998, 62(1):59-64.

85. World Health Organization: Diet, Nutrition and the Prevention of Chronic Diseases. Report of a Joint WHO/FAO Expert Consultation. WHO Technical Report Series no. 916. Geneva: WHO; 2003.

86. U.S. Department of Agriculture, Agricultural Research Service. USDA National Nutrient Database for Standard Reference, Release 27.
[http://www.ars.usda.gov/ba/bhnrc/ndl]

87. National Nutrient Database for Standard Reference
[http://ndb.nal.usda.gov/ndb/foods/show/8256?fg=&man=&lfacet=&count=&max=&sort=&qlookup=&offset=&format=Full&new=&measureby=]

88. Bulley S, Wright M, Rommens C, Yan H, Rassam M, Lin-Wang K, Andre C, Brewster D, Karunairetnam S, Allan AC, Laing WA: Enhancing ascorbate in fruits and tubers through over-expression of the L-galactose pathway gene GDP-L-galactose phosphorylase. Plant Biotechnol J 2012, 10(4):390-397.

89. Hemavathia, Upadhyayaa CP, Younga KE, Akulaa N, Kimb HS, Heungb JJ, Ohc OM, Aswathd CR, Chuna SC, Kima DH, Parka SW: Over-expression of strawberry d-

galacturonic acid reductase in potato leads to accumulation of vitamin C with enhanced abiotic stress tolerance. Plant Science 2009, 177(6):659-667.

90. Mikirova NA, Hunninghake R: Effect of high dose vitamin C on Epstein-Barr viral infection. Med Sci Monit 2014, 20:725-732.

91. Ipsen DH, Tveden-Nyborg P, Lykkesfeldt J: Does vitamin C deficiency promote fatty liver disease development? Nutrients 2014, 6:5473-5499.

92. Kawanaka M, Nishino K, Nakamura J, Suehiro M, Goto D, Urata N, Oka T, Kawamoto H, Nakamura H, Yodoi J, Hino K, Yamada G: Treatment of nonalcoholic steatohepatitis with vitamins E and C: a pilot study. Hepat Med 2013, 5:11-16.

93. Duffy SJ, Gokce N, Holbrook M, Huang A, Frei B, Keaney Jr JF, Vita JA: Treatment of hypertension with ascorbic acid. The Lancet (North American Edition) 1999, 354(9195):2048-2049.

94. Vollbracht C, Schneider B, Leendert V, Weiss G, Auerbach L, Beuth J: Intravenous vitamin C administration improves quality of life in breast cancer patients during chemo-/radiotherapy and aftercare: results of a retrospective, multicentre, epidemiological cohort study in Germany. In Vivo 2011, 25(6):983-990.

95. Gao Z, Spilk S, Momen A, Muller MD, Leuenberger UA, Sinoway L: Vitamin C prevents hyperoxia-mediated coronary vasoconstriction and impairment of myocardial function in healthy subjects. Eur J Appl Physiol 2012, 112(2):483-492.

96. Cristóvão C, Cristóvão L, Nogueira F, Bicho M: Evaluation of the oxidant and antioxidant balance in the pathogenesis of chronic obstructive pulmonary disease. Rev Port Pneumol 2013, 19(2):70-75.

97. El-Kannishy G, Arafa M, Abdelaal I, Elarman M, El-Mahdy R: Persistent oxidative stress in patients with chronic active hepatitis-C infection after antiviral therapy failure. Saudi J Gastroenterol 2012, 18(6):375-379.

98. Takahashi N, Morimoto S, Okigaki M, Seo M, Someya K, Morita T, Matsubara H, Sugiura T, Iwasaka T: Decreased plasma level of vitamin C in chronic kidney disease: comparison between diabetic and non-diabetic patients. Nephrol Dial Transplant 2011, 26(4):1252-1257.

99. Pfister R, Sharp SJ, Luben R, Wareham NJ, Khaw KT: Plasma vitamin C predicts incident heart failure in men and women in European Prospective Investigation into Cancer and Nutrition-Norfolk prospective study. Am Heart J 2011, 162(2):246-253.

100. Oresajo C, Stephens T, Hino PD, Law RM, Yatskayer M, Foltis P, Pillai S, Pinnell SR: Protective effects of a topical antioxidant mixture containing vitamin C, ferulic acid, and phloretin against ultraviolet-induced photodamage in human skin. J Cosmet Dermatol 2008, 7(4):290-297.

101. May JM, Jayagopal A, Qu ZC, Parker WH: Ascorbic acid prevents high glucose-induced apoptosis in human brain pericytes. Biochem Biophys Res Commun 2014, 452(1):112-117.

102. Simon JA, Hudes ES: Serum ascorbic acid and gallbladder disease prevalence among US adults: the third National Health and Nutrition Examination Survey (NHANES III). Arch Intern Med 2000, 160(7):931-936.

103. Dawsey SP, Hollenbeck A, Schatzkin A, Abnet CC, Lee JE: A prospective study of vitamin and mineral supplement use and the risk of upper gastrointestinal cancers. PLoS One 2014, 9(2):e88774.

104. Khaw K-T, Bingham S, Welch A, Luben R, Wareham N, Oakes S, Day N: Relation between plasma ascorbic acid and mortality in men and women in EPIC-Norfolk prospective study: a prospective population study. The Lancet (British edition) 2001, 357(9257):657-663.

7

Fortification of Foods with Micronutrients

Ozge Kahraman

Università Politecnica delle Marche, Dipartimento di Scienze Agrarie, Ancona, Italy

Introduction

Nutritional deficiencies are a serious global problem since they cause detrimental results to humans and also decrease their life quality. The World Health Organization (WHO) has identified iron, zinc, iodine, and vitamin A deficiencies as the most serious risk factors. However, some other minerals and vitamins have also been included in both single- and multiple- fortification programs. Therefore, both developing and developed countries have published legislation to fortify staple foods to ensure that a wide proportion of the population has access to these nutrients (which are deemed essential to the body's metabolism and to reduce prevalence of these deficiencies). Nevertheless, stability, interactions and bioavailability of some fortificants, properties of food vehicles, and fortification levels before and after application are major concerns of fortification strategies. If levels are too high, the overconsumption of some nutrients constitutes a potential public health and safety issue. For this reason, upper intake levels have been determined for a variety of micronutrients. Consequently, good planning and surveys have to be developed before stepping into application. Additionally, good monitoring of results is also needed when collecting and analyzing data to check the success of fortification in populations according to predefined criteria.

Food fortification is in the modified food categories of functional foods, and is defined as the addition of one or more essential nutrients (**forticant**) to a particular food (**food vehicle**), whether or not it is normally contained in the food [1]. While poverty and the lack of access to a variety of foods are major factors for deficiencies in developing countries, high incidence of infections, lack of knowledge towards appropriate dietary practices, and unhealthy diet habits are other impediments for deficiencies in developed countries. Many people in the world, especially school-age children, pregnant women and elderly people, suffer from the consequences of vitamin and mineral deficiencies. Thus, fortification of staple foods has become one of the most-cost effective approaches and long- term strategies to remedy or correct a demonstrated deficiency of nutrients in the population without significant changes tofood habits [2].

For a successful fortification, target population, appropriate level of fortification, processing and preparation methods of the food vehicle, estimated nutrient requirement, cost, and finally, consumer acceptability, have to be taken into consideration [1, 3]. Additionally, monitoring and controlling systems have to be implemented. The selected food vehicle must be technologically and economically fortifiable, have wide and constant consumption, have an appropriate serving size to meet a significant part of daily dietary requirement of the fortificant added, and it must have good stability as well as a low cost [2]. On the other hand, the fortificant must be resistant to dietary inhibitors (either added or naturally present), have good bioavailability, and must retain the desired quality of the food such as flavor, color, odor, texture- and yet is safe to consume [4 -7].

WHO has defined three types of fortification strategies: i) mass fortification, which refers to the fortification of a food that is widely consumed by the general population, ii) targeted fortification, which refers to the fortification of a food designed for a specific population subgroup, and iii) market-driven fortification, which refers to the fortification of foods, voluntarily, that are already in the market. Food fortification can be single, referring to the fortification of a food vehicle with a single fortificant (e.g., either iron or zinc), or multiple, referring to the fortification of a food vehicle with a multiple fortificant to combat multiple deficiencies (e.g., iron and zinc) [7, 8]. Maize flour and meals have been fortified with multiple fortificants such as iron, thiamine, niacin and riboflavin in various Latin American countries [2].

Basic micronutrients, such as vitamin A, thiamine, iron, zinc, iodine, calcium, vitamin D, riboflavin, folic acid, niacin, vitamin B12, and vitamin B6, are generally used in the fortification programs of many national governments as a public health policy, since their deficiencies are widespread. Salt, wheat flour, margarine, sugar or dried skimmed milk have mostly been fortified under mandatory and voluntary fortification legislations in some developing and also developed countries for over seventy years. For example, flour has been fortified in Afghanistan with vitamin A, thiamine, riboflavin, niacin, folic acid and iron through the facilitation of the UN World Food Program [2]. Fortification levels of some fortificants in staple food vehicles are presented in Tables 2-10.

Some Useful Definitions:
Bioavailability: The proportion of an ingested nutrient in a food that is absorbed and utilized through normal metabolic pathways [9]. In other words, bioavailability means how well the human body absorbs and utilizes nutrients [10].

Recommended Dietary Allowance (RDA): The average daily dietary intake level is sufficient to meet the nutrient requirement of nearly all healthy individuals in a particular life stage and gender group [11]. The RDA values are presented in Table 2-10.

Adequate Intake (AL): The recommended average daily intake level based on observed or experimentally determined approximations when the RDA cannot be established and scientific evidence is not available. The AL value of fluoride is presented in Table 1.

Tolerable Upper Intake Level (UL): The highest average level of daily intake that is likely to pose no risk of adverse health effects for almost all people in the general population [1]. The ULs are presented in Table 1-10.

Generally Recognized as Safe (GRAS): GRAS is a term that states which substances are safe to use as food additives by experts and published scientific evidence. The FDA has published a GRAS substance list that categorizes using three terms: substances generally recognized as safe (21 CFR part 182), direct food substances affirmed as generally recognized as safe (21 CFR part 184), and indirect food substances affirmed as generally recognized as safe (21 CFR part 186).

Mineral Fortification

FLUORIDE

Fluoride is a trace mineral in the human body that makes bones stronger by replacing a part of the hydroxyapatite crystal with fluorapatite [12]. Fluoride deficiency causes dental caries, whereas high exposure results in dental fluorosis [13].

Even though fluoride is not a substance on the GRAS substance list, it has been added to drinking water (~1 ppm). Ireland is the country where fluoridated water is mostly used, with a 66% rate; subsequently, USA (60%), Canada (55%), UK (10%), and Australia and New Zealand. Salt has been fortified with fluoride in Switzerland, Hungary, Colombia and Jamaica to prevent dental caries [7, 14, 15]. Nevertheless, there is a dilemma. Even though studies show that water fluoridation decreases tooth decay, it is still low in the countries where fluoridation is not used [15].

Calcium and magnesium decrease absorption of fluoride by forming insoluble complexes. Therefore, these minerals have to be taken separately to prevent insoluble complex formation. In addition, a low dietary intake of chloride has also shown to influence fluoride bioavailability, whereas zinc and iron do not [16]. Table 1 provides information about the RDA for fluoride, and commonly used food vehicles.[17, 18]

Table 1: Fluoride [17,18]		mg/d
AL **(19-30y)**	male	4
	female	3
	pregnancy/lactating	3/3
RDA Europe		3.5
UL		10
Commonly used fortificant		fluoride
Commonly used food vehicles		salt and water

IODINE

Iodine is one of the most attractive minerals for fortification programs because it is a very essential mineral for the synthesis of the thyroid hormones thyroxine and tri-iodothyronine. **Iodine deficiency (IDD)** is a worldwide disorder that results in the impaired synthesis of the thyroid hormones, thereby causing not only goiter but retarding growth, physical and mental development, and functional and developmental abnormalities [19]. Nevertheless, excessive consumption of iodine can lead to iodine-induced hyperthyroidism [20].

Iodine is added to food vehicles as either iodide or iodate. Iodides are more soluble, less resistant to oxidation and evaporation, and have higher iodine content. However, iodates are more stable under conditions of high moisture, high ambient temperature, sunlight, aeration and the presence of impurities [21]. Potassium, calcium or sodium salts of iodine are used as fortificants, namely, calcium iodide (CaI_2), calcium iodate ($Ca(IO_3)2.6H_2O$), potassium iodide (KI), potassium iodate (KIO_3), sodium iodide ($NaI.2H_2O$), and sodium iodate (NaI) [7]. Three of them are included in the GRAS list **(Table 2).**

Table 2: Iodine [18,23]		µg /d
RDA (19-30y)	**male**	150
	female	150
	pregnancy/lactating	220/290
RDA Europe		150
UL		1100
GRAS substances		calcium iodate, potassium iodide, potassium iodate
Commonly used food vehicles (fortification level [24])		salt (30-200 ppm) and fish sauce

Many countries have mandatory iodine fortification policies for salt or the replacement of salt with iodized salt in bread (e.g., Australia, Turkey, and New Zealand etc.). However, in Thailand, iodized salt has not met its expectations, as they have used fish sauce instead of salt while cooking. A study showed that only iodinated fish sauce reduced the goiter rate of women in northeast Thailand [22].

IRON

Iron is an essential trace element as well as an integral part of cytochromes, several iron-sulfur enzymes, and structure and transport proteins, such as: transferrin, lactoferrin, ferritin, hemosiderin, and hemoglobin and myoglobin [23, 25, 26]. Therefore, iron deficiency can result in mental and psychomotor retardation, impaired immune response, and tiredness, thus, contributing to a low work capacity [26, 27]. However, overconsumption of iron increases cancer and cardiovascular risks [27]. For this reason, final levels of fortificants added to a food vehicle must be both safe and efficacious for all population groups consuming the fortified food.

Iron compounds used as fortificants are divided into four categories: i) water-soluble: ferrous sulfate, ferrous gluconate, ferric ammonium citrate, ferrous amonium sulfate, ferrous lactate, ferrous bisglycinate, ii) poorly water soluble but soluble in dilute acid such as gastric juice: ferrous succinate, ferrous fumarate, ferric, and iii) water insoluble but poorly soluble in dilute acid; ferric orthophosphate, ferric pyrophosphate and elemental iron (H-reduced, atomized, CO-reduced, electrolytic, carbonyl), and iiii) experimental compounds: sodium iron EDTA, stabilized–

solubilized ferric pyrophosphate, microencapsulated ferrous sulfate (SFE-171), and ferric ammonium orthophosphate [7, 28-30]. Iron compounds recommended by the World Health Organization (WHO) are ferrous sulfate, ferrous fumarate, ferric pyrophosphate and electrolytic iron powder.

Fortification with an iron-soluble salt, such as ferrous sulfate, is often problematic due to the oxidation from the ferrous form to ferric form; this can cause a metallic taste and a color change of food to brown. Unfortunately, less reactive iron sources lead to low bioavailability and decrease efficiency [27], so new iron compounds have been developed to avoid these problems. Advantageously, NaFeEDTA is stable during storage and processing and has fewer organoleptic problems. Another commercial product, SunActive Fe™, a super dispersed ferric pyrophosphate (SFP), does not affect the flavor of a final product, is stable at high temperatures and salt concentrations, and has a higher bioavailability than ferric pyrophosphate, ferrous sulfate, and sodium ferrous citrate [31]. Table 3 provides information about the Iron RDA and commonly used food vehicles.[18, 23]

Table 3: Iron [23, 18].		mg/d
RDA USA (19-30y)	**male**	16-18
	female	12
	pregnancy/lactating	27/9
RDA Europe		14
UL		45
GRAS substances		ferric ammonium citrate, ferric chloride, ferric citrate, ferric phosphate, ferrous gluconate, ferrous lactate, ferrous sulfate, ferric pyrophosphate, ferric sulfate, ferrous ascorbate, ferrous carbonate, ferrous citrate, ferrous fumarate
Commonly used food vehicles (fortification level (mg/kg)) [42]		Cereal, wheat and maize flours (45-60), pasta (25-35), soy sauce, cocoa products, rice, juice, soft drinks, fish sauce, biscuits, milk and milk powder, dried milk powders, dairy products

In fortification strategies of food with iron, a level between 10- 80 mg Fe/100 g product is generally preferred [27]. Doses selected for iron fortification also depend on the presence of enhancers or inhibitors in the food vehicle. At this stage, the main challenge is to protect iron from potential inhibitors of iron absorption present in commonly fortified foods. Ascorbate (vitamin C) enhances the bioavailability of iron by reducing iron to a ferrous state, which is a more soluble form when dissolved in gastric juice [32, 33]. It was indicated that the addition of ascorbate in a ratio 2:1 increased iron absorption [7]. Additionally, muscle tissue, vitamin A, E, NaFeEDTA, ferrous bisglycinate and folic acid also have a positive effect on iron absorption [26, 31]. On the other hand, Phytate (myoinositol hexaphosphate), polyphenols, calcium, malonaldehyde, phosphorus, proteins, and oxalic acid reduce the bioavailability of iron [27, 33].

Cereal, wheat and maize flours, salt, soy sauce, cocoa products, rice, juice, soft drinks, fish sauce, milk, dried milk powders [7] and dairy products such as cheddar cheese [35-37], domiati cheese [38], mozzarella cheese [39], baker's and cottage cheese [40], and petit suisse cheese [41] are staple foods fortified with iron.

ZINC

Zinc occurs as Zn^{2+} in biological systems. Since it does not exhibit redox chemistry in living organisms, it does not cause oxidative damage. This property makes zinc important in a wide variety of biological processes [43]. Over 300 zinc enzymes, which have structural, regulatory or catalytic roles, have been discovered [44-47]. Also, numerous physiological functions (mitosis, DNA synthesis, neurogenesis, synaptogenesis, neuronal growth, neurotransmission, protein and regulation of gene expression, bone mineralization, and collagen synthesis) require zinc. As a result, zinc deficiency alters protein synthesis besides the nature of RNA polymerase and may affect gene expression. Growth, cellular immunity, fertility, hair growth, wound healing and plasma protein levels are suppressed in the absence of zinc [47]. A genetic disorder called acrodermatitis enteropathica is associated with zinc deficiency, which results in skin parakeratosis and diarrhea. Sickle cell anemia is also associated with zinc deficiency [48].

RDA values of zinc can differ according to zinc bioavailability in a diet. For example, a diet with high zinc bioavailability (i.e., diets high in meat), 3-4.2 mg zinc/day intake is recommended; for a diet with moderate bioavailability, 4.9-7.0 mg zinc/day intake is recommended, and for a diet with low bioavailability (i.e., vegetarian diets) 9.8-14.0 mg zinc/day intake is recommended [43].

Interactions with a number of dietary factors influence zinc uptake. The intestine is the major organ in which variations in bioavailability affect dietary zinc requirements. The environment within the gastrointestinal tract drastically influences zinc solubility and absorptive efficiency [23].

Although zinc deficiency depends on generally low zinc intake, the presence of compounds such as phytic and oxalic acids, tannins, fiber, proteins, selenium, iron, and calcium, inhibit or decrease absorption of zinc as well. Wheat bran, lignin, and some hemicelluloses can also reduce the bioavailability of zinc [49]. Folic acid can also inhibit zinc retention and metabolism, although more recent evidence indicates that folic acid does not adversely affect zinc status [50]. Table 4 provides information about the zinc RDA and commonly used food vehicles. [18, 23]

Table 4: Zinc [18,23].		mg/d
RDA USA (19-30y)	male	11
	female	8
	pregnancy/lactating	12-13
RDA Europe		10
UL		40
GRAS substances		zinc acetate, zinc chloride, zinc gluconate, zinc oxide, zinc sulfate
Commonly used food vehicles (fortification levels (mg/kg)) [42]		cereal flours, breakfast cereals, dairy products, wheat flour (15-30)

The compounds that enhance the absorption of zinc include: picolinic acid secreted by the pancreas, vitamin B6 (that increases picolinic acid secretion), and citrate and amino acids, such as glycine, lysine, histidine, cysteine and methionine [51]. These latter three amino acids remove zinc from the zinc-calciumphytate complexes [50]. Proteins in foods also enhance zinc absorption. But, in general, zinc absorption from a diet high in animal protein will be greater than a diet rich in proteins of plant origin [52]. In regard to chelating agents, EDTA (ethylenediamine tetraacetic acid) was recorded having an enhancing effect on zinc absorption [1].

There are studies on fortification of cereals flours [53] and dairy products such as cheddar cheese [54], Turkish white cheese [55], squacquerone and caciotta cheese [56].

CALCIUM

Calcium is one of the most abundant minerals in the human body. A deficiency of calcium may lead to muscle cramps, heart palpitations, high blood pressure, brittle or soft bones, tooth decay, back and leg pains, insomnia and nervous disorders. Rickets and osteomalacia diseases are associated with a calcium deficiency in children and adults, respectively. However, lack of vitamin D causes a reduction in the absorption of calcium and results in osteoporosis that affects elderly women [57]. Consequently, it has been mandatory to fortify wheat flour in the United Kingdom since 1943. Surprisingly, however, it is optional in United States [7].

Calcium from milk and dairy products is more absorbable and bioavailable than calcium from meats, poultry, fish, eggs, grains, nuts, beans, and green leafy vegetables [57]. Table 5 provides information about the calcium RDA and commonly used food vehicles.[18, 58]

Table 5: Calcium [18,58]		**mg/d**
RDA USA (19-30y)	male	1000
	female	1000
	pregnancy/lactating	1000
RDA Europe		800
UL		2500
GRAS substances		calcium acetate, calcium alginate, calcium carbonate, calcium chloride, calcium citrate, calcium gluconate, calcium hydroxide, calcium iodate, calcium l-ascorbate, calcium lactate, l(+)-calcium lactate, calcium oxide, D- or DL calcium pantothenate, calcium propionate, calcium pyrophosphate, calcium silicate, calcium sorbate, calcium stearate
Commonly used food vehicles (fortification levels (mg/kg)) [42]		wheat flour (2100-3900), juice, milk

SELENIUM

Selenium (Se) is another essential trace mineral, as well as an antioxidant that protects tissues from oxidative stress in the human body. It is crucial for efficient thyroid hormone synthesis and is a constituent for several selenoenzymes such as glutathione peroxidase, iodothyronine deiodinases, thioredoxin reductases, and selenophosphate synthetase [59, 60, 61]. Selenium deficiency has been associated with degenerative diseases and cancer [55]. China is a country where selenium deficiency is endemic and where Keshan disease was first described [7, 62]. Therefore, in China, salts have been fortified with sodium selenite since 1983 [7]. Even though selenium is not included in the GRAS substance list created by the FDA, sodium salts are preferred for fortification (especially sodium selenite) because it has better absorption and stability than sodium selenite [7, 63].

Selenium fortification has been practiced with numerous food vehicles, such as salt, cereal, infant formulas, and dairy products. In a study, Turkish white cheese, which had been fortified with 730 µg Se/kg cheese, when fortified via cheese milk and 550 µg Se/kg, when fortified via brine solution. The recovery ranges have been 58.11 % and 70.91 %, respectively [55]. Table 6 provides information about the selenium RDA and commonly used food vehicles.[18] [23]

Table 6: Selenium [64,18].		µg /d
RDA USA (19-30y)	male	55
	female	55
	pregnancy/lactating	60/70
RDA Europe		55
UL		400
Commonly used fortificants		sodium selenite, sodium selenate
Commonly used food vehicles		salt, cereal infant formulas, dairy products

Vitamin Fortification

VITAMIN D

Vitamin D (calciferol) is a fat-soluble vitamin that regulates calcium and phosphorus metabolism. Vitamin D2 (ergocalciferol) is present in plants and fungi, while another form, vitamin D3 (cholecalciferol), is present in animal skin. Upon exposure to ultraviolet B (UVB) radiation in the wavelength range of 280-315 nm, 7-dehydrocholesterol (provitamin, which is present in the epidermis) changes conformation to form previtamin D3. Biologically inactive vitamin D (cholecalciferol or ergocalciferol) is metabolized to an active form upon consumption in the diet or when synthesized in the skin [7, 65].

Vitamin D deficiencies can develop as a result of insufficient exposure to UVB radiation, living in northern latitudes, aging, obesity, wearing excess clothing and having darkly pigmented skin, as well as having an insufficient dietary intake. Vitamin D deficiency results in soft, thin, and brittle bones, known as rickets in children and osteomalacia in adults. Table 7 provides information about D vitamin RDA and commonly used food vehicles.[18, 69]

Table 7: Vitamin D [18,69].		µg/d
RDA USA (14-70y)	male	15
	female	15
	pregnancy/lactating	15

RDA Europe	5
UL	100
GRAS substances	Vitamin D2 (ergocalciferol), Vitamin D3 (cholecalciferol)
Commonly used food vehicles (fortification levels (mg/kg)) [42]	Margarine (0.02–0.15), milk (0.01), wheat flour (0.014)

Some countries have mandatory fortification regulations for vitamin D (e.g., margarines and milk in Canada; margarine in Australia), while it is optional in the USA [7, 66]. In addition, five countries (Denmark, Spain, Poland, Ireland, and Finland) have been involved in a project called "Optiford" which refers to optimal fortification of vitamin D. The vitamin D status of elderly women and young girls, indigenous or immigrant, has been evaluated, and appropriate levels of fortification have been discussed in this project [67, 68]. However, in Europe, fortification of margarine with vitamin D is not mandatory and fulfills 30% of RDA [7].

Vitamin D is included in the GRAS list, nevertheless, in accordance with 21 CFR 184.1(b) (2). The use of vitamin D as sole source in milk products has limitations;89IU/100 g (2.22 μg). According to the FDA, vitamin D may be added to foods as crystalline vitamin D2 (ergocalciferol), crystalline vitamin D3 (cholecalciferol), and vitamin D2 resin or vitamin D3 resin. Vitamin D2 and D3 have similar biological activities; both are very sensitive to oxygen and moisture, and both interact with minerals. However, a dry stabilized form of vitamin D is generally used for most commercial applications; it protects activity even in the presence of minerals by means of an antioxidant, which is usually tocopherol [7].

B VITAMINS

B vitamins include Vitamin B1 (thiamine), Vitamin B2 (riboflavin), Vitamin B3 (niacin or niacinamide), Vitamin B5 (pantothenic acid), Vitamin B6 (pyridoxine, pyridoxal, or pyridoxamine, or pyridoxine hydrochloride), Vitamin B7 (biotin), Vitamin B9 (folic acid), and Vitamin B_{12} (cobalamin). B complex vitamins are water-soluble and are not stored in the body [70].

Thiamine is involved in the metabolism of carbohydrates as a coenzyme. People consuming alcohol are prone to thiamine deficiency (because it reduces thiamine availability), as well as Wernicke–Korsakoff syndrome resulting in impaired memory [71]. The Thiamine hydrochloride form of Vitamin B1 is more water soluble than the mononitrate form. Thiamine is stable at around pH 6 [7].

Riboflavin is a coenzyme in oxidation-reduction reactions and aids in the conversion of tryptophan into niacin [70]. Symptoms of riboflavin deficiency are bloodshot eyes, a sore and red tongue, dermatitis on the lips, extreme and unusual sensitivity to light and irritability in the eyes [70]. It is unstable in an alkaline pH, and labile in the presence of light and ascorbic acid [7].

Niacin is involved in energy production and is a coenzyme for dehydrogenases. A severe deficiency of niacin results in symptoms including cramps, nausea, mental confusion, and skin problems [70]. Niacin is soluble in an alkaline medium and stable in oxygen, heat, and light [7].

Pantothenic acid contributes to the sugar metabolism and is involved in the energy production as well as the synthesis of hormones and coenzyme A (CoA). Its deficiency is rare; however, a severe deficiency causes the inability to cope with stress and the development of acne, headaches and burning hands and feet [70, 72]. Pantothenic acid is very stable at pH 5-7 [24].

Pyridoxine is involved in the production of insulin, hemoglobin, amino acids, and the glycogen metabolism. Basic symptoms of vitamin B6 deficiency are nausea, a defect in amino acid metabolism (e.g., tryptophan, methionine), dermatitis, changes in leukocyte count and activity, and kidney stones [70, 73]. Pyridoxine is very stable when heated and in the presence of atmospheric oxygen, but is sensitive to UV light [7, 24].

Biotin, also called "Vitamin H" and "Coenzyme R", helps out in the metabolism of fats, proteins and carbohydrates. Intestinal bacteria have the capability to make biotin [70, 74]. **Avidin** (an egg-white glycoprotein resistant to pancreatic proteases) binds biotin in the intestines, thus preventing the bioavailability of vitamin B7 [74]. Deficiency is rare. However, symptoms include loss of appetite, nausea, vomiting, depression, muscle pains, and heart abnormalities [70]. Biotin is reasonably stable in the presence of heat, oxygen and light [24].

Folic acid is involved in the synthesis of S-adenosylmethionine thematabolism of nucleic acids. It is also involved in the synthesis of amino acids as a coenzyme. Deficiency of folate causes folate-deficient erythropoesis and meaining. DNA synthesis is also impaired, and neutrophils hypersegmentation occurs. If there is a deficiency in pregnant women, the baby can have neural tube defects, such as spina bifida or anencephaly [70, 75]. Folic acid is heat-labile and sensitive to light, sunlight, and oxidizing and reducing agents. However, it is very stable in neutral solutions [7].

Vitamin B_{12} is a cofactor for the activity of two enzymes: methionine synthase, which is used for methyl transfer (cofactor, methylcobalamin), and methylmalonyl CoA mutase, which is used to convert L-methymalonyl-CoA to succinyl-CoA (cofactor, adenosylcobalamin). Vitamin B_{12} functions in the building of genetic material as well as maintaining the nervous system. Its deficiency leads to numerous severe impairments, such as reduced purine synthesis, reduced methyl donors, increased methylmalonic acid, and increased homocysteine (which is damaging to DNA in the central nervous system thereby causing degeneration of the nerves) [70, 76, 77]. Vitamin B_{12} is stable in the presence of heat and oxygen in neutral and acid mediums; however, it is unstable in strong acid and alkaline mediums, as well as strong light [7].

Thiamine hydrochloride, thiamine mononitrate, niacin, biotin, pyridoxine, pyridoxine hydrochloride, and vitamin B_{12} are included in the GRAS substance list. Some of these vitamins have been used in developed countries under mandatory fortification regulations to fortify margarines, wheat flour (e.g., thiamine and folic acid in Australia, folic acid in the USA and Canada since 1998), pasta, cereals and cereal products (e.g., thiamine in Austrialia), and bread and cereals in the USA [2, 71]. Folic acid fortification of flour has reduced the incidence of neural tube defects (NTD). Nonetheless, it was reported that a high daily consumption of folic acid could mask vitamin B12 deficiency and neurologic impairment could develop [78]. Table 8 provides information about the B vitamin RDA and commonly used food vehicles.[18, 77]

Table 8: B vitamins [Adapted from references 77 and 18].		Vitamin B1(mg/d)	Vitamin B2(mg/d)	Vitamin B3(mg/d)	Vitamin B5(mg/d)
RDA USA/ RDA Europe	**male**	1.2/1.1	1.3/1.4	16/16	*5/6
	female	1.1/1.1	1.1/1.4	14/16	*5/6
UL		ND	ND	35[b]	ND
Commonly used food vehicles (fortification levels (mg/kg)) [42]		wheat flour (1.5–7.0), pasta (8–10), maize flour (2.4)	margarine (16), wheat flour (1-5), pasta (3-5), maize flour (2.5)	margarine (180), wheat flour (15-55), pasta (35-57), maize flour (1.6)	
		Vitamin B6(mg/d)	Vitamin B7(µg/d)	Vitamin B9(µg/d)	Vitamin B12(µg/d)
RDA USA/ RDA Europe	**male**	1.1/1.4	*30/50	400/200	2.4/2.5
	female	1.1/1.4	*30/50	[a] 400/200	2.4/2.5
UL		100	ND	ND	ND
Commonly used food vehicles (fortification levels (mg/kg)) [7, 42]		margarine (20), wheat flour (2.5)		margarine (2), wheat flour (0.5-3.0)	wheat flour (1.3-4)

ND: Not determinable due to the lack of data on the adverse effects in this age group and concern with regard to lack of ability to handle excess amounts.

* Adequate Intakes (AIs).

[a] As dietary folate equivalents (DFE). 1 DFE = 1 µg food folate = 0.6 µg of folic acid from fortified food or as a supplement consumed with food = 0.5 µg of a supplement taken on an empty stomach.

[b] The UL for niacin applies to synthetic forms obtained from supplements, fortified foods, or a combination of the two.

VITAMIN A (RETINOL)

Vitamin A is one of the fat-soluble vitamins limited by its application, but it still makes a good candidate to fortify margarine, oils and dairy products. Vitamin A is used in acetate or palmitate forms; however, a mixture of phenolic antioxidants or tocopherols are used to stabilize vitamin A [24].

Vitamin A deficiency causes early childhood blindness called xerophthalmia, as well as night blindness, defects in bone growth, defects in reproduction and defects in the growth and differentiation of epithelial tissues [79].

Zambia is the first country to fortify sugar with vitamin A, but Latin America does it as well [2]. Margarines are the most common food vehicles fortified with vitamin A in developing countries, such as the Philippines, Malaysia, Indonesia, etc. Other foods successfully fortified with vitamin A include fats and oils, milk, cereals, tea, rice, salt, infant formulas, wheat flour and noodles [7, 8, 24, 79]. Table 9 provides information about vitamin A RDA and commonly used food vehicles.[18, 23]

Table 9: Vitamin A [18,23]		µg /d
*RDA USA (19-30y)	male	900
	female	700
	pregnancy/lactating	770/1300
RDA Europe		800
UL		3000
GRAS substances		Retinyl acetate and retinyl palmitate
Commonly used food vehicles (fortification levels (mg/kg)) [42]		Sugar (5-15), margarine (5-15), fats and oils (5-15), milk (0.7–1.0), cereals, tea, rice, salt, infant formulas, wheat flour (1-5) and noodles

*Under assumption of minimal sunlight

VITAMIN C (ASCORBIC ACID)

Vitamin C is an essential water soluble vitamin that takes part in several metabolic pathways, the synthesis of connective tissue protein, and the conversion of dopamine to the neurotransmitter noradrenaline. It also takes part in the biosynthesis of the amino acid carnitine, which has a fundamental role in fatty acid metabolism. In addition, it has antioxidant capacity against free radical damage, and helps heal wounds and repair bones and teeth. There is no storage or synthesis of vitamin C in the body, since humans lack the key enzyme, L-3 gulonolactone oxidase [80]. Vitamin C deficiency leads to scurvy, a disease causing general weakness, anemia, gum disease, and skin hemorrhages and in further stages, gingivorragia and loss of teeth. Scurvy generally occurs when access to fresh fruits and vegetables containing vitamin C is limited for 3-6 months [81].

As discussed in the iron section above, the addition of vitamin C enhances the absorption of non-heme iron in a diet. In Chile, the prevalence of iron deficiency has been reduced by the fortification of milk with both iron and vitamin C [7].

L-ascorbic acid and ascorbyl palmitate are used in the fortification of vitamin C and vitamin A, and improve the stability of vitamin C. Vitamin C is sensitive to the presence of oxygen, metals, humidity and/or high temperatures. Therefore, it is better to encapsulate to prevent interactions [7]. Table 10 provides information about vitamin C RDA and commonly used food vehicles.[18, 82]

Table 10: Vitamin C [18,82].		mg /d
RDA USA (19-30y)	male	90
	female	75
	pregnancy/lactating	85/120
RDA Europe		80
UL		2000
GRAS substances		L-ascorbic acid, ascorbyl palmitate
Commonly used food vehicles		breakfast cereals, soft drinks, oils, infant formulae

Fatty Acids Fortification

OMEGA-3

Omega-3 fatty acids are essential for normal brain structure and function. They cannot be produced by the human body, and therefore, have to be gained from foods [83]. In diets, there are three omega-3 fatty acids: eicosapentaenoic acid (EPA, 20 carbons and 5 double bonds), docosahexaenoic acid (DHA, 22 carbons and 6 double bonds) and α-linolenic acid (ALA, 18 carbons and 3 double bonds) [84]. Among these, ALA is found in dark green leafy vegetables, variousnuts and seeds, and seafoods [85]. Omega-3 reduces blood pressure, anti-allergic effects, triglycerides and subsequent cardiovascular diseases. It also improves the function of retina and testis [84, 86]. Omega-3 deficiency is associated with dyspraxia, dyslexia, autism and mood disorders [84].

EFSA, 2012 [87] has published a scientific opinion on recommended dietary intakes and tolerable upper intake levels for eicosapentaenoic acid (EPA), docosahexaenoic acid (DHA), and docosapentaenoic acid omega-3 polyunsaturated fatty acids. This publication stated that the dietary recommendations for EPA and DHA (based on cardiovascular risk considerations for European adults) were between 250 and 500 mg/day. The adequate intake recommended by the USDA for n-3 fatty acids is approximately 1.3 to 1.8 g/d for men and 1.0 to 1.2 g/d for women [13]. In addition, the dietary reference intake of α-linolenic acid is 1.6 g/d for adult males (>19y) and 1.1 g/d for adult females (>19) [83].

However, as to the tolerable upper intake levels, EFSA has stated that the consumption of omega-3 fatty acids at observed intake levels had no adverse effects in healthy children or adults. The panel also indicated that supplemental intakes of EPA and DHA combined at doses up to 5 g/day, and supplemental intakes of EPA alone up to 1.8 g/day, did not raise safety concerns for adults. Supplemental intakes of DHA alone, up to about 1 g/day, did not raise safety concerns for the general population. However, there is no available data for DPA when consumed alone. The Food and Drug Administration (FDA) has also specified that an intake of omega-3 fatty acids (EPA and DHA), which does not exceed 3 g/day, is safe against possible adverse effects of these fatty acids [88].

Short-term studies have shown that food matrices affect the bioavailability of omega-3 LCPUFA, while there are no reported significant effects after a long-term intake of foods fortified with these fatty acids. Lipid structures can also affect the bioavailability of omega-3 LCPUFA, but more studies are required to clarify the long-term effects [88].

Food vehicles recently fortified with omega-3 fatty acids are: juice, breakfast cereals, bread, margarine, yogurt drink, milk, and eggs in markets. Also, there are studies on the fortification of cheeses with omega-3 via fish oil [88] - a new approach to increase omega-3 fatty acids intake. However, there are some challenges due to the sensitivity of lipids in the presence of heat, light and oxygen [86, 89]. Oxidation of fatty acids can lead to the deterioration of foods and can alter some properties such as flavor, texture, shelf life and color. Furthermore, other by-products of lipid peroxidation may be formed which are harmful to human health [86]. The oxidative damage risk is reduced when oxidizable lipids are encapsulated and combined with numerous substances, such as polysaccharides and proteins as well as other oils [89].

SUMMARY

- ➤ The fortificant must be resistant to dietary inhibitors, have good bioavailability, and must retain desired quality of food (flavor, color, texture, and odor) and must still be safe to consume.
- ➤ WHO has defined three types of fortification strategies: mass fortification, targeted fortification, and market-driven fortification. Single and multiple fortifications also exist.
- ➤ Iron deficiency can result in mental and psychomotor retardation, impaired immune response, and tiredness (contributing to a low work capacity). Overconsumption of iron can cause cancer and cardiovascular risks.
- ➤ Iron fortificants are divided into four categories: water-soluble, poorly water soluble but soluble in dilute acid, water insoluble but poorly soluble in dilute acid, and experimental compounds.
- ➤ Vitamin B12 functions in the building of genetic material as well as maintaining the nervous system. It's stable in the presence of heat and oxygen in neutral and acid mediums, but unstable in strong acid, alkaline mediums, and strong light.
- ➤ Omega-3 fatty acids are essential for normal brain structure and function. They can't be produced by the human body, so they have to be gained from foods.
- ➤ Most studies have shown that fortification programs successfully overcome micronutrient malnutrition, and this strategy has been applied in both developed and developing countries with the fortification of wheat flour, breakfast cereals, beverages, milk, etc.

REVIEW QUESTIONS

1. A deficiency in all of the following nutrients would be detrimental, except for:
    a. Iron
    b. Riboflavin
    c. Vitamin A
    d. Zinc
2. These two minerals decrease absorption of fluoride by forming insoluble complexes.
    a. Iron and chloride
    b. Magnesium and zinc
    c. Calcium and magnesium
    d. Iodine and iron

3. All of the following are Omega-3 fatty acids, except for:
    a. Docosahexaenoic acid (DHA)
    b. Eicosapentaenoic acid (EPA)
    c. Linoleic acid (LA)
    d. α-linolenic acid (ALA)

4. Vitamins can be categorized as fat-soluble and water-soluble. Which of the following vitamins is fat-soluble?
    a. Vitamin B1 (thiamine)
    b. Vitamin D
    c. Vitamin C (ascorbic acid)
    d. Vitamin B9 (folic acid)

5. Long periods of insufficient Vitamin C intake can lead to a disease called
    a. Rickets
    b. Keshan disease
    c. Xerophthalmia
    d. Scurvy

6. Which of the following is not a required consideration for selecting food vehicle for fortification?
    a. Shelf-stable
    b. Low cost
    c. Widely consumed
    d. Highly nutritious

7. Fortification of a food that is consumed regularly by the general population is called
    a. Targeted fortification
    b. Mass fortification
    c. Market-driven fortification
    d. Single fortification

8. The presence of Vitamin D increases body's absorption of
    a. Selenium
    b. Iron
    c. Calcium
    d. Zinc

9. The average daily dietary intake level sufficient to meet the nutrient requirement of nearly all healthy individuals in a particular life stage and gender group is known as the
    a. Recommended Dietary Allowance
    b. Adequate Intake
    c. Tolerable Upper Level Intake
    d. Daily Value

10. All of the following are common food vehicles for Calcium fortification, except for?
    a. Juice
    b. Milk
    c. Wheat flour
    d. Salt

Answers: 1. **(B)** 2. **(C)** 3. **(C)** 4. **(B)** 5. **(D)** 6. **(D)** 7. **(B)** 8. **(C)** 9. **(A)** 10. **(D)**

REFERENCES:

1. Hess SY, Brown KH.: Impact of zinc fortification on zinc nutrition. Food Nutr Bull, 2009, 30:79-107

2. Darnton-Hill I, Nalubola R.: Fortification strategies to meet micronutrient needs: sucesses and failures. Proceedings of the Nutrition Society, 2002, 61:231-241.

3. Brown KH, Wessells KR., Hess, SY.: Zinc bioavailability from zinc-fortified foods. Int J Vitam Nutr Res, 2007, 77(3):174-81.

4. Salgueiro, MJ., Zubillaga MB, Lysionek AE, Caro RA, Weill R, Boccio JR.: Fortification strategies to combat zinc and iron deficiency. Nutrition Reviews, 2002, 60, 52-58.

5. Drago SR, Valencia ME.: Effect of fermentation on iron, zinc, and calcium availability from iron-fortified dairy products. J Food Sci, 2002, 67(8),3130-3134.

6. Gómez-Galera S, Rojas E, Sudhakar D, Zhu C, Pelacho AM, Capell T, Christou P.: Critical evaluation of strategies for mineral fortification of staple food crops. Transgenic Research, 2010, 19:165-180.

7. World Health Organization (WHO).: Guidelines on food fortification with micronutrients, Part III. Fortificants: physical characteristics, selection and use with specific food vehicles, 2006, p:97-122, Geneva, Switzerland.

8. Lotfi M, Mannar MGV, Merx RJHM, Naber-van den Heuve P.: Micronutrient Fortification of Foods: Current Practices, Research, and Opportunities. Ottawa. The Micronutrient Initiative (MI), do International Development, Research Centre (IDRC)/International Agriculture Centre (IAC), 1996.

9. Gibson RS, Bailey KB, Gibbs M, Ferguson EL.: A review of phytate, iron, zinc, and calcium concentrations in plant-based complementary foods used in low-income countries and implications for bioavailability. Food Nutr Bull, 2010, 31:134-146.

10. Gerstner G.: How to Fortify Beverages with Calcium. Food Marketing & Technology, 2003, 16-19

11. Trumbo P, Yates AA, Schlicker S, Poos M.: Dietary Referance Intakes: Vitamin A, Vitamin K, Arsenic, Boron, Chromium, Copper, Iodine, Iron, Manganese, Molybdenum, Nickel, Silicon, Vanadium and Zinc. Journal of the American Dietetic Association, 2001, 101(3), 294-301.

12. Whitney E, Rolfes SR.: Understanding Nutrition. Chapter 13: The Trace Minerals. 2009, Twelth Edition. Wadsworth, Belmonth, CA.

13. USDA, National Fluoride Database of Selected Beverages and Foods, Release 2, 2005.

14. Marthaler TM, Petersen PE.: Salt fluoridation – an alternative in automatic prevention of dental caries. International Dental Journal, 2005, 55, 351-358.

15. Kauffman JM.: Water Fluoridation: a Review of Recent Research and Actions. Journal of American Physicians and Surgeons, 2005, 10(2):38-44.

16. Cerklewski FL.: Fluoride bioavailability -nutritional and clinical aspects. Nutrition Research, 1997, 17(5):907-929.

17. Food and Nutrition Board, Institute of Medicine Dietary Reference Intakes for Calcium, Phosphorous, Magnesium, Vitamin D, and Fluoride, 1997, The National Academies, Washington, DC.

18. Commission Directive 2008/100/EC of 28 October 2008 amending Council Directive 90/496/EEC on nutrition labelling for foodstuffs as regards recommended daily allowances, energy conversion factors and definitions.

19. Kapil U.: Health Consequences of Iodine Deficiency. Sultan Qaboos University Medical Journal, 2007, 7(3), p. 267-272.

20. Reid JR, Wheeler SF.: Hyperthyroidism: Diagnosis and Treatment. Am. Fam. Physician, 2005, 72:623-30.

21. FAO/WHO Consideration of iodisation of salt. CX/NFSDU 91/13. 1991, FAO, Rome.

22. Pongpaew P, Saowakontha S, Tungtrongchitr R, Mahaweerawat U, Schelp FP.: Iodine deficiency disorder—an old problem tackled again: a review of a comprehensive operational study in the northeast of Thailand. Nutrition Research 2002, 22(1):137-144.

23. Food and Nutrition Board, Institute of Medicine Dietary reference intakes: vitamin A, vitamin K, arsenic, boron, chromium, copper, iodine, iron, manganese, molybdenum, nickel, silicon, vanadium, and zinc, 2001, The National Academies, Washington, DC.

24. FAO Food Fortification: Technology and Quality Control. FAO Food and Nutrition Paper – 60, 1996, Rome, Italy.

25. Gaucheron F.: Iron fortification in dairy industry. Trends in Food Science & Technology, 2000, 11,403-409.

26. Hunt CD., Nielsen FH.: Advanced Dairy Chemistry Volume 3, 3rd ed. Chapter 10: Nutritional Aspects of Minerals in Bovine and Human Milk. PLH McSweeney and PF Fox (Ed), Springer, New York, 2009, p:420.

27. Martínez-Navarrete N, Camacho MM, Martínez-Lahuerta J, Martínez-Monzó J, Fito P.: Iron deficiency and iron fortified foods. Food Research Interantional, 2002, 35, 225-231.

28. Salgueiro MJ, Arnoldi S, Kaliski MA, Torti H, Messeri E, Weill R, Zubillaga M, Boccio J.: Stabilized–Solubilized Ferric Pyrophosphate as a New Iron Source for Food Fortication. Bioavailability Studies by Means of the Prophylactic–Preventive Method in Rats. Biol Trace Elem Res, 2009, 127,143–147.

29. Lysionek AE, Zubillaga MB, Salgueiro MJ, Pineiro A, Caro RA, Weill R, Boccio JR.: Bioavailability of microencapsulated ferrous sulfate in powdered milk product from fortified fluid milk: A prophylactic study in rats. Nutrition, 2002, 18, 279-281.

30. Hurrell RF.: Preventing iron deficiency through food fortification. Nutrition Reviews, 1997, 55:(6)210–222.

31. Juneja LR.: Improved Solubility, Safety and Bioavailability of Superdispersed Ferric Pyrophosphate-a New Concept of Iron Fortification. IFT Annual Meeting, 2001, New Orleans, LA, USA.

32. Hurrell RF, Cook JD.: Strategies for iron fortification of foods. Trends in Food Science & Technology, 1990, 56-61.

33. Hurrell R, Egli I.: Iron bioavailability and dietary reference values. Am J Clin Nutr, 2010, 91, 1461S–7S.

34. Hurrell RF, Sean L, Thomas B, Héctor C, Ray G, Eva H, Zdenek K et al.: Enhancing the absorption of fortification iron. Int J Vitam Nutr Res, 2004, 74(6):387-401.

35. Zhang D, Mahoney AW.: Effect of iron fortification on quality of cheddar cheese. J. Dairy Sci. 1989, 72:322-332.

36. Zhang D, Mahoney AW.: Effect of iron fortification on quality of Cheddar cheese. 2. Effects of aging and fluorescent light on pilot scale cheeses. J. Dairy Sci. 1990, 73:2252–2258.

37. Zhang D, Mahoney AW.: Iron fortification of process Cheddar cheese. J. Dairy Sci. 1991, 74:353–358.

38. Gamal El-Din AM, Hassan ASH, El-Behairy SA, Mohamed EA.: Impact of Zinc and Iron Salts Fortification of Buffalo's Milk on the Dairy Product. World Journal of Dairy & Food Sciences, 2012, 7(1), 21-27.

39. Rice WH, McMahon DJ.: Chemical, Physical, and Sensory Characteristics of Mozzarella Cheese Fortified Using Protein-Chelated Iron Or Ferric Chloride. in J. Dairy Sci., 1998, 81, 318–326.

40. Sadler AM, Lacroix DE, Alford JA.: Iron Content of Baker's and Cottage Cheese Made from Fortified Skim Milks. J. Dairy Sci., 1973, 56(10), 1267–1270.

41. Janjetic M, Barrado A, Torti H, Weill R, Orlandini, J, Urriza R, Boccio J.: Iron bioavailability from fortified petit suisse cheese determined by the prophylactic-preventive method. Biol Trace Elem Res., 2006, 109(2), 195-200.

42. Flores-Ayala RC.: Food fortification. Encyclopedia of Human Nutrition, 2013, Volume 2, p:296-305.

43. Shrimpton R, Shankar AH.: Nutrition and Health in Developing Countries 2nd ed. Chapter 15: Zinc Deficiency R. D. Semba and M. W. Bloem (Ed.), 2008, Humana Press, Totowa, NJ.

44. Saper RB, Rash R.: Zinc: An Essential Micronutrient. American Family Physician, 2009, 79,768-772.

45. Qin Y, Melse-Boonstra A, Shi Z, Pan X, Yuan B, Dai Y, Zhao J, Zimmermann M.B.: Dietary intake of zinc in the population of Jiangsu Province, China. Asia Pac J Clin Nutr, 2009, 18,193-199.

46. Maret W, Sandstead HH.: Zinc requirements and the risks and benefits of zinc supplementation. J. Trace Elem. Med. Biol. 2006, 20, 3-18.

47. Jeejeebhoy K: Zinc: An essential trace element for parenteral nutrition. Gastroenterology, 2009, 137, S7-S12.

48. World Health Organization (WHO). Environmental Health Criteria 221: 1 Zinc, Geneva: 2001, World Health Organization.

49. Harzer G, Kauer H.: Binding of zinc to casein. Am J Clin Nutr, 1982, 35, 981-987.

50. Scientific Committee on Food - SCF/CS/NUT/UPPLEV/62 Final (5th March 2003) Opinion of the Scientific Committee on Food on the Tolerable Upper Intake Level of Zinc.

51. Salgueiro MJ, Zubillaga M, Lysionek A, Sarabia M, De Paoli RCT., Hager A, Weill R, Boccio J.: Zinc as an essential micronutrient: a review, 2000, Nutr Res, 20, 737–755.

52. Otten JJ, Hellwig JP, Meyers LD.: DRI, dietary reference intakes: the essential guide to nutrient requirements Part III Vitamins and Minerals. The National Academies Press, Washington, DC, 2006.

53. Brown KH, Hambidge KM, Ranum P.: Zinc fortification of cereal flours: Current recommendations and research needs. Food & Nutrition Bulletin, 2010, 31(1):62S-74S.

54. Kahraman O, Z Ustunol. Effect of zinc fortification on Cheddar cheese quality. Journal of dairy science, 2012, 95(6):2840-2847.

55. Gulbas SY, Saldamli I.: The effect of selenium and zinc fortification on the quality of Turkish white cheese. International Journal of Food and Nutrition, 2005, 56, 141-146.

56. Aquilanti L, Kahraman O, Zannini E, Osimani A, Silvestri G, Ciarrocchi F, Garofalo C, Tekin E, Clementi F.: Response of lactic acid bacteria to milk fortification with dietary zinc salts. International Dairy Journal, 2012, 25, 52-59.

57. Mora-Gutierrez A, Farrell JHM, Attaie R, McWhinney VJ, Wang C.: Effects of bovine and caprine Monterey Jack cheeses fortified with milk calcium on bone mineralization in rats. International dairy journal 2007, 17(3):255-267.

58. Food and Nutrition Board, Institute of Medicine Dietary Reference Intakes for Calcium and Vitamin D, 2011. The National Academies, Washington, DC.

59. Rayman MP.: The importance of selenium to human health. Lancet. 2000, 15; 356(9225):233-41.

60. Roy G, Sarma BK, Phadnis PP, Mugesh G.: Selenium-containing enzymes in mammals: Chemical perspectives J. Chem. Sci., 2005, 117(4), pp. 287–30.

61. Zimmermann MB, Köhrle J.: The impact of iron and selenium deficiencies on iodine and thyroid metabolism: biochemistry and relevance to public health. 2002, Thyroid. 12(10):867-78.

62. FAO/WHO Human Vitamin and Mineral Requirements. 2002, Chapter: 15 Selenium.

63. Smith AM, Chen LW, Thomas RM.: Selenate fortification improves selenium status of term infants fed soy formula. Am J Clin Nutr, 1995 61:44-7.

64. Food and Nutrition Board, Institute of Medicine Dietary Reference Intakes for Vitamin C, Vitamin E, Selenium, and Carotenoids, 2000, The National Academies, Washington, DC.

65. Whiting SJ, Calvo MS.: Nutrition and Lifestyle Effects on Vitamin D Status. In Feldman D, Pike JW, Adams JS. (Ed.), Vitamin D (979-1007). 2011, Academic Press.

66. Calvo MS, Whiting SJ, Barton CN.: Vitamin D fortification in the United States and Canada: current status and data needs. Am. J. Clin. Nutr., 2004, 80, 1710-1716.

67. Andersen R, Mølgaard C, Skovgaard LT, Brot C, Cashman KD, Chabros E, Charzewska J, Flynn A, Jakobsen J, Karkkainen M, Kiely M, Lamberg-Allardt C, Moreiras O, Natri A M, O'Brien M, Rogalska-Niedzwiedz M, L Ovesen.: Teenage girls and elderly women living in northern Europe have low winter vitamin D status. European Journal of Clinical Nutrition. 2005, 59, 533–541.

68. Andersen R, Mølgaard C, Skovgaard LT, Brot C, Cashman KD, Jakobsen J, Lamberg-Allardt C, Ovesen L.: Pakistani immigrant children and adults in Denmark have severely low vitamin D status. European Journal of Clinical Nutrition. 2005, 59, 533–541.

69. Food and Nutrition Board, Institute of Medicine Dietary Reference Intakes for Calcium, Phosphorous, Magnesium, Vitamin D, and Fluoride, 1997, The National Academies, Washington, DC.

70. Bellows L, Moore R.: Water-Soluble Vitamins: B-Complex and Vitamin C. Food and Nutrition Series,Health, 2012, Fact Sheet No. 9.312.

71. Martin PR, Singleton CK, Hiller-Sturmhofel S.: The role of thiamine deficiency in alcoholic brain disease. Alcohol Research and Health, 2003, 27(2), 134-142.

72. Jacobs P, Wood L.: Vitamin B5. Disease-a-Month, 49(11), 2003, Pages 664-665.

73. Bender DA.: Vitamin B6: Physiology. Encyclopedia of Human Nutrition (Third Edition), 2013, Pages 340–350.

74. Mock DM.: BIOTIN: Physiology, Dietary Sources, and Requirements. Encyclopedia of Human Nutrition (Third Edition), 2013, Pages 182-190.

75. Neuhouser ML, Beresford SA.: Folic acid: are current fortification levels adequate?, Nutrition, 2001, 17(10):868-872.

76. Walter JH.: Vitamin B12 deficiency and phenylketonuria. Molecular Genetics and Metabolism. 104, 2011, S52–S54.

77. Food and Nutrition Board, Institute of Medicine Dietary Reference Intakes for Thiamin, Riboflavin, Niacin, Vitamin B6, Folate, Vitamin B12, Pantothenic Acid, Biotin, and Choline, 1998, The National Academies, Washington, DC.

78. Agnoletti D, Zhang Y, Czernichow S, Galan P, Hercberg S, Safar M E. Blacher J.: Chapter 40 – Fortification of Vitamin B12 to Flour and the Metabolic Response. Flour and Breads and their Fortification in Health and Disease Prevention, 2011, P:437–449.

79. Klemm, RDW, West Jr, Keith P, Palmer AC, Johnson Q, Randall P, Ranum P, Northrop-Clewes C.: Vitamin A fortification of wheat flour: considerations and current recommendations. Food & Nutrition Bulletin, 2010, 31(1):47S-61S.

80. Thomson B, On S, Mitchell J.: ESR Report on Fortification overages of the food supply, Vitamin C, zinc and selenium, NZFSA, 2007.

81. Fain O.: Vitamin C deficiency, La Revue de medecine interne/fondee... par la Societe nationale francaise de medecine interne, 25 (12), 2004, 872–880.

82. Food and Nutrition Board, Institute of Medicine Dietary Reference Intakes for Vitamin C, Vitamin E, Selenium, and Carotenoids, 2000, The National Academies, Washington, DC.

83. Franzen-Castle LD, Ritter-Gooder P.: Omega-3 and Omega-6 fatty acis. Foods and Nutritions, 2010.

84. Bermúdez-Aguirre D, Barbosa-Cánovas GV.: Fortification of queso fresco, cheddar and mozzarella cheese using selected sources of omega-3 and some nonthermal approaches. Food Chemistry, 2012, 133, 787–797.

85. Richardson AJ.: The importance of omega-3 fatty acids for behaviour, cognition and mood. Food & Nutrition Research, 2003, 47(2), 92-98.

86. Kolanowski W, Weißbrodt J.: Sensory quality of dairy products fortified with fish oil. International Dairy Journal, 2007, 17, 1248–1253.

87. EFSA (European Food Safety Authority) Scientific Opinion on the Tolerable Upper Intake Level of eicosapentaenoic acid (EPA), docosahexaenoic acid (DHA) and docosapentaenic acid (DPA). 2012, EFSA Journal, 10(7):2815.

88. Mu H.: Bioavailability of omega-3 long-chain polyunsaturated fatty acids from foods. AgroFOOD industry hi-tech., 2008, 19(4), 24-26.

89. Ye A, Cui J, Taneja A, Zhu X, Singh H.: Evaluation of processed cheese fortified with fish oil emulsion. Food Research International, 2009, 42,1093–1098.

8

Functional Food Ingredients Market

Swamy Gabriela John[1], and Melvin Holmes[2]

[1]Department of Food Technology, Kongu Engineering College, India; [2]Department of Food Science and Nutrition, University of Leeds, United Kingdom

Introduction

The nutraceuticals industry has created a new identity for functional ingredients linking to their health benefits. Thus, moving from the phase of generic categories (such as antioxidants, vitamins, minerals, and so on), functional ingredients are now being identified as "heart health," "bone and joint health," and "eye health" ingredients. This metamorphosis is designed with a consumer-centric approach, which aids effective marketing while improving consumer awareness. The end-products presented to the consumers are available as both dietary supplements and functional foods. The delivery formats of dietary supplements include tablets, capsules, chewable tablets, and soft gels. At present, functional food ingredients are available as supplements, fortified beverages, premix powders, dairy products, baked foods, and convenience foods. This category is poised for robust growth in the forthcoming years, primarily due to the high degree of scope to penetrate different application sectors.

Classification of Functional Food Ingredients

Functional food ingredients are classified into different categories, as shown in **Figure 1** below:

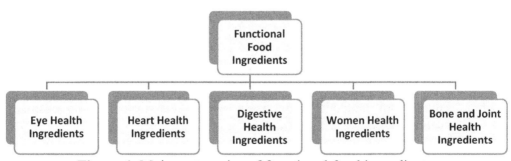

Figure 1. Major categories of functional food ingredients.

Functional food ingredients are discussed in detail below.

Eye Health Ingredients

The visual processing system requires many complex functions to work before achieving visual perception. Eyes form a key component of the visual system and have evolved to dynamically project received light onto a light-sensitive medium (the retina), which is then propagated to the brain via the optic nerve. The structure of the eye is essentially an organic camera with a compound lens controlled by the cornea and lens, projecting an inverted image onto the retina consisting of a large number of photoreceptor cells [1]. This finely tuned process requires a highly synchronized route to adequately transfer optical information to the brain. However, the retinal photoreceptors are compounds rich in polyunsaturated fatty acids, which make them particularly susceptible to oxidation by free radicals resulting in damage to the eye [2]. These radicals are supplied through the abundant blood and oxygen supply and photoelectric exposure within the eye. Such an environment makes the retina subject to oxidative stress, which may be further aggravated if an unbalanced diet is maintained, thereby offering insufficient micronutrients. **Figure 2** illustrates the important components that make of the human eye. Increasing evidence now exists establishing the connection between dietary intake and health. The promotion of functional foods to specifically target health concerns is a major area of research.

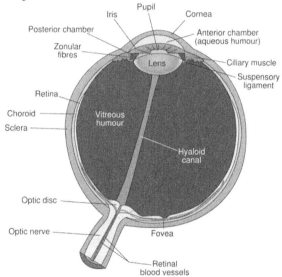

Figure 2. Anatomy of a human eye

A focus on eye health is one such area of concern within the food industry. Traditionally, the market for eye health ingredients has been an issue for healthcare companies, focusing on vitamins and tablets to maintain and improve vision. However, the rise of the dietary supplement and functional food sector has prompted this market to divert towards preventative medicine. For instance, 'xerophthalmia,' a common cause of childhood blindness, is caused by a dietary deficiency of vitamin A [3]. A major area receiving attention has been vitamins and **active pharmaceutical ingredients (APIs)**. Ingredients rich in preventative compounds have been researched in relation to their positive effects against age-related eye conditions, such as **age-related macular-degeneration (AMD)** and cataracts, since these diseases are normally a result of time, environment, tobacco abuse, and inadequate diet.

The market for eye health ingredients addressing various eye diseases is in a stage of growth, spurred by modern lifestyles and unwholesome diets. With the rise in interest from the supplement and natural extract sectors, a new genre of specific eye health ingredients has emerged with proven benefits on eye health. These ingredients include:

- Lutein
- Zeaxanthin
- Astaxanthin
- Beta-carotene
- Bilberry extracts

Lutein

Lutein is a member of the xanthophylls group of carotenoids, commonly found in spinach, kale and other green leafy vegetables, marigold flowers and algae [4, 5]. A small portion of the lutein market has traditionally been used as a colorant in the food industry and is given the E-number E161b [6].

Lutein is present in the macula (central optical) region of the retina, and along with zeaxanthin, it plays a significant role in eye health [7]. The macula is a small area of the retina responsible for central vision. Lutein also acts as an antioxidant to protect the cornea (transparent front portion of the eye covering the pupil) from oxidative stress and high-energy light. Lutein can absorb blue light, and hence appears yellow at low concentrations and orange-red at high concentrations [8]. Traditionally, lutein was used in the meat industry to add colour to chicken feed. This fortification then led to the colouring of the egg yolk for feed fortification. New research has identified the benefits of lutein on eye health with over 300 peer-reviewed studies documenting beneficial effects [9, 10].

Several of these studies found that eating a diet rich in lutein reduces the risk of age-related macular degeneration (AMD) and cataracts and some evidence has shown that lutein can actually reverse prior damage [11]. Lutein ester is converted in the body to free lutein before it can be used.

Kemin Food ingredients patented its extraction method, which resulted in the free or purified form of lutein [12]. Other methods involve the use of solvents or CO_2 for the extraction of lutein esters. Lutein is available as a water-soluble powder, oil and in beadlet form.

Zeaxanthin

Zeaxanthin is recognized as one of the two macular pigments responsible for the yellow color of the macula lutea in the eye. This pigment is found in corn, marigolds and saffron. Zeaxanthin, in combination with lutein, is said to play a role in the protection of the retina against light-induced damage. Chemically, zeaxanthin differs from lutein in the location of its double bond allowing for two chiral centers, while lutein possesses three. In addition, the stereoisomer meso-zeaxanthin is produced in the macula by lutein in the absence of normal zeaxanthin. Zeaxanthin and lutein are distributed within the macula at different locations pertaining to their function within the eye. Lutein is in the periphery while zeaxanthin is placed in the centre in the fovea. Zeaxanthin is concerned with central vision, contrast sensitivity and glare reduction. Lutein helps with night, low light and peripheral vision. Dietary supplementation of zeaxanthin works to maintain pigment levels in the eye and filter out damaging blue light.

The market for zeaxanthin benefits from the wide array of clinical studies documenting the positive effects of a diet supplemented with zeaxanthin at a recommended daily intake of 2-4 milligrams (mg) [13]. However, studies have determined that the European dietary intake of zeaxanthin is less than 0.5mg a day [14].

Astaxanthin

Within carotenoids, astaxanthin falls under the sub-class of xanthophylls known to impart orange color to yellow pigments in a variety of fruits and vegetables. Astaxanthin produces a dark red pigment and is found primarily in marine life forms such as algae, aquatic animals and birds. Well-known astaxanthin-containing species include micro algae, salmon, trout, red sea bream, shrimp and lobster, as well as birds, such as flamingo and quail. However, only phytoplankton, algae, plants and certain bacteria and fungi synthesize astaxanthin [15]. Animals, including humans, must consume carotenoids as part of their diet and rely on this external supply. Marine animals such as salmon consume krill and other organisms that ingest astaxanthin-containing algae and plankton as a major part of their diets. This nutrient therefore moves up the food chain, providing essential nutrition.

Astaxanthin is a potent antioxidant. It is 10 times more potent than beta-carotene and 550 times more powerful than vitamin E [16]. Moreover, these carotenoids possess the unique ability of crossing the blood-retinal barrier in the eyes. Research has revealed that diseases and injuries of the eye such as glaucoma, diabetic retinopathy and age-related macular degeneration (AMD) are primarily caused by the amplified presence of singlet oxygen, as well as other free radicals [17]. These free radicals include compounds such as super oxide, hydroxyl, and hydrogen peroxide. Astaxanthin works in the eye as a potent free-radical scavenger. In addition, the nutrient also aids in the prevention of damage due to ultraviolet (UV) light. Since 2001, astaxanthin has been increasingly used in the food supplement sector with the entry of natural astaxanthin products.

Like beta-carotene, there are two types of astaxanthin; synthetic and natural source variety. The majority of the synthetic variety is used in aquaculture feed. Currently, synthetic astaxanthin is not approved in Europe for human use [18]. The natural variety accounts for up to 2.0% of the market share. The natural version is used in dietary supplements due to its clean label nature and provenance. Natural sources may be extracted from either *Haematococcus pluvialis* or the yeast, *Phaffia rhodozymam*, which accumulates natural astaxanthin as a result of unfavorable conditions. The natural molecule is said to work better than the synthetic molecule due to its conformation. Natural astaxanthin is found paired with a fatty acid resulting in **esterification**. According to a study conducted by the Kyoto University of Medicine, esterification is the primary reason for astaxanthin's ability to pass through the blood retinal barrier, which is not possible for other carotenoids [19].

Astaxanthin is available as a dry powder, a cold-water-soluble powder, or in tablet form. The synthetic variety is only available as a powder and is only offered in 8.0 and 10.0 percent concentrations. The natural source is available as a powder, beadlet or softgel in lower concentrations.

Beta-carotene

Beta-carotene is an active pharmaceutical ingredient and a well-known carotenoid. The ingredient is found in carrots and green leafy vegetables such as spinach, kale and cabbage (**Figure 3**). Beta-carotene is a key eye health ingredient commonly found in multivitamin tablets. This carotenoid is included in the tablets because of its provitamin A activity. The ingredient acts as a precursor of vitamin A, converted to the vitamin by the body. While other carotenoids also perform this function, they can only create one molecule of vitamin A. Beta-carotene, conversely, generates two molecules of vitamin A, which are then broken down into retinol. Additionally, beta-carotene acts as an antioxidant, thereby promoting free radical scavenging, which is the key cause of age-related macular degeneration (AMD).

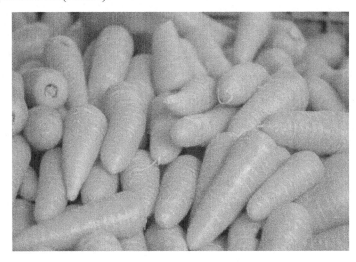

Figure 3. Beta-carotene is a red-orange pigment found in carrots and other vegetables.

Vitamin A, a micronutrient essential to most mammals, is an element of a group of lipid soluble compounds metabolically related to trans-retinol. In diet, vitamin A is found in products of animal origin as retinyl esters, mainly retinyl palmitate. Other esters (oleate, stearate and myristate) and retinol contribute to dietary vitamin A intake. The forms most commonly found in vitamin supplements or enriched food are retinyl acetate, retinyl palmitate and retinol. These vitamin A compounds (together with their metabolites and synthetic derivatives that exhibit the same properties) are called **retinoids**. Vitamin A deficiency is one of the gravest nutritional deficiency problems worldwide. The World Health Organization (WHO) estimated that vitamin A deficiency alone causes blindness in up to 500,000 children each year [20].

Traditionally, beta-carotene has been used as a pigment in food color. However, with rising scientific backing, this ingredient has found increased usage in the dietary supplement sector. There are two kinds of beta-carotene: synthetic, usually referred to as nature identical, and the naturally extracted variety. While synthetic beta-carotene is chemically synthesized, natural beta-carotene can be extracted from carrots, yams and other yellow or orange plant material. It can also be extracted from the alga *Dunaliella salina* or from the fungi *Blakeslea trispora*, which are grown using fermentation technology [21, 22]. Natural beta-carotene is primarily used in eye health supplements.

Bilberry extracts

Bilberry belongs to the family of red fruits known for being rich in natural pigments termed **anthocyanins**, bioactive components that impart pink, red and blue colors to plants and flowers. Bilberry (*Vaccinium myrtillus*) is a short deciduous shrub native to northern Europe, illustrated in **Figure 4**. Bilberry extracts contain a high amount of natural antioxidants, such as flavonoids and phenolic acids. It is known for its eye health potential due to its anthocyanin pigments, which aid in protecting the light-sensitive photoreceptor rod cells present in the retina, called rhodopsin. Balanced rhodopsin levels are imperative to facilitate adequate vision in dim light conditions.

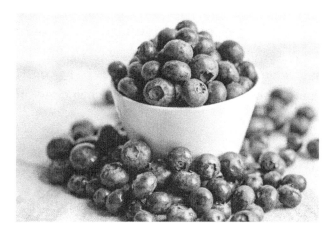

Figure 4. Bilberry is a native European species closely related to blueberries.

Medical practitioners in Europe have used bilberry for over 900 years to treat a variety of disorders, ranging from diarrhea to scurvy (vitamin C deficiency). The leaves and fruits of these shrubs possess powerful astringents and anti-inflammatory qualities. Such positive validation has resulted in manufacturers such as Chr. Hansen supplying bilberry extracts as functional ingredients to enhance the eye health benefits of various foods and beverages [23]. This newly discovered product utility has opened up additional opportunities for the bilberry extracts market, making it one of the most popular emerging eye health extracts today.

Bilberry extracts used for eye health supplements are mostly produced in powder form, whereas extracts used for beverages and dairy products are mainly produced in liquid form. While extracts contain the highest concentration of anthocyanins, bilberries can be consumed with liquids, or eaten fresh or dried.

Industry Challenges

Variant regulation hampers growth

The European Union and US FDA regulations and directives regarding health claims lack clarity and vary from member state to member state. The European Food supplements directive introduced a framework that aims to establish a system of available nutrients for supplements approved by the European Food Safety Authority (EFSA). Eye health ingredients such as lutein and astaxanthin are not covered in the positive list of this directive. This is a major problem for smaller companies populating a large portion of this market. These smaller companies focus primarily on innovation in ingredients and nutritional complexes similar to that in conventional foods. However, a large proportion of these ingredients are absent from the directive and pending approval. Such ambiguity in legislation is particularly apparent where various committees have different interpretations of the positive list. However, the Alliance for Natural Health (ANH) claimed that this opinion had been refuted by the Legal Affairs department within the European Commission [24]. Moreover, there is an immense amount of contrasting information on the methodology involved in legally enforcing maximum and minimum limits of these ingredients in foods. Such situations have a negative effect, lack of credibility and diminish consumer confidence. In addition, there is no agreed measurement for the use of antioxidants, such as bilberry and lutein, and legislation for these products is vague. The lack of standards has led to misleading nutritional information on product packaging and loss of reliability. Consumer confidence cannot be acquired unless manufacturers are in a position to guarantee safety and efficacy of their products and are able to provide scientific support. End users may be less inclined to use bilberry or vitamin A supplements unless manufacturers can provide assurances of its consistent purity and activity. This situation has resulted in much uncertainty, especially since target ingredients are in various modes of commercialization.

Low consumer awareness

In the dietary supplements market, especially those catering to specific health benefits such as eye health, for commercial success, it is imperative that there is significant consumer awareness. Lutein is an exception to this rule due to the efforts of Kemin Foods. Kemin launched an awareness campaign on Age-Related Macular Degeneration (AMD), the leading cause of blindness in the industrialized world [25]. This omnibus campaign significantly raised lutein awareness and has become the benchmark for eye health ingredient manufacturers. However, the situation for other functional ingredients is less than positive. Consumer awareness for products such as bilberry and zeaxanthin are still at very low levels, as consumers are confused about how these active ingredients actually work and their efficacy. This results in such products gaining popularity only for a short term. The level of awareness on eye health ingredients and their potential as functional foods and supplements is extremely low.

Asian competition restricting profit margins

The North American and European market for eye health ingredients is facing fluctuating prices and constant price erosion due to competition from Asian manufacturers. Asian competitors provide low-priced raw material sources and lower exchange rates. Therefore, manufacturers are unable to compete with them in terms of pricing. This has caused considerable price erosion, especially in the cases of bilberry extracts. In the case of vitamin A, such price erosion has greatly reduced profit margins for European manufacturers. Moreover, Asian companies have effective marketing strategies of catering to particular segments of the society, especially that of children and senior citizens.

Substitution obstructing market advancement

The eye health ingredient market is constantly being inundated with new chemical compounds claiming eye health benefits. Other eye health ingredients competing for a portion of this market are quercetin, green tea extracts and omega-3 fatty acids. Moreover, with the trend of globalization, there is a constant stream of new fruit extracts claiming such beneficial effects. It is a major challenge for established premium ingredients such as lutein to maintain their market position and prevent substitution from lesser known ingredients. Manufacturers are concerned that the constant ebb and flow of such ingredients will cause the rise of fads rather than established markets for eye health ingredients, thus retarding revenue growth. This has directly affected the demand for more established eye health ingredients, especially supplements.

Drivers in the Eye Health Ingredients Market

Rising prevalence of eye-related disease promoting demand for eye health ingredients

The global population is faced by a growing incidence of age- and lifestyle-related degenerative eye diseases. Of these, blindness or visual impairment will occur in over 20% of the population in the form of cataracts and AMD, at some point in their life [26]. As mentioned previously, the primary eye diseases are cataracts, glaucoma and AMD. Of these three, AMD can most effectively be improved when correct nutrition is supplied. It is a chronic progressive eye disorder causing partial or complete blindness. Prevalence has increased due to a variety of factors including age, smoking, UV exposure and occupational hazards. As consumers' awareness increases and healthy lifestyles are adapted, prevention of the onset of such diseases through the right nutrition has increased and led to a rising popularity for ingredients such as lutein and zeaxanthin to reduce the risk of AMD and cataracts.

Expanding aging population promotes interest in preventative health care

The global population is aging with better lifestyles accounting for longer life expectancies. Globally, the number of people above 60 years is growing at a faster rate than any other age group. Such an increase in the age of the population greatly drives the demand for eye health ingredients to combat diseases that mostly affect and are a major concern for the elderly. The incidence of eye diseases has been found to compound in humans at a mean age of 43.9 years [27]. Indeed, the risk for the most common sight-threatening eye diseases is set to increase as people live longer. In the Netherlands, for instance, AMD lists as the key cause of blindness, followed in descending order by glaucoma, cataract and diabetic eye disease [28]. While countries in Western Europe have advanced healthcare options, the increasing trend towards preventative medicine has resulted in increased dietary supplementation, such as lutein. In contrast, within Eastern Europe, cataracts are the leading cause of blindness, but due to smaller and less developed economies, the aging populace is often neglected. As such, this sector of Europe is even more in need of preventative medication as consumers desperately seek to avoid what they may regard as inevitable blindness as they grow older.

Solid scientific evidence validates market credibility

In most cases, the market for most natural antioxidants is plagued by a lack of scientific evidence supporting their efficacy. Fortunately, this is not the case for the eye health ingredients market. One of the key positive factors is the abundance of evidence on the beneficial aspects of these ingredients in supporting eye health. Research studies conducted around the world support the benefits of nutrition for eye health. The results of the study entitled 'Age-Related Eye Disease Study' (AREDS) proved that high-dose antioxidant vitamins and minerals (vitamins C and E, beta-carotene, zinc and copper) ingested orally reduced the risk of AMD development by 25 percent

[29]. Antioxidants were also found to improve marginal vision loss by 19 percent. The results of this study were so well accepted that both European and American eye health institutes recommended the intake of AREDS formulations for AMD-susceptible age groups. Similarly, researchers from Wayne State University, Detroit, reported that an antioxidant combination of alpha-tocopherol, N-acetyl cysteine, ascorbic acid, beta-carotene and selenium helped inhibit diabetic retinopathy in rats [30]. Studies have also investigated individual ingredients for their beneficial role in eye health. A pilot study was conducted in the United Kingdom on lutein supplementation, finding that plasma lutein and mean macular pigment optical density (MPOD) were significantly increased with supplemented dietary lutein [31]. Such clinical trials and validation have produced beneficial support for this market.

Formulation advances increases application bases

The increasing discovery of new antioxidants and ingredients for claiming eye health benefits has caused ingredient manufacturers to look into the prospects of newer applications for existing established ingredients. This option guarantees a validated scientific basis while providing a new market opportunity, newer application sectors and a broader customer base. Such a trend is based on advances in formulation and packaging technologies such as micro-encapsulation. This trend is foreseen to increase the demand for existing ingredients and help provide a one-stop shop for customers in terms of their choice of eye health ingredients. For example, Kemin Foods introduced dairy formulations for lutein, thus entering a new application base [32]. Similarly, Cognis (now BASF) uses its lutein esters to fortify a range of products from cake batters to milkshakes [33].

Restraints in the Eye Health Ingredients Market

Fluctuating raw material availability hindering revenues

The availability of raw materials has an impact on pricing in the eye health ingredients market, particularly with respect to vitamin A and bilberry. Availability can be affected by many factors, including unforeseen climate, social, economic and political changes, all of which may influence raw material prices. Furthermore, the raw materials for natural vitamin extraction should come from non-genetically modified (GM) sources such as soya, which is often difficult and is an on-going concern. In the case of other ingredients such as bilberry, bad harvests in Europe result in shortages that allow Asian participants to dominate the market with cheaper products, resulting indramatic price fluctuation. Similarly, astaxanthin manufacturers have been hindered by heavy disease outbreaks in fish, a popular source of astaxanthin, leading toheavy losses in some cases. Such limitations contribute to variations in the prices of ingredients. In some cases, food manufacturers may need to seek more reliable alternative ingredient supplies or reduce their order volumes. Unlike companies involved in specific segments of the supply chain, vertically integrated companies, especially those operating through algal raw material, are protected from these variations. Some manufacturers source their raw materials from a wider geographical spread to lessen the impact of price changes.

Price competition restricts margins

The market for eye health products is extremely price sensitive due to the high rate of substitutions among the ingredients within this market. Lutein is the only ingredient that has firmly established itself as an eye health supplement. Other ingredients, such as astaxanthin and bilberry, are still emerging in the eye health ingredients market and are being threatened by reduced margins in a bid to offer competitive pricing. With lutein, the amount of patent protection will safeguard manufacturers over the next few years. However, as patents expire, Asian manufacturers will invade this market. Bilberry has also faced waning prices. The increasing number of suppliers and cost-effective modes of extraction have also caused a fall in prices. While this erosion of pricing premiums in ingredients will be the largest threat to market growth, the question of quality and good service will nevertheless impede any dramatic declines in ingredient prices.

HEART HEALTH INGREDIENTS

Introduction to Heart Health Ingredients

Currently, the global food industry has been addressing the various disease concerns, with the importance of functional foods and dietary supplements playing a significant role. Increasing prevalence of various chronic conditions (obesity and diseases, such as cardio-vascular disease (CVD) and diabetes) often associated with imbalanced diet have mandated the need for healthy eating. Such a scenario has resulted in the emergence of functional foods, defined as food products that have health benefits over and above their innate nutrition. With its origins in Japan, the most successful functional foods are primarily focused on addressing key health concerns, such as hypercholesterolemia, poor immunity, gut, and bone health issues. Heart health products have become increasingly important in Europe as a reflection of concerns over the high levels of death and illness caused by the disease [34]. The heart health category has been driven by innovations in a number of key ingredient application areas, including phytosterols and stanols, omega-3 fatty acids, soya, and dietary fibre.

Phytosterols

Plant sterols and stanols are inclusively addressed by the term 'Phytosterols'. Plant sterols are naturally- occurring substances primarily found as minor components of vegetable oils, such as sunflower oil. Sitosterol, campesterol and stigmasterol represent some of the most common plant sterols used in the food and beverage industry. Plant stanols are obtained by hydrogenation of the plant sterols. For example, campestanol is the hydrogenated product of campesterol and sitostanol from sitosterol. In general, phytosterols are naturally present at low levels in a variety of plants and plant-derived products including wood pulp, soybeans, vegetable oils, corn oil, rice bran and wheat germ. Plant sterols have a role in plants similar to that of cholesterol in mammals, primarily used in the formation of cell membrane structures and affects its permeability and fluidity. It is estimated that 2500 tons of vegetable oil or tall oil needs to be refined to produce 1 ton of plant sterols [35]. Tall oil, produced in the process of paper production from wood, is used for the manufacture of phytosterols. The advantage of tall oil is that it is GMO free and contains a higher proportion of plant stanols (primarily ß-sitostanol) compared to vegetable oils.

The cholesterol-lowering properties of plant sterols have been known since the 1950s. Over the years, scientific studies have shown that consumption of about 2 to 3 grams of phytosterols per day can reduce LDL-cholesterol levels by 9.0-20.0 percent [36]. The consumption of plant sterols and plant stanols lowers blood cholesterol levels by inhibiting the absorption of dietary and endogenously-produced cholesterol from the small intestine. This inhibition is due to the structural similarities of phytosterols and cholesterol.

An elevated level of blood cholesterol is one of the well- established risk factors for coronary heart disease. Blood cholesterol levels can be decreased by adopting diets low in saturated fat, high in polyunsaturated fat and low in cholesterol. Irrespective of the considerable achievements made in terms of knowledge and education, consumers still find it difficult to follow a healthy diet. Although people consume phytosterols every day in their normal diet, the amount is insufficient to have a significant blood cholesterol lowering effect. In order to achieve a cholesterol lowering benefit, approximately 1g/day of phytosterol needs to be consumed. According to the Institute of Food Science and Technology (IFST), the normal dietary intake of phytosterols in Europe is between 200-400mg/day [32]. The enrichment of foods such as margarines with plant sterols and stanols is one of the recent developments in functional foods to enhance the cholesterol-lowering ability of traditional food products. Cooking oils, margarines and peanut butter containing about 100-500mg/100g have been the main sources of phytosterols in most diets. Other sources include legumes (up to 220mg/100g) and oils of some seeds such as sunflower and sesame containing 500-700mg/100g.

Plant sterols represent one of the most important ingredients in the development and marketing of cholesterol lowering food and drinks. This can be attributed to the generally accepted scientific evidence that plant sterols such as phytosterols can block the intestinal absorption of cholesterol, which can lead to lower blood cholesterol. Though phytosterols provide various other benefits, such as the stimulation of insulin production and anti-aging effects on the skin, they are almost wholly positioned towards heart health. The extensive scientific support coupled with the 'Natural Ingredient' status of phytosterols has made it one of the most marketable bioactive components currently available in the market. As a result, plant sterols are by far the most used ingredient in the cholesterol lowering category accounting for a quarter of all new products launched.

Omega-3 PUFA

Traditionally, the word 'fat' has always been associated with a negative connotation, something which needs to be avoided at any cost. In the last decade, 'Not all Fats are bad' should arguably be the phrase that has managed maximum media attention and the focus of food manufacturers. Fats are a large group of compounds typically being triglycerides and any fatty acids. Fatty acids can be divided into three main categories:

- Saturated fatty acids (SFA)
- Monounsaturated fatty acids (MUFA)
- Polyunsaturated fatty acids (PUFA)

Documented research shows that the regular intake of PUFAs is essential for the general health of the body. The main PUFA groups commonly referred to are;

- Omega-3 fatty acids
- Omega-6 fatty acids

The human body cannot synthesize omega-3 and omega-6 fatty acids, as it cannot produce the precursor to these fatty acids [38]. Hence, they are termed as essential fatty acids (EFA) and must be obtained from dietary sources. The primary omega-3 fatty acid is α-linolenic acid (ALA). In the body, ALA is converted into eicosapentaenoic acid (EPA) and docosahexaenoic acid (DHA) at a conversation rate of just less than 10%. On the other hand, the primary omega-6 is linoleic acid (LA). LA is converted in the body to gamma-linolenic acid (GLA) and arachidonic acid (AA).

Long chain omega-3 fatty acids, DHA, and EPA are found in fish, particularly oily fish, such as tuna, salmon, sardines, mackerel, and swordfish, as well as seaweed. Fish is the best source of physiologically useful long chain omega-3s, although some seeds also contain short chain omega-3s; these are of less significance, as their conversion rate is extremely low in the body. ALA, a shorter chain omega-3 fatty acid, can be found in plants and plant oils, such as linseed, canola, soy, and some vegetables, likespinach, green peas, and beans.

Numerous studies suggested that an increased intake of omega-3 fatty acids reduces the incidence of coronary heart disease and the risk of cardiac arrests [39, 40, 41, 42]. This is accomplished by preventing atherosclerosis (hardening of artery walls and the clogging of arteries), inhibiting inflammation, reducing blood viscosity, stabilizing the heart beat, lowering blood pressure, and improving arterial elasticity. The Omega-3 fatty acids make this possible by reducing the low-density lipoproteins (LDL) and very low-density lipoproteins (VLDL) that deposit cholesterol in the artery walls. They also lower the levels of triglycerides (a fat that contributes to heart disease) and form a different anti-inflammatory pattern of prostaglandin.

The body functions best when an optimum balance is maintained between omega-6 and omega-3 fatty acids. Omega-6 fatty acids are widely found in plant-based oils, chicken, eggs, and grains. European diets provide an adequate level of these fatty acids. However, unlike a typical Japanese diet, European diets fail to include sufficient amounts of omega-3 fatty acids. This leads to an imbalance, wherein omega-6 intake is grossly in excess of omega-3. Since omega-6 fatty acids compete with omega-3 fatty acids for the same enzymes that metabolize them, an imbalance between the two intake levels (where omega-6 levels are far in excess of omega-3) has detrimental effects on health. Omega-6 fatty acids are linked to the stimulation of inflammatory prostaglandin (a hormone-like substance found in body tissue), while omega-3 fatty acids are linked to the stimulation in production of prostaglandin that is anti-inflammatory. Thus, consumer exhortation to increase their omega-3 consumption is at an all- time high, providing enormous scope for food manufacturers to exploit the opportunity.

Omega-3 PUFA oils represent the most aggressively branded ingredient towards heart health. Omega-3 and heart health have become synonymous as a result of these campaigns, and consumer awareness regarding their benefits is at a peak. Although omega-3 and omega-6 PUFA oils beneficially effect the heart, the consumption of omega-6 is generally more than the required amounts, and has resulted in the classic **'Omega Imbalance**.' Thus, the scope for omega-6 fortification is considerably lower as manufacturers are concentrating more on bridging the imbalance. Consequently, the contribution of omega-6 PUFA oils towards the 'Heart Health' market is minimal.

Also, among the various omega-3 types (based on raw material source), algal oils are primarily positioned towards cognitive health, as it contains only DHA, which has established beneficial effects on the brain. In addition, since their volumes are extremely low in comparison with marine oils and they lack the economies of scale, and hence are priced significantly higher. Consequently, they are used only in selective application categories, such as infant nutrition and pregnant women, where marine oils cannot be used due to the blood thinning effects of EPA. Thus, at current volumes, they only satisfy the need for cognitive health, and any impact on the heart health market is highly unlikely. In the case of flaxseed oil, since it only contains the short chain ALA with a minimal conversion rate (into EPA and DHA) in the body, its impact in the heart health market is also restricted. However, on a comparative note, flaxseed oil has a much more significant role in the heart health market compared to omega-6 or algal oil.

Thus, marine oils have maximum impact on the heart health market. On the whole, about 80% of the total omega-3 PUFA ingredients produced globally are positioned towards heart health, and marine oils account for more than 70% of this market, with the remaining 10% being shared between the other sources.

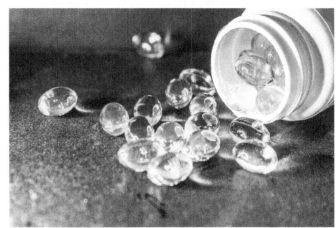

Figure 5. Omega-3 is a common functional food ingredient used by both the food and dietary supplement industry.

Beta-Glucan

The words 'carbohydrate' and 'fiber' have arguably been the most debatable topics of the modern food industry. Consumer awareness regarding 'low-carb' and 'GI' diets has reached new heights, resulting in an increased propensity among consumers towards healthy-eating. Technically, dietary fiber is nothing but carbohydrate polymers with a degree of polymerization (DP) greater than or equal to three, meaning they are neither digested nor absorbed in the small intestine. Since the term "fiber" first began to appear in scientific journals, there has been considerable controversy among food scientists, nutritionists, and medical experts about an exact definition.

Although most experts agree that one of the key defining characteristics of food fibers is that it is derived from the edible parts of plants not broken down by human digestive enzymes, many believe this definition is too ambiguous and that a clearer, internationally acceptable definition is needed to provide and validate data for legal requirements, such as food labeling.

In recent years, various organizations have come out with various definitions for fiber. For example, the American Association of Cereal Chemists (AACC) proposed a new definition for food fibers that included its health benefits. The definition is given as: "Dietary fiber is the edible parts of plants or analogous carbohydrates that are resistant to digestion and absorption in the human small intestine with complete or partial fermentation in the large intestine; dietary fibre includes polysaccharides, oligosaccharides, lignin, and associated plant substances; dietary fibers promote beneficial physiological effects including laxation, and/or blood cholesterol attenuation, and/or blood glucose attenuation" [43]. The Codex Committee on Nutrition and Foods for Special Dietary Uses (CCCNFSDU) defined dietary fiber as "food material, particularly plant material, that is not hydrolysed by enzymes secreted by the human digestive tract but that may be digested by micro flora in the gut." Plant components that fall within this definition include non-starch polysaccharides (NSP) such as celluloses, some hemi-celluloses, gums and pectins, as well as lignin, resistant dextrins and resistant starches.

Dietary fiber is further classified based on its water solubility into soluble and insoluble fiber. Insoluble Dietary Fiber (IDF) includes celluloses, some hemicelluloses and lignin, while soluble dietary fiber (SDF) includes beta-glucans, pectins, gums, mucilage and some hemicelluloses. Foods rich in soluble fiber include fruits, oats, barley and beans, while vegetables, wheat and most grains provide a good source of dietary fiber in general. While IDF aids the bowel movement and enhances the gut-health, soluble fiber has been established with significant heart health benefits; more specifically, the beta-glucans that have approved health claims in Europe and in the US.

There is no exclusive deficiency disease caused by a lack of fiber in the diet. However, research has shown that a low intake of food fibers (less than 20 grams per day) over long periods of time may be associated with the development of numerous health problems, including constipation, hemorrhoids, colon cancer, obesity and elevated cholesterol levels [44]. Due to changing lifestyles and eating habits, most people do not eat enough food fiber. The average intake of fiber is 12g per day (Source: British Nutrition Foundation) and it has been recommended that this should rise to an average of 18g per day for adults, while children need it proportionally less [45]. The major sources of food fibers are whole-grain and high-fiber breakfast cereals, and bread.

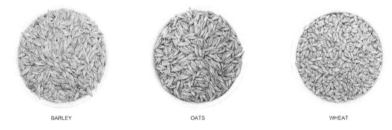

Figure 6. Common sources of Beta-glucan include bran of oats, barley and wheat.

Beta-glucan is a natural soluble fiber that occurs in the bran of oats, barley and wheat, as shown in **Figure 6** above, and can also be extracted from the cell walls of Baker's yeast. Beta-glucan is a polymer of glucose, which is soluble in water and forms a viscous solution upon consumption inside the human alimentary tract. Beta-glucans cannot be digested by human enzymes, but become degraded by the colon bacteria. Beta-glucans reduce the amount of cholesterol produced by the liver while reducing the serum cholesterol by inhibiting its absorption. Beta-glucan forms a complex with the bile acids formed by the liver from cholesterols, resulting in a highly viscous solution in the small intestine that slows down the absorption of cholesterol. In addition, as bile acids are essential for the digestion of fat, the liver produces additional bile acid, resulting in the increased utilization of cholesterol.

Fiber has long been recognized for its health benefits, which include facilitating digestion and bowel movement, and reducing food craving (thus helping with weight management), as well as preventing certain diseases, most notably cardiovascular diseases. As discussed earlier, insoluble fiber is mainly responsible for bowel movement and weight management, while soluble fiber helps in cholesterol reduction. Amongst the soluble fiber, beta-glucans have gained the most significant market share towards heart health products. For many years, soluble fiber from oats has been known to decrease total cholesterol levels when consumed in adequate quantities. The first study linking the relation of oats and cholesterol reduction was published in 1963 [46]. The active components in oats have now been identified as beta-glucans, which make up about 4% of the total weight of oats. In 1997, the FDA approved a health claim for beta-glucans from oats towards cholesterol reduction, as a result of a petition by the Quaker Oats Company. Subsequently, beta-glucans have been used to fortify a wide range of foods and drinks in order to position them towards cardiovascular health. Beta-glucans have been historically derived mainly from oats, and recently from barley. Though beta-glucan can be derived from various sources, oats currently represent almost the entire market. Currently, the regulatory scenario in Europe favors oat beta-glucans, as barley beta-glucans do not have any approved health claim in Europe, although it has one in the US.

In the near future, other soluble dietary fibers such as inulin and oligofructose would also be positioned for heart health, as early studies by ORAFTI have indicated their beneficial heart health effects. These ingredients are currently positioned as prebiotics by ORAFTI under its BENEO brand. Psyllium seed husk has also been shown to reduce cholesterol levels in the human body, and even obtainedan approved claim in the US. However, it has failed to make any great impact in the European market. Thus, beta-glucans currently represent the premier choice among soluble fibers and will remain so for some time in the heart health ingredients market.

Soy protein

Consumption of soy products has many health benefits, including protection against heart diseases, breast cancer, prostate cancer, menopausal symptoms and osteoporosis. Soy is typically made up of:

- 30% carbohydrate
- 38% protein
- 14% moisture

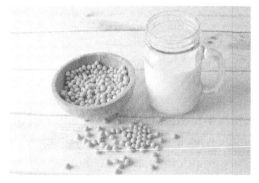

Containing all the essential amino acids, soy protein is the largest plant-based protein market in the world. This market includes soy flour and grits, soy concentrates, and soy isolates and textured soy proteins. Soy flour and grits are produced by grinding and sieving soy flakes to give a protein content of 40%. This can be increased to 50% by removal of fats. Soy flour and grits also contain oligosaccharides, insoluble fibers and soy oil. Full fat products contain about 12% oil while defatted

Figure 7. Soybean is a great source of plant-based protein, and is the main ingredients to products such as soy milk.

products contain only one percent. They are used mainly in the bakery industry for products such as biscuits and cakes, and in animal feed applications. Soy protein concentrates have a minimum protein content of 65% and are made by removing a proportion of the carbohydrate from soy flour. Traditional concentrates are used mainly in animal feed, but there are also a wide range of functional concentrates designed for specific human food applications for its nutritional values. Soy protein concentrates are primarily used in the dairy, meat and bakery applications. Figure 7 illustrates the source of these functional ingredients, soy bean.

Soy isolates have a minimum 90% protein content and are used in meat, bakery and dairy products. They are made by removing nearly all carbohydrates and fat. Textured soy proteins are defatted soy flour or concentrates textured to resemble meat products. **Isoflavones** are secondary vegetable substances, which can act as estrogens in the body and have protective functions. The estrogen effects of isoflavones are much less powerful than the estrogen hormones (its effectiveness represents around 1/1000 of the estrogen hormones). Isoflavones are present in relatively large amounts in virtually all soy products, with the exception of soy-protein concentrate. Whole soy contains about 200 mg isoflavones per 100g. Isoflavones are a component of soybeans that offer health benefits for the heart and circulation.

Soy protein has gained considerable attention for its potential role in mitigating risk factors for cardiovascular disease. The US Food and Drug Administration (FDA) approved labeling for foods containing soy protein as protective against coronary heart disease after reviewing 27 clinical trials. For the claim to be valid, the FDA requires that a serving must contain at least 6.25g of soy protein. The UK followed suit and approved the health claim for soy protein towards healthy heart products. However, the current ambiguities in the legislations towards health claims have not spared the soy market as well. The AHA (American Heart Association) has reported that some claims are not justified due to a lack of well- controlled trial studies, which support its use as cholesterol lowering protein source. Scientific evidence supports soy protein's ability to reduce LDL cholesterol and triglycerides by about 3-6%, at 25g/day consumption, which is in line with the American Heart Association's finding of a 2-7 percent decrease in LDL cholesterol [47]. A 3% reduction in LDL cholesterol from a public perspective translates to a 6% reduction in mortality rate. Studies have also repeatedly established that soy protein's cholesterol and lipid lowering effect is independent of isoflavones, although it can be enhanced when consumed in tandem with isoflavones [48, 49, 50].

Other Ingredients

Apart from the four gold-standard ingredients discussed in research, there are many other ingredients which are being researched for their potential benefits towards a healthy heart. However, much depends on the regulatory acceptance of these ingredients before they could have any great impact in the heart health market. Some of them include:

Green Tea

The use of herb and vegetable extracts for medicinal purposes has long been a practice. Green tea is one such extract that has been gaining popularity. *Camellia sinensis* (green tea) extracts include active polyphenol components, such as flavonoids and epigallocatechin gallate (EGCG). These two active pharmaceutical ingredients (API) are believed to be responsible for its heart health benefits. According to the American College of Nutrition, "EGCG acutely improves endothelial function in humans with coronary artery disease, and may account for a portion of the beneficial effects of flavonoid-rich food on endothelial function" [51].

Flavonoids

Diets enriched with fruits and vegetables can protect against heart disease. Diverse phytoestrogenic compounds important for heart health are found abundantly in soy, flaxseed oil, whole grains, and fruits and vegetables. In addition, other bioactive flavonoids, found in fruits, vegetables and teas, are believed to be beneficial towards a healthy heart. Finnish researchers found among 1,400 middle-aged men that, after taking into account known risk factors for heart disease, those with the lowest intake of flavonoids were at the greatest risk of heart disease [52]. Flavonoids also contain antioxidant activity and may protect LDL-cholesterol from oxidation. Fruits that contain high antioxidant content, or "superfruits", such as açai, mango steen, goji and blueberry, have emerged as popular sources of antioxidant. Increased consumer interest and awareness of the health benefits of flavonoids is likely driving the sales of flavonoid-rich foods in recent years.

Vitamins

Increased consumption of antioxidant vitamins can have a positive effect on CVD risk. They can have an indirect effect by mitigating the major contributors of CVD, such as obesity and diabetes mellitus, or direct effects on the molecular mediators of CVD. For example, several epidemiologic studies have found an inverse association between plasma vitamin C levels and blood pressure [53]. This association was particularly strong among women. In addition to vitamin C, vitamin E is also an important antioxidant, which, in tandem with vitamin C, can help reduce the risk of CVD by preventing free radical damage of LDL-cholesterol.

Pomegranate Extract

There is an abundant mythological and ancient history regarding the pomegranate fruit. In Babylonia, pomegranate was an agent of resurrection and the Persians believed that pomegranate seeds conferred invincibility on the battlefield. Present day nutraceuticals and functional foods have utilized pomegranate extracts in many commercial applications from skin health and aging to diabetic control. Pomegranate is one of the multifunctional fruits which has recently gained momentum towards heart health (**Figure 8**).

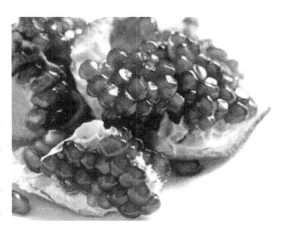

Figure 8. Pomegranate is a superfruit that have shown to have great health benefits.

Glucomannan

Glucomannan is a soluble fiber which has both a cholesterol-lowering and a hypoglycemic influence. It is hypothesized that glucomannan lowers cholesterol concentration by decreasing cholesterol synthesis. Additionally, cholesterol may be influenced as glucomannan swells in the presence of water, forming a highly viscous gel, which delays gastric emptying time and reduces plasma glucose and insulin concentrations. The reduction of insulin may also suppress cholesterol synthesis in the liver. Although glucomannan has primarily been promoted as a possible weight loss agent, the forthcoming years may see a shift towards its CVD applications.

Industry Challenges
Internal Competition among Heart Health Ingredients

Consumers are being bombarded with information regarding various heart health ingredients, resulting in confusion in consumer perception. The various competing ingredients include fiber, phytosterols, omega-3 fatty acids, and various fruit and vegetable extracts. As a result, consumers are unable to distinguish between them, generally resulting in lack of action. This poses a new challenge for the marketers and health organizations, as it is needed to devise strategies for persuading consumers to embrace the heart health concept and to turn that increased awareness into a positive purchasing motivation.

Threat from Asian Manufacturers

Chinese manufacturers provide various ingredients, such as Omega-3, phytosterols and soy protein, at a price 15 - 20% cheaper than those offered by European suppliers. Asian manufacturers have lower overheads, access to cheaper labor, favorable exchange rates, and are sometimes government subsidized. With the increased interest in heart health ingredients, more Asian suppliers are likely to compete in the European market on both cost and quality levels.

Examples of three Chinese suppliers that have already gained Identity Preservation (IP) status in Europe include:

- Shaanxi Tianwei Biological Products gained IP certification from the testing company GeneScan
- Fenchem gained IP certification from the testing company "'SGS" (Switzerland)
- Beijing Gingko Group Biological Technology, which sells its Ginnovay brand through the U.S. company SourceOne Global Partners, gained IP status from GeneScan

The increased activities among Asian manufacturers poses a significant threat to the sales of European manufacturers.

Competition from Pharmaceutical Companies

Pharmaceutical companies with established brands continue to compete indirectly with heart health ingredients. Drugs such as Baycol, Lescol, Lipitor, and Mevacor have established scientific evidence proving their cholesterol-lowering benefits. The higher efficiency of these prescription drugs compared to food ingredients works in their favor. Also, many countries provide reimbursement for these medical drugs, making them more cost effective compared to food ingredients.

Tendency of market cannibalization by products in different segments poses a challenge

Threat of substitution is one of the key challenges in the heart health ingredients market. The market faces a significant threat from external substitutes. Some of these substitutes include other ingredients positioned for cardiovascular health, such as a wide range of antioxidants, herbal extracts and ingredients, including coenzyme Q10. Although these ingredients do not have an approved health claim, they are used in a wide range of supplements and food products, posing a considerable threat in the market. Besides external substitution, heart health ingredients also face stiff competition from ingredients within the category. For example, omega-3 PUFAs compete with other established ingredients such as soy protein, fiber and phytosterols. Though internal substitution has a negligible effect on the overall industry in terms of volume and revenues, it is likely to prove to be disadvantageous to manufacturers active in only specific sectors. Furthermore, wide ranges of food products compete in the heart health ingredient space. For example, food products such as whole grains, olive oil, canola oil, and nuts have gained qualified heart health claims from the U.S. FDA and European Union. Thus, heart health ingredients such as phytosterols, fiber, omega-3 fatty acids, and soy protein are in a highly competitive marketplace, wherein they contend for share not only with other ingredients but also with food products with innate heart health benefits.

Drivers in the Heart Health Ingredients Market

Aging population stimulates demand for heart health products

As the post-war 'baby boomer' generation approaches old age, there will be an increase in the demand for heart health products. An expected increase in the implantation of pacemakers for patients over 60 years old is also likely to drive the market for heart health ingredients and dietary supplements. **Congestive heart failure (CHF)** is already common throughout Europe and its prevalence is increasing in line with the general aging of the population.

Unhealthy lifestyles contribute to increased risks

Cardiovascular Disease (CVD) is currently the main cause of death in Europe. The unhealthy lifestyle of many Europeans is further aggravating the problem of CVD. These include habits such as smoking, high levels of alcohol consumption, incomplete nutrition and lack of physical exercise resulting in obesity and elevated cholesterol levels. These negative aspects will inevitably increase the incidence of CVD and thereby potentially increase the demand for heart health products.

Restraints in the Heart Health Ingredients Market

Legislative Uncertainty

The EU Food Labeling Directive does not currently define the conditions for the use of health claims, thereby prohibiting them. The heart health ingredients market is greatly restrained due to this lack of clear legislation, which prevents health claims being made on products. Manufacturers can be forced to alter the formulations of products, as there are also significant issues relating to safe maximum levels of ingredients. Such requirements often come at a high cost, and small and even medium-sized companies struggle to implement new regulations. Since the legal definitions are not clear in some regions, there can also be a delay in getting approval for products from the regulatory agencies.

Digestive Health Ingredients

Introduction to Digestive Health Ingredients

Due to the increasing public awareness and interest in health and the relationships with dietary choices, health products specific for digestion, heart and bones are now seeingfast growing commercial markets. In previous years, products aimed at digestive health have had significant popularity in Europe when compared tothe United States. However, this market view is changing as global marketing strategies are being implemented. Consumers are accepting the value of maintaining good gut health, and have started purchasing food and beverage products to boost and maintain gut health.

For instance, Actimel®, Groupe DANONE's flagship probiotic brand drink is an extremely popular probiotic product in Europe. However, the brand now exhibits good growth in North American, Asian, and Latin American regions. In the United States, the same product was launched in 2005 under the brand name DanActive®. Since then, the product has seen appreciable growth in both the United States and Canada, though overall, Europe still leads the way in terms of the number of product launches and market value in the digestive health category. In the United States, it is estimated that around 60 million people suffer from heartburn, 50 million from irritable bowel syndrome, and around 20 million from stomach ulcers [54]. Therefore, the potential is huge for digestive health products such as prebiotics, digestive enzymes, probiotics and zinc carnosine to penetrate the largely untapped markets.

Prebiotics

The digestive system of humans and animals plays an important role in immunity against disease and infection. The system is a complex environment which can be populated by hundreds of microbial species. These bacteria can be either harmful (pathogenic) or beneficial. Diseases caused by some of these microbes, such as *E. coli* and *Salmonella*, have fuelled consumer concerns and propelled the market for preventive healthcare, most notably probiotics. Probiotics are beneficial bacteria; its growth helps competitively exclude pathogenic bacteria and strengthen the immune system. It is believed that at least 70% of the immune system's benefits come from probiotics naturally produced in the gut of humans. However, certain non-digestible food ingredients classified as prebiotics act as substrate for the growth of probiotics. The term 'prebiotic' was coined by professors Gibson and Robert Froid in 1995. It is used to refer to ingredients that fit this definition: that a prebiotic is a non-digestible food ingredient that beneficially affects the host by selectively stimulating the growth and/or activity of one or a limited number of bacteria in the colon to improve the host's health. In other words, prebiotic refers to non-digestible carbohydrates, usually fibers that stimulate the growth and activity of beneficial bacteria in the gut. They pass through the small intestine undigested and are fermented in the large intestine or colon. Generally, prebiotics are believed to stimulate growth and activity of bifidobacteria and lactic acid bacteria. Generally, any product that stimulates bifidobacteria is considered as a bifidogenic factor, so prebiotics can also be referred to as bifidogenic.

Recent research also shows that prebiotics have benefits in other areas, such as improved mineral absorption and beneficial effects on blood lipid levels [55]. Their close association with probiotics (the beneficial bacteria) has led to their increased use in conjunction with probiotics in synbiotic products. In addition, prebiotics such as inulin and fructo-oligosaccharide (FOS) are also non-cariogenic and low calorie. The low-GI properties of inulin enable its usage in food and beverages suitable for diabetic consumers. Both inulin and FOS exhibit beneficial properties toward immune health, cancer prevention and decreasing liver toxins. They have similar effects on animals. Benefits of inulin and FOS consumption in animals include immune modulation leading to increased resistance to disease, increased calcium and mineral absorption for stronger muscles and bones, reduction of mortality due to digestive disorders, and optimum growth and performance. This has helped manufacturers offer their customers a higher value proposition than a simple fiber claim or benefit.

Prebiotic carbohydrates are found naturally in chicory, bananas, asparagus, garlic, wheat, tomatoes, Jerusalem artichoke, onions, soybeans, flax seeds and whole and unrefined grains. Even breast milk naturally contains prebiotics. Due to the aforementioned phenomena, prebiotics are mostly used as digestive health ingredients. However, some of the prebiotic ingredients may also be used for other functional or technical properties. For example, inulin is commonly employed in processed food for fat replacement, fiber enrichment or for improving texture or mouth feel. Some ingredients that are prebiotic by nature are; inulin, FOS, mannan oligosaccharide (MOS) and galacto-oligosaccharide (GOS). Some prebiotics like inulin and FOS have been in the market longer than others. Many others, such as soy oligosaccharides, are still in the development stage in the market.

Probiotics

According to the most widely accepted definition of probiotics given by the Food and Agricultural Organization (FAO) of the United Nations in 2002, probiotics are live micro organisms administered in adequate amounts, which confer a beneficial health effect on the host. While all probiotics are considered live active cultures, not all live active cultures are probiotic; starter cultures, *Lactobacillus bulgaricus* and *Streptococcus thermophilus* used in the fermentation of yogurt are generally not considered probiotic.

Figure 9. Probiotics is a functional food ingredient found in foods such as yogurt.

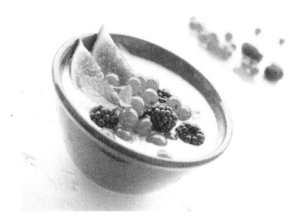

The role of probiotics in health is often associated with the GI system to aid digestion, or as a means to maintain good digestive health. Most brands of probiotic products of food and supplements sold in the market are communicated to address this concern (**Figure 9**). However, numerous other findings and scientific documentation have been published on several other health benefits associated with the consumption of probiotics. More research through carefully designed clinical trials is needed in order to arrive at firmer conclusions [56, 57]. Some of the popular health benefits attributed to the consumption of probiotics include:

- Potential to influence different IBS disease mechanisms
- Modulation of the immune system
- Prevention of select allergies (for example, atopic dermatitis)
- Help with lactose intolerance
- Treats vaginitis

Among these aforementioned health benefits, IBS and lactose intolerance are directly related to the digestive system.

Digestive enzymes

Enzymes are biological catalysts that assist speeding up biochemical reactions in the human body. There are thousands of biochemical reactions that take place in all living organisms. High temperatures help accelerate these reactions. However, as all complex life forms have metabolic temperatures below 40°C, it is the enzymes which act as biological catalysts and intermediaries or facilitators to hasten biochemical reactions [58]. These enzymes are protein molecules, which act on a specific substrate and remain unmodified at the end of each reaction in which they participate.

However, the aforementioned phenomenon is the ideal scenario. There are many cases where these enzymes (secreted by the respective organs such as the pancreas) that mainly assist in food digestion are either subjected to damage or get excreted during the process of digestion, absorption, and elimination, and are therefore not recycled to function continuously. There are also cases where enzymes are excreted in the body in insufficient quantities [59]. In addition, enzymes normally supplied through the ingestion of raw or mildly cooked foods may be depleted when the food is over-cooked, since the enzymes may be denatured under extreme cooking and processing conditions. The aforementioned reasons accordingly increase production demands on the organs which secrete enzymes such as the pancreas and duodenum. This creates the need for enzyme supplementation to avoid digestive disorders.

Digestive disorders cover ailments that range widely in severity. These encompass occasional discomforts such as gas, heartburn, and indigestion to more serious illnesses: namely gastritis, pancreatitis, irritable bowel syndrome (IBS), hepatitis, ulcers, Crohn's disease, celiac disease and gallstones.

The supplementation of every enzyme that our body produces is not currently possible as only a few among them can be synthesized or extracted at affordable costs. There are primarily four areas where enzyme therapy is used. These include:

- Acute injury (trauma)
- Chronic inflammation and allergies
- Digestive disorders
- Cancer treatment

Enzymes consumed as supplements for maintaining proper digestion are discussed below. These include mainly proteases, lipases, carbohydrates (such as glycases and amylases), that assist in digesting proteins, fat and carbohydrates respectively. Evidence supports the benefits of supplemental digestive enzymes in maintaining a healthy digestive system. For example, a British clinical study established that taking a digestive enzyme supplement notably assuages the symptoms of **dyspepsia** [60]. Dyspepsia is a medical condition, typically characterized by chronic or recurrent pain in the upper abdomen, upper abdominal fullness, and feeling of satiety much earlier than expected with eating.

Based on the source, digestive enzymes can be categorized into:

- Plant-derived enzymes
- Animal-derived enzymes
- Microbial enzymes

Plant-derived enzymes

There are two key plant-derived digestive enzymes available: papain and bromelain. Both papain and bromelain are proteases obtained from papaya and pineapple, respectively. In addition to its usage in conjunction with multi-enzyme digestive supplements, there are a few papain-sweetened chewable tablet brands promoted as natural products in the marketplace. However, people allergic to papaya latex (from leaf or unripe fruit), which is generally used as the source of papain, may have some allergic cross-reactions [61].

Apart from being used in digestive enzyme supplements, plant-derived sources may confer additional benefits. For instance, bromelain can be also employed in seasonal allergy treatment to reduce swelling of the throat, sinuses, and nasal passages and thinning of mucus so that it may be more easily expectorated [62]. In addition, a lesser known property of bromelain is that it is highly effective in thinning the blood preventing blood clots that can otherwise lead to thrombophlebitis and heart attacks. Papain, on the other hand, has many industrial uses apart from being used as a digestive enzyme supplement, such as breaking down proteins for medical research, stain removal, food processing and drug manufacturing.

Animal-derived enzymes

Pancreatin is the key digestive enzyme extracted from bovine or swine pancreas. It is a natural blend of proteases, amylases and lipases in pre-defined proportions. In addition to pancreatin, there are certain enzymes sourced from the stomach or intestine of various livestock. These enzymes include pepsin, trypsin, and chymotrypsin. Certain thymus enzymes (digestive enzymes) from calves and lambs also form part of the animal-derived digestive enzymes. Also, the enzymes known as lactase (derived from both animals and microbial sources) are used to digest the lactose present in milk and milk products. People who are lactose intolerant can resort to dairy products that contain added lactose. Lactase is also added to dietary supplements.

Microbial enzymes

Microbial enzymes offer protease, peptidase, lipase, amylase, glucoamylase, invertase, malt diastase, lactase, alpha-galactosidase, cellulase, hemicellulase, pectinase, and phytase activities. Digestive enzymes derived from microbes have a number of advantages over those derived from animals. These are:

a) Since microbial enzymes are active in a broader pH range of 3.0 to 9.0, they can facilitate the digestion of much larger amounts of protein, carbohydrates and fat before hydrochloric acid is secreted in sufficient quantities to neutralize their activity [63]. In contrast, animal-derived digestive enzymes are easily destroyed by the low pH within the stomach, unless they are enterically coated. Studies reveal that non-enteric coated products can be more effective than coated products in influencing digestion [64].

b) Animal-based enzymes are active only at narrow pH ranges found at specific anatomical sites. For example, pepsin is only active in the highly acidic environment of the active stomach, while pancreatin, trypsin, and chymotrypsin are exclusively active at the alkaline pH of the duodenum. In contrast, supplemental microbial enzymes have the capability to exhibit activities throughout the entire digestive process, which enables them to play a key role in improving food nutrient utilization.

c) Microbial enzymes can be customized according to the end-point requirement, whereas animal-derived enzymes, such as pancreatin, comprise of a pre-defined blend of amylase and lipases restricting their flexibility in usage with often only a proportional increase in total activity available, which may not be the desired aim.

Zinc Carnosine

Zinc carnosine is a patented ingredient manufactured by Hamari Chemicals Ltd in Japan. The ingredient is targeted for stomach health in Japan, Europe, Asian countries, and the United States. It provides relief in stomach disorders, such as heartburn, indigestion, stomach irritation, and ulcers. There are two primary causes of ulcers in humans: first, individuals who suffer from stomach and intestine infections with the spiral-shaped bacterium helicobacter pylori often have ulceration problems. This type of ulcer is generally referred to as H. pylori-associated non-ulcer dyspepsia (NUD). It is believed that this bacterium is present in more than 50% of the global population and almost 20% of the U.S. population [65]. Statistics also reveal that more than 75% of the people globally with gastric ulcers are diagnosed to be infected with H. pylori [66]. Therefore, these people are most likely to act as vectors for causing H. pylori-associated non NUD. Zinc-carnosine has been shown *in vitro* to inhibit H. pylori and in being effective in treating ulcerations.

A second key cause of ulcers is the use of non-steroidal anti-inflammatory drugs (NSAIDs), such as aspirin and similar Over-The-Counter (OTC) substances [67]. This is because these drugs inhibit the activity of the enzyme cyclo-oxygenase, which performs significant functions in maintaining the integrity of the upper GI tract and in promoting blood flow to the stomach. During animal trials, zinc carnosine has been shown to reduce or prevent gastric erosions in animals exposed to hydrogen peroxide, ethanol, or NSAIDs [68]. In addition, zinc carnosine has been shown to prevent stress-induced ulcers [69]. In the backdrop of the high frequency in which NSAIDS are consumed worldwide and the risk of associated ulcerations with their use, zinc carnosine could be an effective healthcare option in preventing peptic ulcers.

Zinc carnosine is a combination of L-carnosine and elemental zinc. L-carnosine is a naturally occurring di-peptide found in muscle and brain tissues. When this combines with elemental zinc, it gives rise to a complex that is a potential antioxidant with tissue-healing and mucosal-supporting capabilities. Zinc carnosine exhibits exceptional biological activity compared with either the individual components or a simple mixture of the ingredients. In addition, certain human trials conducted to test zinc carnosine's capability demonstrated promising improvements not only in the objective outcomes but also subjective symptoms related to stomach disorders. These include heartburn, nausea, vomiting and bloating. For example, in humans with either peptic ulcers or H. pylori-associated NUD, zinc carnosine has been shown to boost the response to combination H. pylori eradication therapy and is an effective tool in supporting the natural defense mechanisms of the stomach [70]. Primarily, zinc carnosine aids in maintaining the protective mucosal lining in the stomach and intestines and thus guards against attack from harmful bacteria and acid exposure.

Hamari Chemical Ltd's zinc carnosine has been marketed in the United States under the PepZin GI brand name. In Japan, the same supplement has gained immense popularity since 1998, under the commercial brand Polaprezinc. Apart from the key ingredient in PepZin GI, which is responsible for supporting good digestive health, other ingredients present in minor quantities include rice powder and magnesium stearate. It has been shown to improve the stomach lining integrity by stimulating the production of mesenchymal insulin like growth factor (IGF-1) and by curbing the expression of gastric epithelial NF-kB and IL-8. In addition, PepZin GI has antioxidant properties that play a direct role in reducing the extent of cellular damage generally caused by reactive oxygen species (ROS) in the human body. These antioxidant properties are mostly attributed to the presence of elemental zinc (chelated with L-carnosine) in the supplement.

Industry Challenges

High cost of clinical trials poses challenge to the industry

Clinical trial is one of the best ways to prove the efficacy of any product. Consumers are increasingly requiring evidence and the level of research completed at each stage of the product evolution. Digestive health products require clinical trials to prove their efficacy and to be provided with product information. Furthermore, the proposed health claim regulations seem to emphasize the need of well- documented research support in order to make any claim on the product label. The main problem with such trials is the high cost involved in conducting them, while the return on investment could be uncertain. Thus, manufacturers of ingredients, dietary supplements and functional foods are highly skeptical in conducting clinical trials. There is a limited amount of research on enzymes because of the high costs in running clinical studies.

Access to raw material

Access to reliable and quality raw material is becoming increasingly important in this market. There are numerous examples of vertical integration. Many top manufacturers in the fructans market are owned by leading sugar and starch producers. Even these companies have been affected by recent external pressures such as climate change, which have resulted in a shortage of raw materials. Although some companies have taken steps to address this imbalance, other companies may take a longer time to recover. Other new markets like Mannanoligosaccharide (MOS) have witnessed manufacturers integrate backward, and set up captive production plants to guarantee the supply of reliable raw material that meets their own standards. Both access and control of raw material are considered to be the key factors for success in this market, especially as the demand is still growing at a steady pace.

Awareness level of enzyme deficiencies

The awareness level of enzyme deficiencies among the general population is very low. A very small fraction of the population appreciates the relationship of enzymes with digestion. Health food consumers tend to have higher education and are more aware of enzymes and the role they play, but still lack complete understanding that enzymes are essential for cellular function. Educating these consumers about this basic concept of health a major challenge.

Competing with large pharmaceutical drugs

According to Brandweek magazine, the third and fourth best-selling drugs in the world are for digestive health problems (**Figure 10**). The leading products are Nexium and Prevacid. These types of drugs pose tough competition to functional foods with digestive health ingredients. Consumers look for short-term relief while ignoring the long-term consequences of some of the most popular medicines. Consumers make decisions based on price and doctors' recommendations to get short- term relief. Some of these products neutralize stomach acid and thus result in the production of more acid, because the body requires acid to break down protein. This, in turn, drives consumers to take greater amounts of over-the-counter (OTC) remedies. Finally, the use of products that shut down this production are taken as the acid level becomes high. Eventually, this process inhibits proper digestion of proteins and becomes increasingly difficult to correct. In this scenario, digestive health products experience strong competition from pharmaceuticals, and there lies a huge gap in sales between these two categories. Educating consumers about superior benefits and offering prices close to over-the-counter (OTC) products are the main challenges faced by digestive health or dietary supplement companies.

Figure 10. Pharmaceutical drugs are strong competitors against functional food ingredient in the digestive health sector.

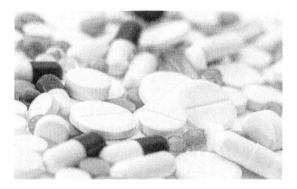

Difference in consumer perception on the efficacy of different types of probiotics
The awareness of the efficacy of probiotic products is varied. In Europe, consumers perceive dairy probiotics as being much more effective than supplements. In the United States, it is the reverse situation, with more emphasis placed on the efficacy of dietary supplement probiotics as opposed to dairy products. This situation requires an investment in consumer education in order to influence consumers and convince them the efficacy of alternative probiotic products.

Innovation and technological advancement required to tap maximum application potential
The probiotics market is in different stages of growth in a range of diverse food and beverage applications and in an emerging phase with reference to dietary supplements. Food and beverage manufacturers have an increasingly wide array of potential product applications. This forces probiotic manufacturers to come up with new product developments, which may require different types of encapsulation procedures in a very limited time frame. The diversity of applications in the market and the timelines for efficacious product developments with probiotics will limit growth in the market to a medium extent throughout the course of the forecast period due to the product development requirements.

Scarcity of patented enzyme products and little scope for innovation limit growth
Considering the extent to which companies are investing in researching newer health benefits of enzymes, apart from those used as digestive aid, it is expected that there is a huge potential for the systemic category of enzymes to flourish. However, there are two major challenges which the digestive enzymes industry faces. There is very little scope for any innovation within the digestive enzymes apart from extracting a few unique enzymes or enzyme complexes from unexplored sources.

Creating awareness and educating customers

It is essential to effectively and clearly communicate scientific evidence relating to the findings of studies conducted in functional foods and supplements. Ingredient manufacturers must be able to communicate the benefits effectively to end users, food and beverage producers, and consumers. In the past, the burden lay on the food and beverage producers to promote the product to the consumer and create awareness. However, this responsibility has now shifted to the ingredient manufacturer/promoter within the product. This trend is increasingly being witnessed in the digestive health ingredients market. Examples of manufacturers that have been successful in this area abound in the industry - Kemin with their FloraGlo® lutein; within the prebiotics market, and Orafti with its Beneo™ program. These companies specifically target consumers and end users by developing effective marketing and communication strategies. For example, Orafti developed considerable scientific evidence to support its inulin and FOS products. The company then changed the product name to Beneo™ and created a branding programme, specific to end users who incorporate a minimum amount of Beneo™ into their products. This strategy enabled products to display the Beneo™ logo on the product. Similarly, Orafti promoted scientific evidence and created a brand logo, and helped to set up an independent scientific committee to ensure that products meet certain standard criteria with regard to appropriate claims and dosage. This programme has been extremely successful. It is estimated that more than 150 products carry the Beneo™ logo at present.

Drivers in the Digestive Health Ingredients Market

Aging population and increasing healthcare costs driving digestive enzymes consumption

One of the factors helping the reinforcement of enzyme supplementation's benefits is the growing aging population in the United States. With age, several digestive factors become increasingly less efficient. For instance, the production of gastric acid starts diminishing, leading to a reduction in the amount of effective gastric protease (pepsin) available and a decrease in the amount of intrinsic factor. This intrinsic factor is essential for the absorption of vitamin B12. Additionally, intestinal wall integrity begins to break down in aging people that can cause absorption of larger molecules that might be detrimental within systemic circulation. Most importantly, the development that has a crucial negative impact on the efficiency of digestive process inside the body is the decrease in productivity of the enzymes normally produced within the brush border of the intestinal wall. There is also a negative influence on the functioning of the pancreas with increasing age in an individual. Since the feedback, mechanisms from the gastrointestinal tract get disrupted, the pancreas itself becomes less competent at digestive enzyme production and secretion, and pancreatic enzyme production to an extent becomes less efficient. Also, if there is an onset of type 2 diabetes in the individual, it can even more affect its capacity to produce and secrete enzymes. With such problems encountered in the aging population in the United States, healthcare costs are also on the rise. People find taking supplemental digestive enzymes a better and more cost-effective option. Mostly, multi-enzyme supplements are consumed as they contain several different types of enzymes that can aid in compensating for those enzymes unavailable due to the aging process.

Increasing demand for multi-enzyme supplements

Multi-enzyme supplements are the most important application of digestive enzymes. These supplements contain all the enzymes to digest the basic constituents in any food item, such as protein, fat, and carbohydrates. Hence, a major chunk of protease, lipase, and carbohydrases find their use in such supplements. Some lactases are also used, but these are mostly consumed as single enzyme tablets or are employed in making lactose-free dairy products. Factors such as aging population and increased consumer awareness about digestive health problems act as drivers for the growth of digestive health supplements. Therefore, increased demand of multi-enzyme supplements can be considered as a combined effect of drivers that are separately discussed in this document.

Spiraling market of lactase enzyme targeting lactose-intolerant people

Lactose intolerance is a genetic disorder caused by a deficiency of the enzyme lactase, which is needed to digest lactose (milk sugar). In patients, undigested lactose lingers in the intestine and upon fermentation causes intestinal discomfort, including abdominal pain, bloating, gas, and diarrhea. The prevalence varies by race and ethnicity. In the United States, the Hispanic population specifically is very fond of consuming dairy products, so when they cannot digest milk, they prefer either taking lactase enzyme supplements or switching to lactose-free alternatives. Consumers prefer taking enzyme supplements, as they perceive this as a more convenient and cost-effective option (taking a tablet after consuming dairy products) instead of buying and taking all lactose-free dairy products (such as cheese and milk).

Increasing awareness about the importance of digestive health fuels the usage of digestive enzymes

There has been an increased awareness about the need for maintaining proper gut health to achieve an overall optimum health. Continued research on the benefits of enzymes as potential digestive supplements has also been helping in attracting the Americans to consume digestive enzyme supplements. Though enzyme usage in systemic applications is witnessing a tremendous growth rate, enzymes for digestive purposes still hold a major chunk of the enzyme supplement market in the United States. Digestive problems can happen to anyone and usually arise when the quantity of food ingested is beyond the capabilities of the gastrointestinal system or when outside pressures and stresses disrupt the quality of the digestive process. Increasing incidences of digestive disorders, such as gas, bloating, heartburn, and constipation, among the Western population provide evidence of the fact that there is a limit to the resilience of the human digestive system and digestive health problems can occur to any individual.

Aggressive and smart marketing promoting consumer awareness about probiotics' benefits

As a result of continued advertising and combined marketing schemes (mainly from processors of finished goods), the level of consumer awareness has greatly improved in the last five years. Effective guerilla tactics (such as from Stonyfield Farm) included on-site sampling in nontraditional places, like rallies, subway stations, and so on. These samplings have afforded consumers the opportunity to try probiotic products for free. This approach helped to reduce the level of perceived risk associated with new products and encouraged impulse purchasing.

A second example is the aggressive campaign of The Danone Company that accompanied the multi-million-dollar launch of Activia® in the United States. This campaign employed in-store sampling as well as point of sale materials and frequent trade promotions. For instance, Danone has been visiting supermarkets and hypermarkets with free samples of their probiotic products as part of its promotion strategy.

Other examples include marketing initiatives by Yakult, educating consumers in the United States about the benefits of consuming probiotics as part of a daily diet. Innovative food and beverage probiotic products have also been launched by certain companies, which have helped to increase market awareness. California-based Attune Foods has already released various health food products and cereal bar combinations, featuring probiotics within the last few years with a heavy promotional campaign. These marketing programs are widely regarded as being the primary driving factor for continued growth in the probiotics market. The public has been exposed to a greater level of advertising campaigns on probiotics in television and other media. However, organizations such as the International Scientific Association of Probiotics and Prebiotics (ISAPP) have also played a strong part in bringing together both academic and industry expertise and opinion on the subject. This drives forward growth in the market.

Restraints in the Digestive Health Ingredients Market

Inconsistent quality standards hampering reputation

The market for some prebiotics, particularly inulin, has suffered because of inconsistent quality standards among manufacturers. Stability and functionality issues continue to prove problematic for manufacturers of certain prebiotics. These factors are important when formulating fructans for use in functional food. The incidence of such cases, however, has reduced in recent years.

Unfavorable side effects drawing away consumers

Although there exists no maximum limit for the consumption of fructans laid down by regulations, manufacturers generally recommend an adult not to consume more than 20 grams per day. This is due to the production of carbon dioxide and hydrogen as a result of fermentation. Although this is harmless, it can be unpleasant. In some cases, where the consumer suffers from irritable bowel syndrome (IBS) or any other digestive disorders, tolerance levels may be lower. Although research has led to the development of fructans where this effect is minimized, it is still a cause for concern for a few consumers.

Increased competition exerts price pressure

Though there are not many participants in the key digestive enzyme segments (proteases, lipases, and carbohydrases), the degree of competition is high, keeping the price under control. On the other hand, the lactase segment witnessed the entry of a few new participants within the United States, which has already started showing its impact on the enzyme price.

Increased promotion of nutrition and health through food

The consumption of wholesome, natural, and organic food to provide nutrients considered essential to maintain good health is expected to have some negative impact on the usage of dietary supplements.

Bone and Joint Health Ingredients

Introduction to Bone and Joint Health Ingredients

The market for bone and joint health ingredients is growing due to a widening customer base. Traditionally, osteoporosis is recognized as a condition affecting mostly women and the elderly, although this disorder is increasingly affecting a wider population including men and young adults. According to the Bone and Joint Decade, individuals over 50 years old are the primary group affected by bone and joint disorders [71].

With the aging population, it is expected that the numbers suffering from the condition will increase significantly. The WHO expects that the number of hip fractures, for example, will rise from 1.7 million in 1990 to 6.3 million by 2050 [72]. The baby boomer generation, all of whom are now between 40–60 years of age, constitutes a large potential market for joint health products.

Consequently, a large number of innovative functional beverages, foods, and cereals fortified with bone and joint ingredients have entered the market. Dietary supplements and functional food and drinks are the most popular format for consumption. There are over 50 well-established manufacturers, including multinational corporations and medium sized companies who comprise the market facilitators for bone and joint health products.

Calcium

Calcium is the primary bone health ingredient. It plays a significant role in the structure and strength of teeth and bones, blood clotting and nerve and muscle function. The calcium mineral market represents the most established category and constitutes the most widely recognized ingredient amongst consumers for bone health. The success of calcium in the bone health ingredients market can be ascribed to established health benefits and a high level of consumer awareness.

In addition, the market growth is fueled by legislative endorsement of calcium's bone health benefits. For example, the European Food Safety Authority (EFSA) affirmed the significance of calcium and vitamin D for bone health by approving Article 14 children's health claim submitted under the EU health and nutrition regulation by Danone's Spanish arm [73]. Examples of products that may employ the claims include cream cheese, ricotta, cottage cheese, farmer's cheese, fromage frais, mascarpone, mozzarella, curd-cheese or quark and queso blanco. EFSA's approval would promote market growth by reinforcing consumer confidence based on the health claim approval.

The key application areas of calcium are dietary supplements and fortified food and drinks. The calcium market is broadly classified as inorganic and organic categories. In terms of volume, inorganic salts including calcium carbonate and calcium phosphate dominate the market. These are followed by organic salts, such as calcium citrate, calcium lactates and calcium gluconate. In addition, calcium is obtained from various sources, such as milk and algae. However, the use of milk calcium is limited to dairy applications. Inorganic salts such as calcium carbonate and calcium phosphate, though widely used, are less soluble, which limits their application prospects in functional foods. However, they exhibit greater calcium content than organic salts. Organic salts of calcium have a higher solubility, bioavailability and better taste profile, but lower elemental calcium content. Organic forms are more soluble, bioavailable and have a better taste profile, and hence are used in beverages and food supplements.

Inorganic

In terms of market share, 85% is attributed to inorganic calcium sources, and typically includes calcium carbonate and calcium phosphates, such as di- and tri-calcium phosphates. Inorganic calcium sources have a lower bioavailability and solubility in comparison with organic sources, but inorganic calcium represents the most widely used form in the market due to low cost, long history of safe use and high elemental calcium content of these salts. Calcium supplement products often contain calcium carbonate, because it is inexpensive and contains approximately 40% elemental calcium. This property enables the delivery of larger doses with the ingestion of fewer capsules, and consequently its key applications include its use in dietary supplements.

Organic

The bioavailability of organic calcium is much higher in comparison with inorganic calcium. Typically, the bioavailability of organic calcium is two to five times higher than that of calcium carbonate. Organic salts include calcium citrate, calcium lactate and calcium gluconate. The organic calcium salts exhibit approximately the same level of bioavailability with a slight advantage to calcium citrate. The taste profile of calcium citrate is neutral, calcium lactate slightly bitter and calcium gluconate dry, slightly bitter and bland. Organic calcium sources have a better solubility and organoleptical characteristics. Calcium citrate is one of the most effective sources and is the most widely used organic salt in the market despite having the least solubility. It is the only organic calcium source that does not influence the taste of fortified products, and is also the most cost effective among other organic calcium salts.

Vitamin D

Vitamin D is a fat soluble vitamin that contributes to the maintenance of normal levels of calcium and phosphorus in the bloodstream. It is often known as calciferol. Forms of Vitamin D are:

- Vitamin D2: Ergocalciferol (made from ergosterol)
- Vitamin D3: Cholecalciferol (made from 7-dehydrocholesterol)

The commercial production of vitamin D3 is completely dependent on the availability of either 7-dehydrocholesterol or cholesterol. This is obtained via organic solvent extraction of animal skins (cow, pig or sheep) followed by extensive purification. Cholesterol is extracted from the lanolin of sheep wool, which is converted by chemical synthesis into 7-dehydrocholesterol. Vitamin D is essential for promoting calcium absorption in the gut and maintaining adequate serum calcium and phosphate concentrations. This enables normal mineralization of bone. It is also needed for bone growth and bone remodeling by osteoblasts and osteoclasts. Without sufficient vitamin D, bones can become thin, brittle, or misshapen. Vitamin D sufficiency prevents rickets in children and osteomalacia in adults. Together with calcium, vitamin D also helps protect older adults from osteoporosis. Most supplementation trials of the effects of vitamin D on bone health also include calcium. However, there is a growing body of scientific evidence that suggests the importance of vitamin D in maintaining optimal bone health [74, 75]. In addition to indicating the need for an increased dosage, these studies also illustrate the importance of vitamin D as a stand-alone supplement [76, 77].

The Food and Nutrition Board has established an AI (Adequate Intake) for vitamin D, which is sufficient to maintain bone health and normal calcium metabolism in healthy people. AI for vitamin D is listed in both micrograms (mcg) and International Units (IU). The biological activity of 1mcg of vitamin D is equal to 40IU of the ingredient. The AI for vitamin D is based on the assumption that the vitamin is not synthesized by exposure to sunlight. Current recommended daily intakes (RDI) of vitamin D are 200IU for people up to 50 years of age, 400IU for people between 51 and 70, and 600 IU for people over 70. Most brands on the market contain 200 to 400 IU of Vitamin D per capsule [78]. Nevertheless, presently, the scientific community is seeking to increase the RDI for vitamin D. The approval of children's bone health claims for Calcium and Vitamin D by EFSA from Danone's Spanish subsidiary is likely to further increase sales and consumption of this ingredient.

Vitamin K

Vitamin K primarily promotes carboxylation of osteocalcin, an abundant protein in bone involved in its mineralization. It also helps in decreasing calcium excretion. Naturally occurring K vitamins can be classified into two groups: Vitamin K1 (phylloquinone), which occurs mainly in plants, and vitamin K2 (menaquinone), which is synthesized by bacteria. Natural sources rich in vitamin K1 are green leafy vegetables such as spinach, broccoli and lettuce with the optimum level of consumption set at 80-200µg day^{-1} (according to studies pertaining to bone health). Dairy products such as cheese are a major source of vitamin K2, and intestinal bacteria also produce vitamin K2. It has become obvious in recent years that the contribution of intestinal-derived vitamin K2 to overall vitamin K status has been overestimated in the past.

A wealth of epidemiological studies have investigated the association of vitamin K status and various markers of bone health including clinical endpoints, such as bone mineral density and fracture rate. They consistently suggest a beneficial effect of vitamin K on bone health. The largest published epidemiological study on the association of vitamin K intake and fracture rate was initiated by DSM Nutritional Products [79]. In the Nurses' Health Study, a prospective study comprising of 72,327 women aged within the range 38-62 years found the adjusted relative fracture risk was significantly reduced by 30% in those women with a vitamin K1 (lettuce, broccoli etc) intake greater than 109µg per day [80]. These findings were later confirmed by other epidemiological studies, such as the Framingham Heart Study.

Osteoporosis is one of the leading health care concerns of developed societies. Research has found improved bone density and reduced fracture rates, and alludes to a combination of vitamin K with vitamin D appearing to provide superior benefits compared with the effects of either vitamin administered individually. DSM Nutritional Products has been involved in the first human study, which used nutritional doses of vitamin K1. This placebo-controlled, randomized clinical study in 244 postmenopausal women reported increased distal radius and improved bone mineralization after a 2-year intervention period [81].

Glucosamine

Glucosamine and chondroitin are the leading ingredients for bone and joint health. They also constitute the ingredients which consumers are most aware of in preventing osteoporosis and osteoarthritis treatments. Glucosamine has been present in 48% of joint health supplements launched since 2000, and chondroitin in 24%. Glucosamine is derived from chitin, the hard outer shells of shrimp, lobsters, and crabs, as shown.

Glucosamine is safe and effective in relieving joint pain. The market is expected to grow as the population ages and other major risk factors, such as obesity, raise the number of patients vulnerable to arthritis. In addition, awareness that the leading prescription drugs that previously helped arthritis sufferers may not be available in the future are giving joint health ingredients a further boost. These include unsuccessful drugs such as Vioxx.

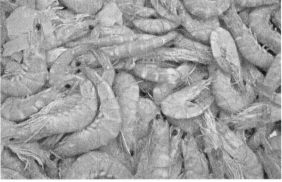

Figure 11 The outer shell of shrimp is a primary source for glucosamine.

Asian countries such as China provide the primary sourcing ground for glucosamine. China exports approximately 80% of its glucosamine output to overseas markets, with the major destinations being the US, Europe, South Korea and Japan. In recent years, China's glucosamine output and exports have been growing with an annual rate of about 10%.

While the number of glucosamine manufacturers has been decreasing, the average capacity of each producer in China has considerably increased in recent times. The glucosamine industry is highly sensitive to the supply of raw materials like shrimp and lobster shells, and pricing competition from the Chinese competitors with the largest producers' concentration being on coastal regions.

Dietary supplements formed the largest end-user segment for glucosamine with functional foods representing a relatively new application segment for joint care ingredients. This segment has gained significance with the emergence of condition specific trends in the functional foods sector. Glucosamine is widely used in combination supplements with other joint health ingredients, such as chondroitin, MSM, and hyaluronic acid. It is one of the most well- established ingredients for joint health in terms of market growth and consumer awareness.

Glucosamine is available in two main forms: e glucosamine hydrochloride and glucosamine sulfate. Glucosamine sulfate is more widely used, as it is priced lower than glucosamine hydrochloride. It is believed to be the best source because it provides the sulfur necessary for making and repairing cartilage. Glucosamine is also available as an injectable form physicians can insert directly into the arthritic joint.

Some of the available formats of glucosamine as an oral supplement include:

- Glucosamine sulfate: 500, 750, and 1,000 mg capsules and tablets
- N-acetyl glucosamine: 500 and 750 mg capsules and tablets
- Glucosamine hydrochloride (HCL): 500, 750, and 1,000 mg capsules and tablets

Glucosamine (which rebuilds cartilage) and chondroitin (which gives cartilage elasticity) are often used in conjunction. An example of a product available in the market is the Leiner Health Products' - Lifesmart Beneflux glucosamine and chondroitin supplement chews. An example of an innovative product available in the United States is 'Logic Nutrition Just 4 Joints' Glucosamine and Chondroitin Liquid Supplement. Packaging information states that it is an all-natural liquid dietary supplement for joint health containing 1,250mg of glucosamine HCl, which is non-shellfish derived along with 250mg of chondroitin sulfate and 60mg Vitamin C. The product is also free from artificial flavors, preservatives, colors or sweeteners.

Chondroitin

Chondroitin sulfate (CS) is an essential component of the connective tissue that provides elasticity. CS further draws water into the extracellular matrix, maintaining the hydration status of joints. CS is usually manufactured from avian, bovine, porcine or marine cartilaginous material with the avian-sourced chondroitin being the most widely harvested source. The GAIT [Glucosamine/Chondroitin Arthritis Intervention Trial] study demonstrated the beneficial properties of chondroitin when combined with glucosamine [82, 83]. However, chondroitin is a powerful and effective joint health ingredient in its own right. A recent meta-analysis of chondroitin based on clinical trials demonstrated chondroitin to be a safe and effective treatment for joint pain [84]. Though chondroitin occurs naturally in the body, the type sold in health-food stores and pharmacies is derived from animal products. Both glucosamine and chondroitin sulfate have been used for several years with few reported side effects [85], and the supplements also have some anti-inflammatory effects that may account for pain relief. The trend is towards developing new applications of chondroitin supplementation. The customer base for these supplements is increasing to encompass men apart from the women and elderly. It is widely available as combination supplements with glucosamine and other joint health ingredients, such as collagen peptides and hyaluronic acid. Food application of chondroitin is restricted by the current regulatory status of chondroitin which is classified as a drug in countries such as France and Spain. However, in the UK, the Netherlands and Italy, chondroitin and glucosamine come under food regulations. With the growing popularity of functional foods, it is anticipated that CS will be increasingly used in functional foods going forward. Bioiberica is a leader in the joint health ingredients line with offerings such as a bioactive line of chondroitin sulfate amongst other joint health ingredients it offers. Quality is a growing concern in the market. The move of manufacturing companies, such as Inter Farma and TSI Health Sciences, reflects an increasing trend towards certification as a means of lending credibility within a highly competitive market.

There are no significant dietary sources of chondroitin. Dietary supplements are the most popular format in terms of applications, followed by functional foods for chondroitin. It is often consumed as a combination supplement along with other joint health ingredients such as glucosamine, Methylsulfonylmethane (MSM) and collagen peptides. Chondroitin is commonly sold as chondroitin sulfate in capsule or tablet form. The dosage administration for adults is 400mg three times a day or 600mg two times a day, taken orally [87].

Methylsulfonylmethane (MSM)

Methylsulfonylmethane is a good source of bioavailable sulfur, a nutrient that the body needs to keep connective tissues such as cartilage and tendons in a healthy condition. Sulfur provides the chemical links needed to form collagen; the protein found in connective tissue. MSM is found in the tissues and fluids of plants, animals and humans and is a naturally occurring sulphur compound. MSM is contained in many foods in trace amounts, and combines with glucosamine and chondroitin to feed joint cartilage and help maintain its strength and elasticity. MSM has a much smaller, biologically active sulphur molecule than any of the glucosamines and can be used for consumers who have tried various glucosamine forms and found them unsuitable. MSM is not known to cause allergic reactions.

MSM is currently sourced from USA, Canada and the Far East. High quality forms of MSM will appear as mini crystal/flakes, whereas cheaper forms are in a fine white powder format. MSM is also faced with significant quality issues; for example, the addition of bulking agents, such as silica, talc and magnesium stearate, have a similar appearance. This has led to a reduced consumer and company trust in product sourcing and quality. The absence of established regulatory standards surrounding MSM products, their raw source material, production and supply is affecting market growth. There are concerns about the purity of synthetic MSM imported from the Far East. Most varieties of MSM available in the United States come from synthetic sources.

Collagen Peptides

The primary protein in cartilage, Type II Collagen (CII), is crucial to joint health and function. Yet the involvement of Collagen Type II in the process of joint inflammation has proven difficult to substantiate. Collagen peptide is a gelatine which is broken down into smaller molecules so that it functions better in the digestion and absorption processes. 28 types of collagens have been found (so far) in humans. The major types are;

- Collagen Type I. The chief component of tendons, ligaments, and bones; 90% of collagen in the body is type I
- Collagen Type II. Represents more than 50% of the protein in cartilage
- Collagen Type III. Reticular found normally with Type I

Hydrolyzed collagen (Types I & III) protein is composed of 19 amino acids, including an unusually high proportion of glycine, proline, hydroxyproline and hydroxylysine. These are essential elements for the production of lean muscles, healthy bones and firm skin. Type II collagen is significant for joint support and maintenance. Furthermore, high molecular collagen or gelatine turns into gel when cooled, which is used in manufacturing.

In contrast, collagen peptide does not gel readily. This characteristic makes it possible to be used in low-viscous drinks and many other processed foods. Some of the application areas of collagen peptides are:

- Health foods, snacks, other general food
- Beauty drinks, health drinks
- Cosmetics, bath goods
- Medicine for intestinal disorders & medical supplies

Characteristics of collagen peptides, which make it useful for food and beverage applications, are:

- Easily digested and absorbed into the body
- Easily dispersed and dissolved in water
- Low odor and high transparency
- Low viscosity
- Low allergen component
- High moisture retention

Fish collagen peptide is a fine powder, white or pale yellow in color, obtained by extracting collagen from the skin of wild catch seafish. Recently, livestock-based collagen peptides have been developed. These are superior to macromolecules such as collagen and gelatin in terms of solubility and digestibility, and have enabled new applications to be devised in the fields of health food and functional beverages. However, since Bovine Spongiform Encephalopathy (BSE) has become a concern, fish collagen peptides extracted from fish and shellfish have been attracting attention as an alternative to livestock-based collagen peptides. Fish collagen peptides have a variety of functions, the most representative ones being improving skin quality and preventing increases in blood pressure. In particular, it has been found to improve skin dryness and roughness, and is already being used widely in health and beauty applications.

In total, there are 28 different kinds of collagen with the most abundant form being collagen type I. Collagen Type II forms the main component of cartilage. If Collagen Type II is derived from chicken sternal cartilage from chicks 6 to 8 weeks old, it contains the greatest number of anti-inflammatory and joint supporting proteoglycans. These proteoglycans include glucosamine sulfate, which helps rebuild the cartilage in arthritis joints. This is supported with over 30 years of double blind, placebo-controlled studies [88]. Chicken sternal cartilage also contains a high concentration of chondroitin sulfate A, a powerful anti-inflammatory compound which also supports the joint tissue.

Collagen Type II also contains a powerful, newly discovered antioxidant proteoglycan called cartilage matrix glycoprotein (CMGP), which can help reduce oxidative damage to the joints. In addition to these new discoveries, other ingredients in Collagen Type II make it more effective than just taking glucosamine or chondroitin.

Fortigel from Gelita AG is a Type 1 Collagen peptide. It is derived from the chicken sternum cartilage and has clinical research backing in its effectiveness in joint health and cartilage regeneration. Diana Naturals has a branded bone health ingredient: ChondrActive, which consists of Type 2 Collagen peptide, chondroitin sulphate, and hyaluronic acid. The French-based Rousselot is a notable manufacturer of collagen peptides and hydrolyzed collagen peptides in Europe.

InterHealth USA are suppliers of UC-II undenatured Type II Collagen. BioCell Technology is the exclusive supplier of patented BioCell Collagen II®, a natural Type II Collagen ingredient that provides a naturally occurring matrix of bioavailable hyaluronic acid (10%), chondroitin sulfate (20%), and Collagen Type II (70%). BioCell Technology, LLC has branded its patented dietary ingredient under the BioCell Collagen II® registered trademark logo. The ingredient is only available to licensed companies who market under their own brand name or formulas.

Hyaluronic Acid

Hyaluronic acid (HA) is a glycosaminoglycan (GAG), which is a substance that attaches to collagen and elastin to form cartilage. HA maintains cartilage strength and flexibility, but also helps increase supplies of joint-lubricating synovial fluid. Research has shown that hyaluronic acid is an effective treatment for both rheumatoid and osteoarthritis [89]. A study showed over 80% of participants had significant relief from painful arthritic symptoms immediately after treatment with HA injections [90]. Hyaluronic acid is available by injection and oral supplements at health food stores and pharmacies. Studies show improvement for most participants after only two to four months of oral supplementation, and some patients are able to decrease their dose after the desired results are achieved [91].

HA or high-molecular weight HA hyaluronan is similar to the synovial fluid that surrounds joints and acts as a lubricant and shock absorber. It is typically injected into the joints, but has become popular as a nutraceutical competing with the likes of chondroitin sulphate and glucosamine as a non-pharmaceutical or surgical means to deal with joint discomfort.

Devil's Claw (Harpagophytum)

Studies show that "devil's claw" may be effective for maintaining joint mobility. In Europe, there is currently use of standardized devil's claw for mild joint pain. It is taken as capsules, tincture or powder. As tablets, 600 to 1,200 milligrams (standardized to contain 50 to 100 milligrams of harpagoside) are advised to be taken orally three times per day. It is believed that harpagosides and other chemicals in devil's claw block enzymes that initiate and prolong inflammatory responses. The medicinal ingredient of the devil's claw plant is extracted from the dried roots. There is increasing scientific evidence suggesting that devil's claw benefits joint health by the inhibition of COX-2, an enzyme linked to the inflammatory process and the stimulation of hyaluronic acid in human cartilage cells [92].

Olive polyphenols

Olives contain a large amount of polyphenolic compounds (**Figure 12**). One of the main polyphenols found in olives is hydroxytyrosol. Hydroxytyrosol is believed to have the highest free radical scavenging capacity of any antioxidant. Polyphenols are scientifically recognized for their tremendous antioxidant capacity. Recent studies have shown olives may promote joint function and mobility [93]. Oleuropein is currently used in dietary supplements marketed for their reported benefits for blood pressure and blood glucose levels. Olive leaf extract is available as a powder and can be used in supplements and some functional foods depending on the food matrix involved, since olive leaf extracts have an inherent bitter taste.

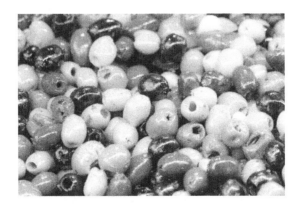

Figure 12. Olive is a great source of antioxidants.

Boswellia serrata

Boswellia serrata has a long history in Ayurvedic medicine popular in India. Its gum resin is reputed to have anti-inflammatory, anti-arthritic and analgesic activities. Extracts of Boswellia serrata have been clinically studied for osteoarthritis and joint function particularly for osteoarthritis of the knee. Boswellic acids have been shown to help control the inflammatory response in several ways. For example, as reported in the Journal of Indian Pharmacology, Boswellia serrata extracts performed well as a selective COX-2 inhibitor in a controlled clinical study to assess its effect on relieving osteoarthritis pain [94].

Rose hip

Rose hips contain vitamins C, D and E, essential fatty acids and antioxidant flavonoids, and in powder form is used as a remedy for rheumatoid arthritis. Rose hips from the dog rose have antioxidant values higher than berries. Researchers have found that a powder made from Rosa canina (a wild variety of rosehip) is three times more effective than standard paracetamol at relieving pain and 40% more effective than glucosamine according to study results of meta-analyses of randomized controlled trials in 2008 [95, 96]. The study was carried out by Frederiksberg Hospital in Denmark, the University of California and the University of Copenhagen. An example is Litozin® Joint Health, a unique patented food supplement with high levels of GOPO®- a key component in rose-hip that may play an important role in the care of joints and joint tissues available in the United Kingdom. It contains a 10% rosehip extract. DSM is involved in the production of a rosehip-based ingredient under the brand i-flax that is targeted towards joint health market. Please see Rose hip image below (**Figure 13**):

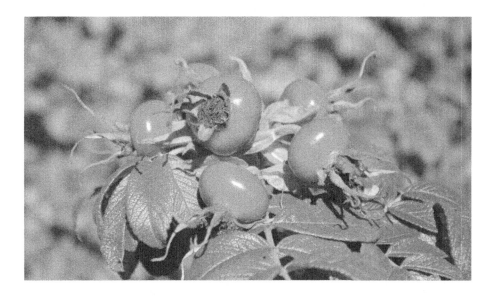

Figure 13. Rose hip image (from Pixabay)

Horsetail Extract

Horsetail Extract is naturally rich in readily absorbable silica. Silica's function is to maintain healthy connective tissue and bone health [97]. Silica also helps the body store more calcium. Horsetail extract helps promote proper joint function and has anti-inflammatory properties.

Omega-3

Much of the research on omega-3 fatty acids found in oily fish has focused on their benefits for the heart, mental health and anti-inflammatory effects [98, 99, 100]. However, omega-3 is increasingly being recognized for its bone health properties. Getting the right balance of omega-3s and omega-6s in diet may reduce the bone loss seen with post-menopausal osteoporosis, according to research by scientists in the United States [101]. A team of Penn State researchers carried out the first controlled diet study of these fatty acids contained in such foods as flaxseed and walnuts [102]. It was found that plant-based omega-3 polyunsaturated fatty acids (PUFA) have a protective effect on bone health.

Industry Challenges

Uncertain regulation scenario

There has always been a debate on the quantity of the functional ingredient included in product health claims. This is in view of the required amount of the active ingredient to experience quantifiable benefits or satisfying recommended daily intake values. The EFSA has already rejected several claims across various categories. This has led to an anticipated frenzy amongst manufactures and developers of ingredients, and those making health claims. The Calcium and Vitamin D claim for children's bone health was approved by EFSA as submitted by Danone Spanish subsidiary. It remains to be seen if the other ingredients pass EFSA's gold standards and make it to the positive list and affect overall market growth.

Competition from substitute ingredients

There are a large number of ingredients addressing bone and joint health. The market is filled with different combinations of complementary ingredients, each addressing similar aspects of bone and joint health. Thus, there is high competition within the ingredients; for example, glucosamine, chondroitin, hyaluronic acid, collagen peptides and devil's claw. In addition, new ingredients with beneficial bone and joint health properties are being discovered.

Lack of clear marketing messages challenging consumer confidence

A large number of bone and joint health ingredients, including glucosamine, chondroitin and MSM, need to be consumed for a minimum course of 6 to 8 weeks. This varies according to individuals based on their requirement and extent of the disorders apart from the supplement concentration. Most consumers complain of lack of benefits due to early termination of their supplements, which is an issue to be addressed by physicians and product marketing campaigns. Clear communication of the length of consumption of the foods and supplements is necessary to win consumer confidence.

Drivers in the Bone and Joint Health Ingredients Market

Rise in Incidence of osteoporosis and osteoarthritis

According to the International Osteoporosis Foundation, the number of osteoporotic fractures was estimated at 5.0 million, of which 1.0 million were hip fractures [103]. The total direct costs were estimated at $31.3 billion (£21 billion), which are expected to increase to $76.0 billion (£51 billion) in 2050. It is estimated that only around 10.0 percent of people suffering from osteoporosis are diagnosed and this usually occurs during the late stage of the disease, where most of the bone loss has occurred (20-50.0 loss), leading to multiple fractures. It is estimated that in Europe, 179,000 men and 611,000 women will suffer a hip fracture each year and that the cost of all osteoporotic fractures in Europe is provisionally $37.3 billion [103]. Thus, the facts and statistics are a clear indication of growth in the joint and bone health ingredients market.

Rising aging population

With the world's increasing aging population, the incidence of osteoporosis is growing at an alarming rate. Similar to many other developed countries, EU member states are experiencing an increase in aging population due to increasing life expectancy and declining birth rates. For instance, according to the United Nations Population Division, the proportion of population over 65 years of age is increasing in Europe [104]. Germany has the highest percent of people affected with osteoporosis, with 21% of it female and 4 percent male. It is followed by Italy, UK and Spain [105]. According to research published by the UK Food Standards Agency (FSA), awareness of healthy eating is high among older people. Two thirds of respondents to the FSA survey said that they know which foods they should eat in order to keep healthy [106]. Thus, the elderly have buying power, and this factor would propel market growth.

Rising awareness about preventive medicine focusing on bone health

Consumers' increasing interest in self-medication and a greater emphasis on disease prevention are driving the management of today's chronic diseases. The food and pharmaceutical industries are attracted by the large and growing market potential of these chronic diseases, but tackle them from different standpoints. The pharmaceutical industry uses traditional drug discovery approaches to develop new medicines to both treat and prevent these diseases. At the same time, the food industry looks to functional foods that assist in preventing disease to help them secure a place in the management of health and wellness. Increasing healthcare costs have caused an upsurge in consumer interest towards preventive healthcare. An increasing number of consumers rely on nutritional supplements and fortified foods as an alternative means to prevent disease afflictions.

Expanding Customer Base

Though the majority of those affected by osteoporosis are women, emphasis of bone health among children and men is also increasing, due to increasing incidences of bone health issues triggered by lifestyle changes. Low intake of milk and dairy products, rich sources of calcium, a reason for low calcium levels among children. Males are also affected by osteoporosis due to excessive intake of alcohol or smoking or due to low testosterone levels. Higher awareness among these two consumer segments has resulted in the opening up of new markets for bone health supplements.

Restraints in the Bone and Joint Health Ingredients Market

Asian competition for ingredients glucosamine and chondroitin

Manufacturers face stiff competition from Asian manufacturers in certain market segments, particularly in the glucosamine and chondroitin sectors. This is accompanied with pricing pressure; they are unable to match the supply and low prices. Asian manufacturers and suppliers today have GMP and other certifications that ensure quality. Thus, increased price pressure has translated to declining profit margins for domestic manufacturers.

Women Health Ingredients

Introduction to Women Health Ingredients

Women's health has remained a major health issue in the United States, Europe, and other countries. Over the years, people have employed the use of traditional herbs and medicines containing therapeutic compounds that help in curbing diseases and curing ailments. Women are prone to particular diseases, such as osteoporosis, osteoarthritis, anemia, menstrual health disorders, obesity, depression, and fibromyalgia. They are also prone to certain autoimmune conditions, such as Sjogren's syndrome, Lupus and Hypothyroidism. Vitamin D and calcium are used in nutritional applications to support bone health. Iron, soy isoflavones, folic acid, and cranberry extract are used in maintaining general women's health to some extent. Aging populations and increasing prevalence of osteoporosis are the key drivers for nutritional solutions to women's health. Functional foods and beverages are still an emerging application for these ingredients, presenting an immense future potential.

Vitamin D

Vitamin D is a fat-soluble vitamin mainly available as a dietary supplement and found naturally in very few foods. Vitamin D is essential for calcium absorption. It also enables normal mineralization of bone and prevents hypocalcemic tetany. Vitamin D also aids in maintaining normal blood levels of calcium and phosphorus. An acceptable daily intake is 200IU for all individuals below 50 and 400IU for all individuals from 50 to 70 years old. Vitamin D2, and Vitamin D3 are the two primary analogues of vitamin D. Research has shown that vitamin D3 is more potent than vitamin D2, and hence, there is a shift of demand in the market towards vitamin D3. To some extent, vitamin D has penetrated the dairy market, which is already witnessing numerous vitamin D2 and D3 supplements and fortified foods. Authorities in Europe have been active in passing legislations in this sector in favor of vitamin D intake.

Iron

Iron, as an essential mineral, has a vital role in carrying oxygen to the lungs and throughout the body. It also helps to store and use oxygen. Iron is commonly taken as a supplement, as it can be available to the body when chelated with amino acids. Iron (II) fumarate is a form of iron supplement that is generally used. Rich sources of dietary iron are legumes, broccoli, dry fruits, lentils, beans, leafy vegetables, red meat, tofu, fortified bread, breakfast cereals, and so on. Iron deficiency might result in fatigue, anemia, general weakness and related ailments. Iron deficiency is estimated to affect approximately two billion people worldwide both in the developed and developing countries [107]. Recent developments include Unilever exploring vegetarian iron for fortification, and a new inorganic iron source by Nestlé, with the use of phytase enzyme to breakdown phytic acid to enable a low-dose iron supplement to be more effective.

Calcium

Calcium is the foremost ingredient with a significant role in deciding the strength and structure of bones, blood clotting, nerve, and muscle function. Calcium has been widely recognized by consumers for its health benefits in the European market with fortified products of calcium receiving considerable support. The mainstay is calcium-fortified juices and cereals, and there is an increasing demand for calcium-fortified chews, functional waters, and confectionaries. The driving factors for the increasing calcium demand are the aging population, low dietary calcium intake, and the high incidence of osteoporosis in women. The calcium market is broadly classified in two segments; namely, the organic and inorganic calcium ingredients market. Organic calcium includes calcium citrate, calcium lactate, and calcium gluconate. Inorganic calcium ingredient includes calcium carbonate and calcium phosphate.

Soy Isoflavones

Soy and soy-based products have beneficial roles in the management of heart diseases and osteoporosis, and have the ability to enhance women's health. Soy isoflavones have the ability to improve bone health and they perform a vital role in preventing bone loss. The major types of isoflavones include genistein, daidzein, and their metabolites. Soy isoflavones have a similar structure of estrogen in maintaining bone mass in premenopausal women. It is observed that soy isoflavones reduce the leaching of calcium into the blood stream, and thus conserve bone mineral density. Isoflavone consumption is also known to result in a moderate decrease in the urinary excretion of calcium, resulting in decreased bone loss. Isoflavones are either naturally derived from soy or produced synthetically. Typically, synthetically produced isoflavones are sold as pure isolated compounds, whereas natural soy isoflavones are a combination of various isoflavones. The market for soy isoflavones is highly competitive, and there is a growing demand for bone health supplements and the trend towards combination ingredients.

Folic acid

Vitamin B9, known as folic acid, is an important vitamin in the B-complex group. Folic acid is reduced to dihydrofolate with the help of folate reductase enzymes in order to be absorbed effectively in the body. The vulnerability of the elderly population to anemia has encouraged the use of folic acid supplements and the consumption of foods fortified with folate. Folic acid is widely used in many pharmaceutical products aimed at treating anemia. It is also used for the treatment of megaloblatic and macrocytic anemia. In addition to being an anti-carcinogen, this vitamin also has anti-atherogenic, neuroprotective and anti-depressant effects.

Cranberry extracts

In Europe, cranberries are processed into products such as juice, sauce, sweetened dried cranberries, and cranberry capsules. Cranberry extracts have been valued for their ability to reduce the risk of urinary tract infections. Evidence suggests their anti-adhesion property may also be useful in preventing periodontal disease inhibiting the co-aggregation of oral bacteria [108]. Cranberry extracts also have antioxidants, known as anthocyanins, and there is a possibility that it reduces the risk of cardiovascular disease. The quality of cranberry extract is measured against the percentage of Proanthocyanidin (PAC) contained in the sample. Among the standard methods for measuring PAC percentage is the BL-DMAC method, which is the recognized method of PAC measurement and may become the universal standard.

Regulations

The regulatory scenario in Europe and North America is becoming increasingly vague and stringent. Strict laws pertaining to infant formulas/nutrition prevent ingredient penetration in this application market. Moreover, the cost of submitting dossiers involves considerable expense, and the future of many companies and manufacturers is uncertain, discouraging innovations in this market.

High degree of competition

A threat of substitution in the Nutritional Solutions in Women's Health Market due to the high degree of competition is a main challenge. The increasing demand for health ingredients has resulted in a burgeoning number of ingredients competing for market share in this arena. The categories presenting competition are fatty acids, vitamins and mineral supplements, antioxidants, botanicals, and herbs. For example, vitamin D and calcium are competing against each other to a great extent to survive in the bone health ingredients market. Folic acid and cranberry extract are facing the same challenge. Although several ingredients across all categories have the advantage of a fair scientific background and proven efficacy, the threat from competing ingredients cannot be negated. In addition, consumers become confused with a plethora of these ingredients in the marketplace.

Limited consumer awareness

Presently, scientific evidence is not enough to ensure success for any ingredient. Another prerequisite is effective communication. Ingredient manufacturers must be able to communicate the benefits of women's health ingredients to end users and consumers. Unfortunately, there is low consumer understanding of the exact mode of action and specific health benefits of various women's health ingredients. Hence, the main challenge for ingredient manufacturers is to create enough awareness concerning their ingredient and its benefits to achieve maximum consumer demand.

Drivers in the Women Health Ingredients Market

Rising prevalence of women's health related disorders

The aging population is at a greater risk of cognitive and brain function disorders. Awareness of the implications of age on the above-mentioned disorders has been on the rise. This awareness leads to a search for preventive solutions, rather than therapeutic intervention after the onset of disease. Supplementing diets with a daily dose of healthy ingredients with preventive or therapeutic value, is, therefore, a key driver for this market.

Escalating healthcare costs

Healthcare costs in regions such as Europe are augmenting, especially during the past few years. This factor has forced Europeans to opt for preventive healthcare means (such as health ingredients), which can keep them healthier. There is a growing consumer realization that women's health needs more attention, especially in reproductive and bone health. Also, the aging population is more prone to disorders such as osteoporosis and osteomalacia.

Augmenting scientific evidence and research efforts

Continued research initiative in terms of providing scientific-backing to benefits of women's health ingredients has beenone of the most vital factors fueling the market, and is likely to remain so. Such efforts have resulted in the unleashing of multi women health benefits of a single ingredient.

Restraints in the Women's Health Ingredients Market

Declining ingredient price affects revenue sales

Key ingredients, such as calcium and iron, have long been available in the market. These markets have experienced falling prices, due to lack of new innovations. Research has peaked in increasing their bioavailability and efficacy, which has reduced the scope for market participants to introduce new innovations. The availability of raw materials for these ingredients has also been on the rise, with a large number of manufacturers from different parts of the world developing supply capacities. Therefore, penetration is high while prices fall. This major factor affects market revenues during the forecast period. Price, however, will keep in trend with the prevailing inflation. Manufacturers are also geared to offer complete solutions and formulations with multiple ingredients rather than stand-alone ingredient solutions. This is expected to either position the ingredients at a premium price or increase the margins available for manufacturers.

Global Functional Food Ingredients Market

According to Frost and Sullivan, the functional food ingredients market in North America stands at $2,186.6 million. 60% of the ingredient sales occur in the beverage sector. 45% of total global sales of functional food ingredients are expected to be earned in the United States in 2013. The European market is estimated to have reached $1.89 billion in 2013 and is expected to garner $3.28 billion by 2018. Similarly, the Asia-Pacific market is estimated to have reached $1.17 billion in 2013 and is expected to reach $1.86 billion by 2018.

Major Companies Active in This Market

A list of companies manufacturing functional food ingredients is listed below in Table 1.

Table 1: List of Major Companies operating in the functional food ingredients segment

Eye Health Ingredients	Heart Health Ingredients	Digestive Health Ingredients	Women Health Ingredients	Bone and Joint Health Ingredients
Kemin Foods	Cognis	Beneo Orafti	BASF	DSM
BASF	Raisio	Sensus	DSM	Cargill
DSM	CreaNutrition	Cosucra Groupe Warcoing	Charles Bowman	Huber and Solvay
Kalsec	Cargill	Probi AB	Parchem trading	Gelita AG

Chrysantis	ADM	Chr Hansen A/S,	LycoRed	Marigot
Naturex S.A.	Solae	Danisco A/S	FortiTech	Frutarom
Indena	Epax	BioGia AB	Albion	Rousselot
LycoRed	Pronova	Novozymes A/S	Purac	BASF

SUMMARY

➤ AMD is a chronic progressive eye disorder causing partial or complete blindness. It can be most effectively improved when correct nutrition is supplied. .

➤ Omega-3 fatty acids prevent atherosclerosis, inhibit inflammation, reduce blood viscosity, stabilize heart beat, lower blood pressure, and improve arterial elasticity. Therefore, consumption of omega-3s can reduce the risk of coronary heart disease and cardiac arrests.

➤ Fiber has long been recognized for its health benefits, which include facilitating digestion and bowel movements, reducing food cravings (helpful for weight management), and prevention of certain diseases (specifically, cardiovascular disease).

➤ The supplementation of every enzyme that our body produces is not currently possible. There are primarily four areas where enzyme therapy is used, including acute injury (trauma), chronic inflammation and allergies, digestive disorders, and cancer treatment.

REVIEW QUESTIONS

1. Xerophthalmia, a common cause of childhood blindness, is caused by a dietary deficiency of:
    a. Vitamin C
    b. Vitamin E
    c. Vitamin K
    d. Vitamin A

2. The reason astaxanthin has the ability to pass through the blood retinal barrier is due to:
    a. Hydrolysis
    b. Esterification
    c. Condensation
    d. Saponification

3. Beta-glucan is a soluble fiber that are commonly sourced from all of the following, except for
    a. oat bran
    b. cell wall of Baker's yeast
    c. wheat bran
    d. soybean

4. Omega-3 and Omega-6 fatty acids are essential fatty acids that belong to a group of fatty acids called
    a. Polyunsaturated fatty acids
    b. Monounsaturated fatty acids

c. Saturated fatty acids

d. Polysaturated fatty acids

5. All of the following popular functional food ingredients targeting heart health, except for

a. Phytosterols

b. Vitamin K

c. Omega-3 fatty acid

d. Soy protein

6. Cranberry extract is a functional food ingredient found in the women's health sector that is primarily used to treat

a. Osteoporosis

b. Anemia

c. Urinary tract infections

d. Hypothyroidism

7. Which of the following is not a characteristic of collagen peptides that make it useful for food and beverage applications?

a. High viscosity

b. Low allergen component

c. High moisture retention

d. Easily dispersed and dissolved in water

8. The leading functional food ingredient in the bone and joint health market, commonly sourced from the outer shells of shrimp, and lobster, and crabs, is called

a. Glucosamine

b. Zinc carnosine

c. Glucomannan

d. Astaxanthin

9. All of the following are examples of prebiotics, except for?

a. Inulin

b. Fructo-oligosaccharide

c. Pectin

d. Galacto-oligosaccharide

10. Which of the following is not a challenge for the heart health functional ingredient industry?

a. Threat from asian manufacturers

b. Internal competition

c. Competition from pharmaceutical companies

d. Low demands for heart health ingredients

Answers: 1. **(D)** 2. **(B)** 3. **(D)** 4. **(A)** 5. **(B)** 6. **(C)** 7. **(A)** 8. **(A)** 9. **(C)** 10. **(D)**

REFERENCES

1. http://www.biology.uoc.gr/courses/BIOL493/documents/book.pdf [Accessed on 2 May 2013]

2. Jerzy Z. Nowak: Oxidative stress, polyunsaturated fatty acids derived oxidation products and bisretinoids as potential inducers of CNS diseases: focus on age-related macular degeneration.

3. Tielsch JM and Sommer A: The Epidemiology of Vitamin A Deficiency and Xerophthalmia, Annual Review of Nutrition 1984, Vol. 4: 183-205.

4. Alves-Rodrigues A and Shao A: The science behind lutein. Toxicology Letters 2004, 150(1): 57-83.

5. Stahl W: Macular Carotenoids: Lutein and Zeaxanthin, Nutrition and the Eye. Dev Ophthalmol 2005, vol 38, pp 70-88.

6. http://www.food.gov.uk/multimedia/pdfs/publication/guidelinessotonsixcolours.pdf [Access on 8 May 2013]

7. Roberts RL, Green J: Lutein and zeaxanthin in eye and skin health. Clinics in Dermatology 2009 27(2): 195-201.

8. Ripoll G, Joy M: Meat and fat colour as a tool to trace grass-feeding systems in light lamb production. Meat Science 2008, 80(2): 239-248.

9. Abdel-Aal ES, Akhtar H, Zaheer K, R. Ali R: Dietary Sources of Lutein and Zeaxanthin Carotenoids and Their Role in Eye Health, Nutrients, 5 (2013), pp. 1169–1185.

10. Richard L. Roberts: Lutein, Zeaxanthin, and Skin Health, American Journal of Lifestyle Medicine 2013, vol. 7 no. 3: 182-185.

11. Ata SM: The Effects of Egg Lutein on Age-related Macular Degeneration and Cardiovascular Disease Risk Factors: A Randomized Placebo-Controlled Trial (2013). Doctoral Dissertations. Paper 96.

12. http://www.nutrafoods.eu/Detail.aspx?id=139 [Accessed on 15 May 2013]

13. Dieter Hartmann, Petra A Thürmann, Volker Spitzer, Wolfgang Schalch, Birke Manner, and William Cohn: Plasma kinetics of zeaxanthin and 3′-dehydro-lutein after multiple oral doses of synthetic zeaxanthin, Am J Clin Nutr March 2004, 79: 410-417.

14. http://lup.lub.lu.se/luur/download?func=downloadFile&recordOId=2343714&fileOId=24 36313 [Accessed on 15 May 2013]

15. Shinichi Takaichi: Tetraterpenes: Carotenoids, Natural Products 2013, pp 3251-3283

16. http://articles.mercola.com/sites/articles/archive/2013/02/10/cysewki-discloses-astaxanthin-benefits.aspx [Accessed on 15 March 2013]

17. Liang FQ and Godley BF: Oxidative stress-induced mitochondrial DNA damage in human retinal pigment epithelial cells: a possible mechanism for RPE aging and age-related macular degeneration. Experimental Eye Research 2003, 76(4): 397-403.

18. http://articles.mercola.com/sites/articles/archive/2013/04/13/salmon-confidential.aspx [Accessed on 13 May 2013]

19. http://www.naturalnews.com/files/astaxanthin.pdf [Accessed on 10 April 2013]

20. http://www.who.int/nutrition/topics/vad/en/ [Accessed on 4 May 2013]

21. Rodríguez-Sáiz M, Paz B, J. L. de la Fuente, López-Nieto MJ, Cabri W and Barredo JL: Blakeslea trispora Genes for Carotene Biosynthesis, Appl. Environ. Microbiol. 2004, vol. 70 no. 9

22. Nelis HJ and De Leenheer AP: Microbial sources of carotenoid pigments used in foods and feeds. Journal of Applied Bacteriology 1990, 70: 181–191.

23. http://www.chr-hansen.com/news-media/singlenews/nutriphyR-bilberry-a-visible-difference.html [Accessed on 14 May 2013]

24. http://www.foodmagazine.eu.com/pdfs/food5.pdf [Accessed on 22 May 2013]

25. http://www.nutraingredients.com/Research/Looking-at-lutein [Accessed on 20 May 2013]

26. http://www.who.int/chp/chronic_disease_report/full_report.pdf [Accessed on 6 May 2013]

27. http://www.nutraingredients.com/Industry/Unravelling-the-market-for-eye-health [Accessed on 7 May 2013]

28. Sanjay S, Neo HY, Sangtam T, Ku JY, Chau SY, Rostihar AK and Au Eong KG: Survey on the knowledge of age-related macular degeneration and its risk factors among Singapore residents. Clinical & Experimental Ophthalmology 2009, 37: 795–800.

29. http://www.nei.nih.gov/amd/summary.asp [Accessed on 12 May 2013]

30. Renu A. Kowluru and Qing Zhong: Beyond AREDS: Is There a Place for Antioxidant Therapy in the Prevention/Treatment of Eye Disease?, Invest. Ophthalmol. Vis. Sci. 2011, vol. 52 no. 12.

31. Koh HH., Murray IJ: Plasma and macular responses to lutein supplement in subjects with and without age-related maculopathy: a pilot study. Experimental Eye Research 2004, 79(1): 21-27.

32. http://www.dairyfoods.com/articles/opportunities-for-lutein-in-dairy?v=preview [Accessed on 9 May 2013]

33. http://www.preparedfoods.com/articles/fortifiers-and-nutraceuticals [Accessed on 9 May 2013]

34. http://www.euro.who.int/__data/assets/pdf_file/0005/98438/e81384.pdf [Accessed on 3 May 2013]

35. Taşan M, Bilgin B, Geçgel U, AND Demirci AS: Phytosterols as Functional Food Ingredients, Journal of Tekirdag Agricultural Faculty 2006.

36. http://egembrs.com/wp-content/uploads/2012/08/EGEs-Food-and-Nutraceutical-Products-and-Competitive-Advantages.pdf [Accessed on 15 May 2013]

37. http://www.food.gov.uk/multimedia/pdfs/d02_018.pdf [Accessed on 2 May 2013]

38. Simopoulos AP: Omega-3 fatty acids in health and disease and in growth and development, Am J Clin Nutr September 1991, vol. 54 no. 3 438-463.

39. Chenchen Wang, William S Harris, Mei Chung, Alice H Lichtenstein, Ethan M Balk, Bruce Kupelnick, Harmon S Jordan, and Joseph Lau: n−3 Fatty acids from fish or fish-oil supplements, but not α-linolenic acid, benefit cardiovascular disease outcomes in primary- and secondary-prevention studies: a systematic review, Am J Clin Nutr 2006, vol. 84 no. 1 5-17.

40. Penny M. Kris-Etherton, William S. Harris, Lawrence J. Appel, and for the AHA Nutrition Committee: Omega-3 Fatty Acids and Cardiovascular Disease: New Recommendations From the American Heart Association, Arterioscler Thromb Vasc Biol. 2003, 23: 151-152.

41. Harris WS and C von Schacky: The Omega-3 Index: a new risk factor for death from coronary heart disease?, Preventive Medicine 2004, 39(1): 212-220.

42. Arja T Erkkilä, Seppo Lehto, Kalevi Pyörälä, and Matti IJ Uusitupa: n−3 Fatty acids and 5-y risks of death and cardiovascular disease events in patients with coronary artery disease, Am J Clin Nutr 2003, vol. 78 no. 1 65-71.

43. http://www.aaccnet.org/initiatives/definitions/Documents/DietaryFiber/DFDef.pdf [Accessed on 17 May 2013]

44. http://gnnwl.ca/resources [Accessed on 19 May 2013]

45. http://nutrition.org.uk/attachments/105_Dietary%20calcium%20and%20health.pdf [Accessed on 19 May 2013]

46. De Groot AP, Luyken R, Pikaar NS: Cholesterol-lowering effect of rolled oats, Lancet, 2 (1963), pp. 303–307.

47. Jones PJH, MacDougall DE, Ntanios F, and Vanstone CA: Dietary phytosterols as cholesterol-lowering agents in humans, Canadian Journal of Physiology and Pharmacology 1997, 75(3): 217-227.

48. Francene M Steinberg, Nicole L Guthrie, Amparo C Villablanca, Kavita Kumar, and Michael J Murray: Soy protein with isoflavones has favorable effects on endothelial function that are independent of lipid and antioxidant effects in healthy postmenopausal women, Am J Clin Nutr 2003, vol. 78 no. 1 123-130.

49. Xing-Gang Zhuo, Melissa K. Melby, and Shaw Watanabe: Soy Isoflavone Intake Lowers Serum LDL Cholesterol: A Meta-Analysis of 8 Randomized Controlled Trials in Humans, J. Nutr. 2004, vol. 134 no. 9 2395-2400.

50. Weggemans RM and Trautwein EA: Relation between soy-associated isoflavones and LDL and HDL cholesterol concentrations in humans: a meta-analysis, European Journal of Clinical Nutrition 2003, 57, 940–946.

51. Widlansky ME, Hamburg NM, Anter E, Holbrook M, Kahn DF, Elliott JG, Keaney JF Jr, Vita JA: Acute EGCG supplementation reverses endothelial dysfunction in patients with coronary artery disease, J Am Coll Nutr. 2007, Apr; 26(2):95-102.

52. http://www.nutritionaloutlook.com/1109/cardio/fortitech [Accessed on 29 May 2013]

53. Gladys Block, Christopher D Jensen, Edward P Norkus, Mark Hudes, and Patricia B Crawford: Vitamin C in plasma is inversely related to blood pressure and change in blood pressure during the previous year in young Black and White women, Nutr J. 2008, 7: 35.

54. http://www.prweb.com/releases/2013MXICorpXocaiTeamElite/05KualaTerengganuMalaysia/prweb10694319.htm [Accessed on 15 May 2013]

55. http://chriskresser.com/articles/prebiotics.pdf [Accessed on 29 May 2013]

56. Charlotte Hedina, Kevin Whelana and James O. Lindsaya: Evidence for the use of probiotics and prebiotics in inflammatory bowel disease: a review of clinical trials, Proceedings of the Nutrition Society / Volume 66 / Issue 03 / August 2007, pp. 307-315.

57. Kukkonen, K., E. Savilahti, et al. (2007). "Probiotics and prebiotic galacto-oligosaccharides in the prevention of allergic diseases: A randomized, double-blind, placebo-controlled trial." Journal of Allergy and Clinical Immunology 119(1): 192-198.

58. http://www.ancientsuninc.com/digestiveenzymes_article1.htm [Accessed on 14 May 2013]

59. http://www.healthcentral.com/encyclopedia/408/195.html [Accessed on 21 May 2013]

60. Karani S, Kataria MS, Barber AE: A Double blind Clinical Trial with a Digestive Enzyme Product, The British Journal of Clinical Practice 1971, Vol. 25, No, 8, 375-377.

61. www.ogtr.gov.au/internet/ogtr/publishing.nsf/.../papaya-4/.../papaya.rtf [Accessed on 22 May 2013]

62. http://www.thorne.com/altmedrev/.fulltext/5/5/448.pdf [Accessed on 25 May 2013]

63. http://rawlivingfoods.typepad.com/1/studies_and_research/ [Accessed on 5 June 2013]

64. http://www.goodpet.com/microbial-vs-animal-enzymes [Accessed on 5 June 2013]

65. Barik AS : Helicobacter pylori Infection in Developing Countries: The Burden for How Long? Saudi J Gastroenterol. 2009, 15(3): 201–207.

66. http://www.cdd.com.au/pages/disease_info/heliobacter_pylori.html [Accessed on 29 May 2013]

67. http://www.wiley.com/legacy/college/boyer/0471661791/cutting_edge/aspirin/aspirin.htm [Accessed on 2 June 2013]

68. http://www.ethosplan.com/l-carnosine-information.aspx [Accessed on 2 June 2013]

69. Mei X, Xu D: Gastroprotective and antidepressant effects of a new zinc(II) curcumin complex in rodent models of gastric ulcer and depression induced by stresses, Pharmacology Biochemistry and Behavior 99(1): 66-74.

70. Hawkey CJ: Personal review: Helicobacter pylori, NSAIDs and cognitive dissonance, Aliment Pharmacol Ther 1999, 13(6):695-702.

71. http://www.arthritis.org/about-us/bone-joint-decade/ [Accessed on 5 June 2013]

72. http://www.who.int/nutrition/topics/ageing/en/index.html [Accessed on 5 June 2013]

73. http://www.nutraingredients.com/Regulation/EFSA-approves-Danone-children-s-bone-health-claim [Accessed on 5 June 2013]

74. Pettifor JM and Prentice A: The role of vitamin D in paediatric bone health, Best Pract Res Clin Endocrinol Metab. 2011,25(4):573-84.

75. William BG and Michael FH: Benefits and Requirements of Vitamin D for Optimal Health: A Review, Alternative Medicine Review 2005, Volume 10, Number 2.

76. Robert P. Heaney: Vitamin D in Health and Disease, CJASN September 2008 vol. 3 no. 5 1535-1541.

77. http://www.theheart.org/article/1315347.do [Accessed on 7 June 2013]

78. https://www.grc.com/health/.../nih_gov_dietary_supplement_fact_sheet.pdf [Accessed on 7 June 2013]

79. Diane Feskanich, Peter Weber, Walter C Willett, Helaine Rockett, Sarah L Booth, and Graham A Colditz: Vitamin K intake and hip fractures in women: a prospective study, Am J Clin Nutr January 1999, vol. 69 no. 1 74-79.

80. Black DM, Cummings SR: Randomised trial of effect of alendronate on risk of fracture in women with existing vertebral fractures." The Lancet 1996, 348(9041): 1535-1541.

81. http://www.plosmedicine.org/article/info%3Adoi%2F10.1371%2Fjournal.pmed.0050196 [Accessed on 7 June 2013]

82. Yves Henrotin, Mariane Mathy, Christelle Sanchez and Cecile Lambert: Chondroitin Sulfate in the Treatment of Osteoarthritis: From in Vitro Studies to Clinical Recommendations, Ther Adv Musculoskelet Dis. 2010, 2(6): 335–348.

83. Jörg Jerosch: Effects of Glucosamine and Chondroitin Sulfate on Cartilage Metabolism in OA: Outlook on Other Nutrient Partners Especially Omega-3 Fatty Acids, International Journal of Rheumatology 2011, Article ID 969012.

84. Richy F, Bruyere O, Ethgen O, Cucherat M, Henrotin Y, Reginster JY: Structural and symptomatic efficacy of glucosamine and chondroitin in knee osteoarthritis: a comprehensive meta-analysis, Arch Intern Med. 2003, 14;163(13):1514-22.

85. http://nccam.nih.gov/research/results/gait/qa.htm [Accessed on 7 June 2013]

86. http://www.naturalhealthmag.com/health/ultimate-guide-healthy-joints?page=2 [Accessed on 7 June 2013]

87. http://www.livestrong.com/article/444794-normal-dosage-of-glucosamine-chondroitin/ [Accessed on 7 June 2013]

88. Carey-Beth James and Timothy L Uhl: A Review of Articular Cartilage Pathology and the Use of Glucosamine Sulfate, J Athl Train. 200, 36(4): 413–419.

89. Chou CL, Li HW, Lee SH, Tsai KL, Ling HY: Effect of intra-articular injection of hyaluronic acid in rheumatoid arthritis patients with knee osteoarthritis, J Chin Med Assoc. 2008, 71(8):411-5.

90. Kopp S and Carlsson GE: Long-term effect of intra-articular injections of sodium hyaluronate and corticosteriod on temporomandibular joint arthritis, Journal of Oral and Maxillofacial Surgery 1987, 45(11): 929-935.

91. http://www.vitaminstuff.com/supplements-hyaluronic-acid.html [Accessed on 7 June 2013]

92. http://www.nutraingredients.com/Research/Burgundy-builds-science-behind-Devil-s-Claw-ingredient [Accessed on 7 June 2013]

93. http://umm.edu/health/medical/altmed/condition/osteoarthritis [Accessed on 9 June 2013]

94. Nahid Akhtar and Tariq M. Haqqi: Current nutraceuticals in the management of osteoarthritis: a review, Ther Adv Musculoskelet Dis. 2012, 4(3): 181–207.

95. http://www.nhs.uk/news/2008/05May/Pages/Rosehipforosteoarthritispain.aspx [Accessed on 9 June 2013]

96. Vijitha De Silva, Ashraf El-Metwally, Edzard Ernst, George Lewith and Gary J. Macfarlane: Evidence for the efficacy of complementary and alternative medicines in the management of osteoarthritis: a systematic review, Rheumatology 2010.

97. http://www.wildflavors.com/NA-EN/innovations/hits/bone-joint-health/ [Accessed on 9 June 2013]

98. Lee JH, O'Keefe JH: Omega-3 Fatty Acids for Cardioprotection, Mayo Clinic Proceedings 2008, 83(3): 324-332.

99. Yashodhara M, Umakanth S, Pappachan JM, Bhat SK, Kamath R, Choo BH: Omega-3 fatty acids: a comprehensive review of their role in health and disease, Postgrad Med J 2009; 85:84-90

100. Ruxton CHS, Reed SC, Simpson MJA, and Millington KJ: The health benefits of omega-3 polyunsaturated fatty acids: a review of the evidence, Journal of Human Nutrition and Dietetics, 17:449–459.

101. http://umm.edu/health/medical/altmed/supplement/omega6-fatty-acids [Accessed on 11 June 2013]

102. http://news.psu.edu/story/198072/2007/02/19/plant-derived-omega-3s-may-aid-bone-health [Accessed on 10 June 2013]

103. http://www.iofbonehealth.org/facts-statistics [Accessed on 10 June 2013]

104. http://www.un.org/esa/population/publications/worldageing19502050/pdf/81chapteriii.pdf [Accessed on 11 June 2013]

105. http://en.wikipedia.org/wiki/Demographics_of_the_European_Union [Accessed on 11 June 2013]

106. http://www.nhs.uk/livewell/healthy-eating/Pages/Healthyeating.aspx [Accessed on 11 June 2013]

107. http://www.who.int/nutrition/topics/ida/en/ [Accessed on 11 June 2013]

108. http://www.cranberryinstitute.org/news/CI_Antiadhesion_Fact_Sheet.pdf.

9

Sensory Evaluation of Functional Foods

S. Sreelatha

Singapore-MIT Alliance for Research and Technology, Singapore

Introduction

Sensory science is the essential sensory analysis of products in food and beverage development. Sensory evaluation is a scientific measurement that analyzes and measures human responses to the characteristics of food and drink. The evaluations are based on appearance, smell, taste, aftertaste, and mouth feel; the key sensory perception dimensions. Sensory science employs trained panelists and sensitive instruments to guide the food manufacturers on product development [1].

Consumers are increasingly demanding the high quality of functional foods (foods which contain ingredients that provide additional health benefits beyond basic nutritional requirements) [2]. The development and consumption of such functional foods not only improves the nutritional status of the general population, but also helps those suffering from degenerative diseases associated with today's changing lifestyles and environment [3].

Sensory evaluation is concerned with precision, sensitivity, accuracy, and optimizing factors such as test designs, instrumentation, and interpretation of results [4]. Sensory methods require the following inputs: perception of stimulus, elaboration of sensation, and communication of sensation.

Objectives of Sensory Evaluation

The sensory response deals with a three-step mechanism, where the sensation results from stimulus detected by the sense organs. The characteristics of food are perceived by five senses: sight, smell, taste, sound and touch. Sight, controlled by the eyes, initially evaluates the food's quality with factors such as color, consistency, size, shape, texture, and opacity.

The desirability and acceptability of certain foods are evaluated by color; this indicates ripeness, strength of dilution, and the degree of heating. Color also triggers an expectation of richness. Regardless of what one believes or has been told, responses to a product are the result of interactions between various sensory messages, independent of the source.

Smell also plays a role in the evaluation of foods. For example, chemical compounds, like aromatic compounds, reach the olfactory region as gases when sniffing occurs and as vapors when swallowing occurs. The sensory experience of eating is essentially a combination of taste and smell. Say one tries to eat while their nose is shut, closing off their sense of smell. Immediately, they should notice a difference in taste. Smell is a crucial factor that works hand-in-hand with taste.

Taste is the most significant factor in selecting food. It is the ability to perceive aromas and tastes as well as building palates in a consistent manner. One area important in selection is the ability to distinguish between the four basic tastes: bitter, sour, salty, and sweet.

Taste buds are primarily located on the surface of the tongue. They have numerous **sensory cells** that are, in turn, connected to many different nerve fibers. The sensory cells are renewed once a week and transmit information based on the intensity of stimulus and the brain translates the nervous electrical impulses into sensation, which is recognized as taste [5].

Flavor is fundamentally the integration of chemical stimuli; a perceptual phenomenon that not only relies on the presence of certain aspects of a product, but also on the physiological status of the individual, memory, and the particular context it is presented. Therefore, flavor is a combined sense of taste, aroma and mouthfeel, where aroma plays approximately 75% impression of the flavor [5].

The sound food makes when it has been bitten or chewed is another sense used when evaluating food quality, like the water content in the food. This indicates characteristics of food like freshness and ripeness.

The ear perceives sound; the organs of the inner ear, like the cochlea (the decoder of every sound we hear) and the vestibule (the center for sensory integration and motor control), can convert sound to electrical signals in the brain.

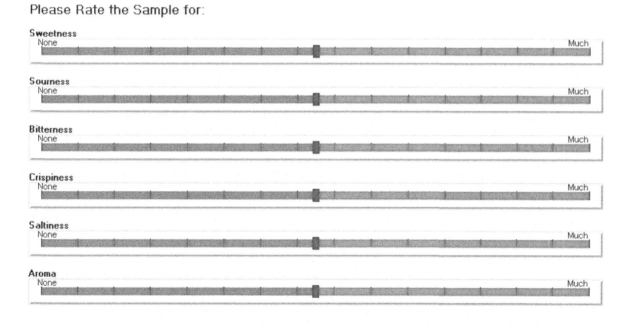

Figure 1. Line scaling, image courtesy Sensory Society 2014. www.sensorysociety.org

Figure 1 is an example of how one would rate some of the characteristics of a food they may be testing. Various categories are shown here, like flavor (such as sweetness and sourness) and textural properties (such as crispiness).

Food texture is delivered by the sense of touch. It encompasses mouth feel, masticatory properties, residual properties and even visual and auditory properties of a food. While often overlooked, touch is an important component of the food we eat, which can assist in decision-making. Tenderness is the only characteristic that is typically measured by a machine [5]. Therefore, all the senses play a key role in the sensory evaluation of food.

Methodology in Sensory Analysis

To achieve full use of sensory evaluation, it is necessary to follow the methodology closely. The steps consist of: selecting a proper panel, maintaining suitable environmental conditions, using standardized equipment for the test, obtaining representative samples, preparing and presenting samples for evaluation in a manner that ensures the uniformity and representation of the samples, and selecting proper statistical techniques.

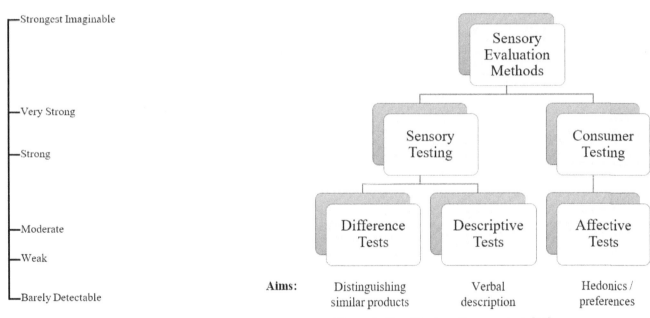

Figure 2. Labeled magnitude scale [7].   **Figure 3.** Classification of sensory tests [11].

Selection and Types of Panels

The development of sensory evaluation techniques is based on a selection of **sensory panels**. It is normally carried out under proper environmental conditions by both trained and untrained panels; difference in degrees of training are required for different types of sensory analysis.

To produce reliable and valid data, the sensory panel must be treated as a scientific instrument. It is therefore necessary that panelists are free from any bias and physical conditions which might affect human judgments. Panelists must have an ability to perform the task and to repeat their judgments. The panel members should be recruited based on various criterias such as interest, motivation, attitude, knowledge and aptitude, health, ability to communicate, and personality characteristics.

When training panelists, it is necessary to first teach them about the products and then take into account the differing quality expectations. There are three types of panels: trained panels, discriminative and communicative panels (semi-trained panels) and untrained panels (consumer panels). The trained panel should be able to fully establish the intensity of sensory characters of the overall quality of a food. The semi-trained panels are capable of discriminating differences and communicating their reactions; they are not to be trained formally but should be capable of following instructions given at the evaluation session. According to **Figure 3**, these panels perform sensory testing. The untrained panel should be selected at random from the potential consumers in a market are; according to **Figure 3**, they perform consumer testing. Prior to the start of the sensory evaluation process, the steps accomplished are screening, training and briefing of panels [6].

Environmental and Product Controls

Samples should be prepared in a way that standardizes their flavor. All variables like temperature, time of boiling, water volume and blending should be controlled to ensure the identical method of preparation for all samples. Care should be taken so that no loss of flavor occurs and no foreign tastes or odors are imparted by the procedure during preparation, storage, and serving [7]. Panelists and tasters should be in a controlled environment as well.

Measurement and Scaling in Sensory evaluation

In sensory evaluation, nominal, ordinal, interval, and ratio measurements are calculated. **Nominal** is the measurement that identifies unique attributes with non-ordered or ranked numerical values. **Ordinal** is the measurement where the attributes are ordered but the *differences between levels are not equal.* **Interval** is the measurement where the attributes are ordered and the *differences between levels are equal.* **Ratio** is the measurement where the attributes are ordered and the *differences are equal, as well as the fact that there is a true zero.*

The common scales used in testing are category scaling, line scaling and magnitude scaling. Category scaling (also known as hedonic scales) is the oldest method of scaling. It measures the extent of like and dislike of the sensory characteristic of food. Line scales may also be referred to as graphic ratings or visual analog scales. When the personal choice is more continuous and less limited, it is line scaling. Magnitude scaling estimates the magnitude of physical stimuli by assigning numerical values proportional to the magnitude of stimulus they perceive. Figure 2 illustrates a labeled magnitude scale. Sensory characteristics such as brightness, loudness, or tactile stimulation can be achieved by this type of scaling [7].

Figure 4 evaluates different characteristics of sensory attributes. In this particular graph, the main attributes are aromas, like fruity and alcohol aromas. But this graph also takes into account viscosity and appearance.

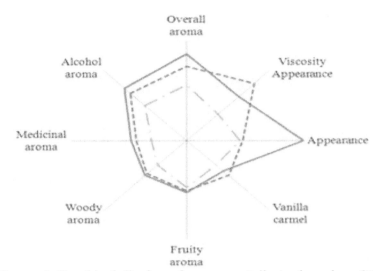

Figure 4. Graphical display of sensory attributes based on QDA [12].

Statistical Techniques

When conducting a taste panel, the food is uniformly prepared and presented to panelists in isolated booths. They record evaluations of the product on a **sensory evaluation sheet** that is decoded and analyzed by statistical procedures to determine significance and effect size.

Types of Sensory Test

Sensory tests can be categorized into three basic categories. The first category of tests includes traditional tools such as USDA grading and ADSA scorecard judging, which were developed in the early twentieth century to ensure product quality and consistency. These scorecard judgments are unsuitable in product and market research. They are used today only as a quick, rough estimate for the manufacturing quality control environment. Therefore, sensory tests are developed based on the psychological, physical, and physiological science of human responses to external stimuli that meet the specific sensory research objective. These sensory tests may be analytical or affective [8].

Analytical Test

The best-known analytical sensory test is the difference or discrimination test. The sole objective of the difference test is to determine if an overall sensory difference or an attribute difference exists between two products. The two types of different tests are the overall difference test and attribute difference test. The simplest test is the overall difference test, which includes the triangle test and duo-trio test.

Triangle Test and Duo-Trio Test

To determine if differences exist between a product and a control, the triangle test is often used with a trained panelist. In a duo–trio test, three samples are given to a panelist. One is marked as "reference" and the other two samples are marked with a random three-digit number. The objective of the panelist is to choose which sample is identical to the reference. Selection of the appropriate difference test to use is often determined by amount of sample, number of samples, testing conditions, nature of the potential difference (e.g., known or unknown), and specific test objectives. These tests are easy to setup and administer and the results are easily determined using a simple binomial calculation or published tables [9].

Attribute Difference Test

Attribute tests are often used to evaluate the qualitative differences in taste, color and mixture. There are three types of tests under this category: paired comparison test, ranking test, and rating difference test. For a paired comparison test, two samples are presented and the one with a particular characteristic is selected. For a ranking test, more than two samples are presented, ranked from lowest to highest on a specific characteristic. For a rating difference test, the panelists differentiate among multiple samples while using a rating scale.

Analytical Descriptive Testing

Descriptive analysis is used to identify and quantify some or all of the sensory attributes of a food with the help of trained individuals. The panel and their training can be adjusted to meet the specific project requirements in a process called profiling, which is used to detail the specific flavors or textures of the food or beverage [10].

Consumer Test

Consumer tests are otherwise called the affective test when a large array of specific and sensitive tools fit in this category. The affective test is used for product maintenance, product improvement, optimization, development of new products, determination of market potential, product comparisons in a category, and to make advertising claims. While this group of tests are expensive, diverse, and very complex, both qualitative and quantitative tests are available.

Quantitative Consumer Test

The most widely-used quantitative consumer tests are the preference and acceptance tests. They are distinct but interchangeable tests. The preference test determines the preference among the samples and includes paired preference tests (two samples), rank preference (three or more samples), and multiple paired preference tests (three or more samples). Rating the difference in the acceptance between two samples is called an acceptance test and is also known as the degree of liking [11].

Qualitative Consumer Test

This tool is the most widely-used test for insights into consumer perceptions, needs, and desires, which can then be probed for the product development and advertising, as well as the development of quantitative screeners and questionnaires. The primary tests in this group are the focus group and the interview. As these are qualitative in nature, the results are interpreted with caution and a quantitative test is conducted as a follow-up to confirm the findings [12].

Sensory Application in Functional Foods

Sensory evaluation tests are commonly used in the food industry. Input of sensory science has expanded significantly beyond the "product development phase" to understand both products and consumers where it reduces the risk in corporate decision-making for both researchers and marketing managers. Therefore, sensory evaluation has become an integral part in defining and controlling product quality. The main applications are new product development, product improvement and cost reduction, quality control, storage stability studies, and product grading or rating [13].

Table 1. Evaluation of an indigenous food blend fermented with probiotic organisms [15].

Fermentation	Colour	Appearance	Flavour	Texture	Taste	Overall acceptability
Single culture fermentation						
L. casei	6.9 ± 0.07	6.0 ± 0.06	7.0 ± 0.08	6.9 ± 0.07	6.8 ± 0.14	7.0 ± 0.15
L. plantarum	7.3 ± 0.70	7.3 ± 0.05	7.3 ± 0.05	7.3 ± 0.06	7.3 ± 0.06	7.1 ± 0.16
Sequential culture fermentation						
S. boulardii + L. casei	8.0 ± 0.07	6.6 ± 0.07	6.6 ± 0.07	6.8 ± 0.03	6.9 ± 0.05	6.9 ± 0.06
S. boulardii + L. plantarum	6.9 ± 0.06	7.3 ± 0.06	6.9 ± 0.06	6.8 ± 0.08	6.8 ± 0.06	7.1 ± 0.04
S.E. (mean) ±	0.11	0.07	0.07	0.06	0.08	0.11
CD ($p<0.05$)	0.33	0.21	0.21	0.18	0.24	0.33

Note: Values are mean ±SD of ten panelists

In **Table 1**, the results of participants' evaluations in rating food blends with probiotic organisms of different factors are projected. These results are used to determine which food blends will be better to market.

Examples

Fermented Foods: Probiotic fermented foods are gaining popularity. Cereals and legumes constitute the staple diet in developing nations, but recently, sources have been scarce. The consumption of such food mixtures may be useful in controlling pathogens/antibiotics that induce diarrhea, as well as in controlling hypercholesterolemia [15].

Meat: The most important sensory properties for most meat products are tenderness, juiciness, and flavor. These are dependent on the meat's chemical characteristics such as pH, content, aging time, and antemortem factors such as nutrition, stress, and breed of the animal. The majority of meat products have a characteristic flavor that is species-dependent [16].

Sensory properties of milk: Milk is an essential component of many diets. Milk and cereal products fortified with iron, as well as a combination of other micronutrients, are more likely to help reduce iron-deficiency anemia in children than foods fortified with iron alone [17].

Several other applications of sensory analysis to dairy products have been completed recently. A few examples include development of a flavor lexicon for chocolate milk, flavor variability in skim milk powder, and development of lexicons for cheese texture to enhance understanding of its rheological and functional properties [18]. Therefore, sensory analysis is a key element in food industry product development. The human sensorium is applied to quality control, taint identification, recipe change, evaluation and benchmarking.

SUMMARY

➤ Sensory methods require the following inputs: perception of stimulus, elaboration of sensation, and communication of sensation.

➤ Sensory cells transmit information based on the intensity of stimulus and the brain translates the nervous electrical impulses into sensation, which is recognized as taste.

➤ Sensory evaluation has become an integral part in defining and controlling product quality. The main applications are new product development, product improvement and cost reduction, quality control, storage stability studies, and product grading or ranking.

➤ Sensory evaluation is the primary means of evaluating food products. This is achieved by analysis of the sensory methods combined with the market research department.

REVIEW QUESTIONS

1. Nominal measurements used in sensory evaluations:
   a. The attributes are ordered, but the differences between the levels aren't equal.
   b. The attributes are ordered and the differences between the levels are equal.
   c. The attributes are ordered and the differences are equal and there is a true zero.
   d. Identify unique attributes with non-ordered or ranked numerical values.

2. The four basic tastes perceived by the human tongue are
   a. Sour, salty, and sweet, and spicy
   b. Bitter, sour, salty, and sweet
   c. Salty, sweet, spicy, and bitter
   d. Sour, spicy, bitter, and salty

3. Which of the following is not an example of an attribute difference test?
   a. Paired comparison test
   b. Ranking test
   c. Rating difference test
   d. Duo-trio test

4. When conducting sensory evaluation using a triangle test, the sensory panel used are
   a. Trained panelists
   b. Semi-trained panelists
   c. Untrained panelists
   d. All types of panelists

Answers: 1. **(D)** 2. **(B)** 3. **(D)** 4. **(A)**

REFERENCES:

1. Lawless HT, Heymann H. Sensory Evaluation of Food: Principles and Practices. 2nd ed. New York: Springer; 2010: 563, 565& 566.

2. Ndife J, Abbo E. (2009). Functional Foods: Prospects and Challenges in Nigeria. J. Sci. Technol., 1(5): 1-6.

3. Jideani V, Onwubali F. (2009). Optimisation of wheat-sprouted soybean flour bread using response surface methodology. Afr. J.Biotechnol., 8(22): 364-6373.

4. Drake MA. (2007). Invited review: Sensory analysis of dairy foods. *J Dairy Sci* 90:4925–37.

5. Drewnowski, A. (1997). Taste preferences and food intake, in Annual Reviews in Nutrition 17: 237–253.

6. British Standard Institution. (1980). Methods for sensory analysis of food. Part 1. Introduction and general guide to methodology, BS 5929:Part1:1980.

7. Meilgaard CC. (1999). "Sensory Evaluation Techniques 3rd Edition," CRC Press, Boca Raton.

8. Ennis DM. (1993). The power of sensory discrimination methods. *J Sens Stud* 8:353–70.

9. Brown A. (2008). Understanding Food: Principles and Preparation. 3rd ed. Belmont, CA: Thompson-Wadsworth.

10. Meilgaard M., Civille GV. Carr BT. (2007). Sensory Evaluation Techniques. 4th ed. Boca Raton, FL. CRC Press.

11. Stone H, Sidel J, Oliver S, et al. Sensory evaluation by quantitative descriptive analysis. *Food Tech.* 1974; 28:24–29, 32, 34.

12. Lawless HT. Heymann H. (1998). Sensory Evaluation of Food: principles and practices. New York, NY. Chapman &Hall; Press.

13. Lawless, H. T., and H. Heymann. (1999)b. Discrimination testing. Pages 116–138 in Sensory Evaluation of Food. 1st ed. Chapman and Hall, New York, NY.

14. Kreuger, R. A., and M. A. Casey. (2000). Focus Groups: A Practical Guide for Applied Research. 3rd ed. Sage Publications, Thousand Oaks, CA.

15. Sangeeta C. Sindhu, Neelam Khetarpaul. (2005) "Development, acceptability and nutritional evaluation of an indigenous food blend fermented with probiotic organisms", Nutrition & Food Science. 35:20–27.

16. Djaafar RA. Mohamed G. Ipek & Jianmei Y. (2009). "Extrusion parameters and consumer acceptability of a peanut-based meat analogue. International." Journal of Food Science and Technology. 44:2075-2084.

17. Drake, M. A. 2004. Defining dairy flavors. J. Dairy Sci. 87:777–784.

18. Thompson JL, Drake MA, Lopetcharat K, & Yates MD. (2004). Preference mapping of commercial chocolate milks. Journal of Food Science. 69:S406-S413.

10

Biotechnology and Functional Food

Thomas Reynolds[1] and Danik M. Martirosyan[2]

[1]University of San Francisco, San Francisco, CA, USA; [2]Functional Food Center/Functional Food Institute, Dallas, TX, USA

Introduction

Few scientific developments of the last 50 years have had as resounding an impact on human society as biotechnology. Manipulating the nucleic acid information medium and its expression in living organisms has redefined the bounds of basic laboratory research, delivered complex macromolecular therapeutics to the clinic, and enabled material commodity production from engineered biological systems. Additionally, from a commercial perspective, the US biopharmaceutical industry's $110+ billion in revenue indicates that biotechnology is a lucrative proposition, as well as a transformative one [1].

While embracing the novel therapies that biotech treatment offers, medical practices and institutions are also reevaluating a very old concept: the therapeutic benefits of functional food. Precisely what constitutes a functional food depends on the definition's source, but the generally accepted definition is that a functional food, when consumed in the regular course of a person's diet, confers a well-defined health benefit beyond basal metabolic needs. The Functional Food Center's current definition [2] posits that functional foods are:

> *Natural or processed foods that contains known or unknown biologically-active compounds; which, in defined, effective non-toxic amounts, provide a clinically proven and strong documented health benefit for the prevention, management, or treatment of chronic disease.*

This prophylactic and therapeutic potential has been drawing an increasing number of like-minded researchers, dieticians, and food producers, especially in light of chronic disease proliferation in developing and industrialized populations [2]. They also benefit from the public's positive perception and an attitudinal shift away from 'avoidance' of specific foods to 'positive eating', allowing the food industry to successfully improve the potential for 'healthy eating' [3]. The world of dietary disease treatment is growing, and the functional food concept may be a lever of sufficient length to move it.

However, the *practice* of functional food usage leaves much to be desired. An idealized goal for functional food, in which the consumer-patient would be able to achieve therapeutic benefit from unprocessed foods, is severely hindered by natural produce variation. A basic variable such as water availability can significantly affect the production of bioactive compound and bulk biomass, making the "defined, effective" amount of a functional food neither [4]. And even if growth characteristics could be precisely controlled for each tuber and sprig, many food items are simply not feasible bioactive compound sources in the first place. For example, quercetin is a bioactive flavonoid that has demonstrated beneficial lipidemic effects in small-scale clinical trials [5]. But these trials used concentrated *Allium cepa* extracts containing 100 mg quercetin per daily dose–equivalent to 400 g of boiled onion, which is more than 16 times the average American's daily onion consumption as recorded in 2011 [6, 7]. Since a functional food cannot be a supplement or pill–it *must* be recognized as a food article and contribute to the consumer-patient's basal metabolism–many bioactive compound sources cannot provide enough bioactivity to be considered functional foods.

Therefore, many functional foods are manufactured, compounded, or otherwise processed to circumvent these limitations. A recent paper in the *Journal of Cereal Science* described development of a wheat pasta product functionalized with probiotic *Bacillus coagulans* culture, which lessened glycemic index impact in consuming subjects compared to nonfunctionalized pasta [8]. This effective functionalization hints at greater health benefits that could achieved by deliberately compounding bioactive agents in dietary staples–but why should food developers limit themselves to nature's preexisting pantry? This literature review will examine the successes and failures of food bioengineering, a few promising techniques and organisms for bioactive compound production, and the challenges still remaining in the biotechnological development of functionalized foods.

Genetic Modification in Food Products

A Golden Dream Deferred: As Western society entered the 21st century, the insufficient dietary intake of vitamin A and the resulting collection of pathologies that ensued cost the eyesight of 500,000 children in developing countries and the lives of an additional 670,000 [9]. Additionally, the optimal strategy to alleviate vitamin A deficiency (VAD) is a matter of scientific debate. Unfortunately, the vitamin A deficiency epidemic is not dire enough to rally the scientific community together and come to a consensus over decades of arguing. However, the VAD epidemic also provides a prototypical case of functional food usage to treat chronic conditions, and a stage for the introduction of a prototypical bioengineered functional food: Golden Rice, an engineered cereal capable of endogenous β-carotene synthesis. By functionalizing this pervasive dietary staple, provitamin-A could be feasibly cultivated in the local community and provided to afflicted children [10]. Although there are many dietary natural sources of provitamin-A in the world, they frequently require industrial processing and transport (e.g. palm oil) or are otherwise too expensive for the affected population to procure (e.g. animal meat).

The genetic engineering that produced Golden Rice (GR), and its more potent successor Golden Rice 2 (GR 2), was elegantly simple–partially because very little genomic information needed to be added. The more-refined transformation element (T-DNA) used in GR 2 (see Figure 1) contains only three expressed genes: a *SSUcrtI* carotene desaturase-RuBisCo chloroplast transit peptide fusion, a phytoene synthase (*psy*) gene from *Zea mays*, and a phosphomannose isomerase (*pmi*) gene that did not participate in pro-vitamin A synthesis, but was used for transformed rice calli selection [11]. The addition of *Z. mays psy* greatly improved pro-vitamin A production in

GR 2, a benefit that can be visibly appreciated compared to GR transformed with *psy* from *Narcissus pseudonarcissus* (see Figure 2). Transforming the plant pathogen *Agrobacterium tumefasciens* with the T-DNA element, to effect gene transfer to the rice through the bacterium's infectious capacity, is a relatively blunt instrument compared to more modern genetic engineering techniques (see below). Nonetheless, *A. tumefasciens* is still an effective vehicle for plant transformation, and sees use today [12].

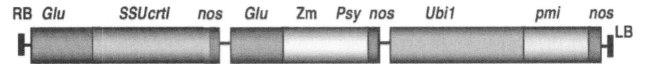

Figure 1: A schematic of the Golden Rice 2 T-DNA construct. This artificial DNA sequence combines the necessary genes for endogenous provitamin-A synthesis in Golden Rice. Glu and Ubi1 genes are promoters that help initiate gene expression, and nos is a terminator gene that signals the end of the gene sequence. SSUcrtI, Psy, and pmi are catalytic genes described in the text. [11]

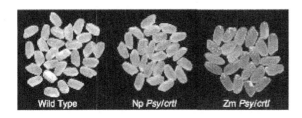

Figure 2: Visual comparison of carotenoid production in WT rice, and rice transformed with the respective N. pseudonarcissus and Z. mays psy transgenes. The Z. mays psy/crtI transgenic rice's higher color saturation indicates its proportionally greater saturation in β-carotene. [11]

Unfortunately, the Golden Rice story is also an ill portent of genetic modification's sociopolitical palatability, despite its explicit benefits to human health. Global regulatory attitudes towards the production of genetically modified crops vary, from generally receptive in the United States to hostile in the European Union. Between 1992 and 2014, US regulators approved 156 applications to plant GM crops and 170 to sell GM-derived food products, while their counterparts across the Atlantic approved 67 products and 6 cultivations [13]. The greatest encumbrance on the process is perhaps that any endorsement of a transgenic crop's safety by the European Food Safety Authority must be approved by the European Parliament–and one in three of its members vote on an explicit platform against genetic modification of *any* food source [14].

Nevertheless, the European Parliament's voting record is only one legislative reflection of global society's mixed opinion on transgenic food cultivation, ranging from the supportive to the antagonistic. Fear, uncertainty, and doubt have been spread by NGOs and competing agribusiness interests, portraying the acceptance of transgenic foods as reckless and predatory, and elected policymakers have complied with this portrayal [15, 16]. Although the rice would have been made freely available to impoverished farmers, the fact that it was developed under license with a major agricorporation gave it the cursory appearance of unethically exploiting vulnerable populations. Additionally, the recent retraction and censure of Tang *et al.*'s study on pro-vitamin A supplementation with Golden Rice in Chinese children, possibly the single best support for its humanitarian use as a functional food, has had crippling effects on further academic interest in GM functionalization (despite the distinct taint of political motivation behind Tufts University's ethical inquest) [17]. The potential benefits of Golden Rice have been suppressed for now, by a weakness to social pathogens rather than biological.

In an important exception, regulators in Japan–the place of origin for the formal functional food concept–have apparently become much more open to genetically modified foods. Between 1992 and 2003, 58 products and 5 plantings were approved there, and has increased to 129 products and 115 plantings between 2004 and 2014 [13]. However, very few globally approved transgenic crops have been designed with the intent of improved nutritional content; producers are more interested in increased production and pest resistance. This will likely change as interest in functional food applications continues to grow.

Newer Options for Genetic Engineering: In the time since GR was developed, more refined approaches to genetic engineering have been applied to crop plants with varying degrees of success. However, the three most prominently applied methods all make use of the target organism's own DNA-repairing pathways for effecting a stable and lasting transformation. The current greatest advance in engineering, the CRISPR/*Cas*9 complex, is a widely-applicable platform quickly being used in multiple domains of life. A DNA plasmid bearing the *Cas*9 nuclease and a guiding RNA sequence can affect genomic edits with high specificity and efficiency, but the guide RNA is much easier to alter for different targets than the peptide-based DNA-recognition sites of previous methods (see Fig. 3) [18]. CRISPR/*Cas*9 has already demonstrated its utility in a wide variety of plants, especially for multiple simultaneous gene insertions [19, 20]. Precisely adding synthetic or accumulative genes to food items, to grow designer functional foods in the soil, is becoming a much more *scientifically* feasible proposition than it was even five years ago.

It also has been suggested that, if the guiding RNA and *Cas*9 nuclease are introduced directly into a cell without a DNA intermediate, a resulting organism can be considered genetically unmodified under current laws and enjoy greater public support. [21] This contention is only relevant in the EU, where transgenic regulation focuses on the processes to introduce the transformative element used, rather than on the product yielded [22].

The relevant regulation in the US, 7 CFR 340, only gives the Department of Agriculture power over "the introduction of organisms and products altered or produced through genetic engineering which are plant pests or which there is reason to believe are plant pests." The only way 7 CFR 340 would apply to CRISPR/*Cas*9 engineering is if the introduced gene material comes from a plant pest, or if a plant pest such as a virus is used as the transformative agent [23]. Moreover, without an additional DNA template Kanchiswamy *et al.*'s ribonucleoprotein method can only silence a target gene, not augment or replace it, thereby severely reducing CRISPR/*Cas*9's usefulness.

Furthermore, it seems unlikely that the nuance between genetic editing and genetic modification will be appreciated, as the end result is still an organism whose genome has been altered by direct intervention. As long as elements of the public remain hostile to bioengineered agriculture, every GM crop will grow in a minefield of inflamed controversy. As a result, concluding that CRISPR/*Cas*9 will usher in a new era of genetic engineering for food functionalization is entirely premature at this stage, due to its novelty and public reticence, but the prospect is an unquestionably tantalizing one.

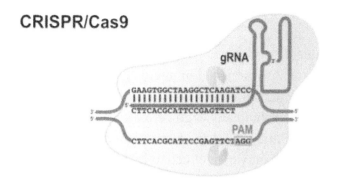

Figure 3: A simplified diagram of the CRISPR/Cas9 complex acting on a DNA strand. The red gRNA construct directs the nuclease activity to sequences with complementarity, provided they are immediately downstream of a protospacer adjacent motif (PAM) sequence specific to Cas9 from a given bacterial species. [21]

Future Direction: Transgenic Producers, Not Products

Algae for A Better Life: Embryophyta, or land plants, are by no means the only genetically engineered templates in development. Microalgal species have been favorite subjects for commodity production, realizing commercial and material value from fatty acid synthesis pathways [24]. The rich energy content of algal fatty acids, and their supposedly-sustainable production compared to fossil fuels, made biofuels the primary drivers of algal biotech development. However, the genetic engineering of microalgae to produce fuel compounds (including alcohols) represents a "fourth generation" of biofuel production methods, and still has yet to fulfill biofuel's promises of environmentally-conscious and economically competitive energy [25]. To expand the platform's utility, and provide alternative revenue streams in the meantime, engineers now offer a portfolio of microalgae-produced substances; these compounds find applications such as industrial lubricants, livestock feed, and consumer foods and cosmetics. In many circumstances compounds destined for different applications can be selectively isolated from the same culture, reducing the overall cost of production (see Fig. 4a) [24, 26].

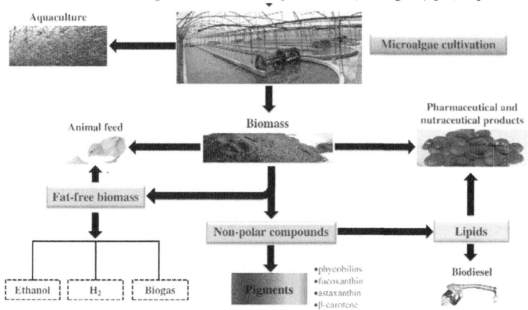

Figure 4a: A high-level conceptualization of the microalgal economy, where high-value compounds and bulk products can be produced and extracted in the same culture. The functional food community would most likely be interested in the production of biomass for pigments, lipids, and miscellaneous bioactive compounds. [23]

Polyunsaturated fatty acids (PUFAs, see Table 1), and the functional food researcher's host of bioactive compounds (see Table 2) are not only readily produced in microalgae but can also be produced in greater quantity per culture by biotechnological means [24]. Nevertheless, the entire point of algal culture for functional food production, metabolically engineered or not, is to improve consumer diet and health *en mass*. The cultivation of microalgae for consumption is still a niche market, despite its historical precedence, and a public already disinclined to eat microalgae is even less likely to be enticed by genetically modifying it.

Table 1: Useful Fatty Acids [26]	Structure	Example Microalgal Source
γ-Linolenic acid	18:3 ω6, 9, 12	*Arthrospira*
Arachidonic acid	20:4 ω6, 9, 12 ,15	*Porphyridium*
Eicosapentaenoic acid	20:5 ω3, 6, 9, 12, 15	*Nannochloropsis, Phaeodactylum, Nitzschia*
Docosahexanoic acid	22:6 ω3, 6, 9, 12, 15, 18	*Crypthecodinium, Schizochytrium*

Table 2: Other Microalgal Products	Properties and Uses	Example Microalgal Source
Phycoerythrin peptide [26]	Anti-inflammatory, antitumor, antiviral	Blue-green algae (Cyanobacteria, not considered a true algae but similarly cultivated)
Astaxanthin pigment [26]	Powerful antioxidant	*Haematococcus pluvialis*
β-carotene pigment [27]	Antioxidant, pro-vitamin A	*Dunaliella salina*
Fucoxanthin pigment [28]	Cytotoxicity, antioxidant, antiproliferative, proapoptotic	*Dunaliella salina*

This presumes that direct consumption, like with Golden Rice, is the only way to partake of microalgal health benefits. Part of the appeal of engineered microalgal food *ingredients* comes from their incorporation into food products already familiar to the consumer. A 2010 patent assigned to the microalgal biotech company Solazyme lists numerous prototypical recipes for common items such as a miso salad dressing, biscuits, pasta, and whole egg liquids; the use of algal flours, proteins, and oils improved these items' nutritional profiles and bioactive compound content without significant detriment to the consumer experience [29]. Bioactive compounds can also be added to foodstuffs by "natural" means–farmed fish fed a PUFA-enriched diet are a demonstrated vehicle for PUFAs to human consumers, although not necessarily in controlled amounts [24].

Defatting and other processing also ensures that the source organisms, engineered or wild type, do not reach the consumer. Many products are from completely unmodified algal strains, and the genetically modified microalgal source for Solazyme's AlgaWise cooking oil is as removed from the final product as any conventional oil-producing crop [30]. Microalgae-produced bioactive compounds added to products of conventional, or even "organic" provenance, creates functionalized foods that can curtail the concerns GM products instigate (philosophically- and politically-motivated objections notwithstanding). Isolating the engineered microalgae from the environment in contained growth conditions, and from the consumer by harvest and extraction of compounds, makes algal bioengineering the better biotechnological method of food functionalization.

Wilting the Algal Bloom: But even with Brooks *et al.*'s patent past its fifth anniversary, and the benefits of microalgae-derived functional foods repeatedly demonstrated, they have a practically non-existent presence in the market. Dietary microalgal cultivation suffers from the same issues that hampers its use in all its other applications. The main challenge continues to be the production of high-value compounds in a manner which is both economical (to maintain the company's viability) and sustainable (to maintain the microbial culture's) [25]. Biofuels have a theoretical environmental incentive by sequestering CO_2 greenhouse gas in carbon compounds, and microalgae are especially potent agents by consuming almost twice as much CO_2 to produce

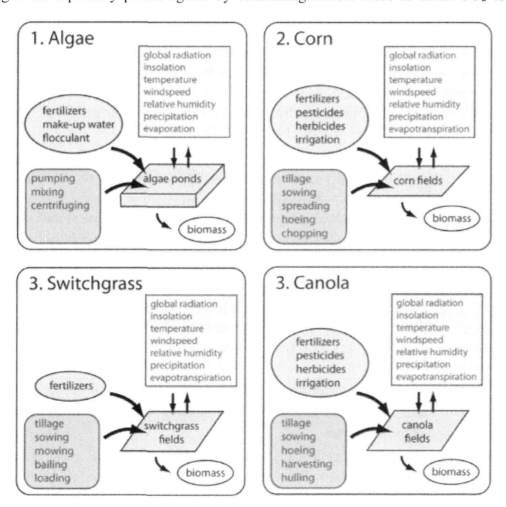

Figure 4b: Processes and materials involved in lgaculture, compared and contrasted with other bioenergy crops. Terms in red are physical materials, terms in green are environmental concerns, and terms in blue are mechanical processing steps. Although microalgal cultivation is radically different in handling its biomass, many of the same physical materials are necessary-especially nitrogen and phosphorus fertilizers-and all are subject to the same environmental effects. [30, coloration added by author]

biomass by weight [31]. The savage irony however is that current algaculture *produces* more CO_2 than it consumes–a bootstrapping problem as mechanical agitation, artificial light sources, fertilizer supplementation, biomass harvesting, and compound extraction still depend on cheaper fossil fuels. Simply put, microalgal cultivation is still agriculture, participating in its complex flux of nutrients and energy and hobbled by the same systematic shortcomings (see Figure 4b [32]).

This is less of a concern for bioactive compound production, since the energy the algae consumes is not the intended output (although it does still factor into economic feasibility). Instead bioactive compound makers have to contend with the secondary nature of the secondary metabolites. The natural rate of microalgal lipid production is too slow for producers to get around by simply scaling up operations, or by judiciously selecting their growing systems [33]. Bioactive compound producers are instead turning to genetic engineering like their biofuel colleagues, to make a given volume of culture more productive than the wild type alone [34].

Photosynthetic augmentation can improve both microalgal growth rate and pigment compound content, and the intricacies of microalgal fatty acid metabolism present numerous trajectories for scientists to pursue [35]. The less-than-stellar success of fatty acid engineering *so far* indicates the rudimentary understanding of this Gordian knot, which will be necessary for mass microalgal production of anything of value.

Current functional food application is frequently hampered by a dearth of foods suitable to the purpose. The concurrent advent of biotechnology means that producers and clinicians are not constrained by limited and precarious natural development. Biotechnology has already produced altered dietary staples that can safely induce real health benefits, but the social approval of genetically modified foodstuffs is inconsistent at best.

Modifying microalgae to produce micro and macronutrients, for harvest and incorporation into functional food products, provides the ideal specificity and reliability for bioactive compound use. However, its application in biomedical science is impeded by technical difficulty. It remains to be seen if microorganism engineering will be able to meet the needs of its many stakeholders, including the functional food community. Nonetheless, the prospect of a flourishing functional food market, and the healthier population it will bring about, certainly makes it worth a try.

SUMMARY

- ➤ Advances in genetic engineering have provided methods of purposefully designing functional foods and bioactive compound-producing organisms to combat nutrient-deficient and chronic diseases.
- ➤ The usage and benefits of genetically modified foods have been limited by the negative perception from the general public, raising concerns about the safety of foods labeled GMO.

➢ New gene editing techniques, such as CRISPR/Cas 9, offer a simple and efficient method for modifying the genome of targeted organisms to introduce desirable traits in a food ingredient or other organisms.

➢ Techniques of genetic modification have been applied to microorganism to mass produce various bioactive compounds found in functional foods.

REVIEW QUESTIONS

1. The Golden Rice is a genetically modified rice variety that increases the biosynthesis of
   a. Vitamin C
   b. Beta-carotene
   c. Calcium
   d. Magnesium

2. Which specific gene was changed to drastically increase the amount of the targeted nutrient in Golden Rice 2 compared to Golden Rice?
   a. Phytoene synthase (*psy*) gene from
   b. Phosphomannose isomerase (*pmi*) gene
   c. *SSU crtI* gene
   d. Ubi 1 gene

3. Which of the following is not a functional food ingredient produced by genetically engineering microalgae species?
   a. Beta-carotene
   b. Astaxanthin
   c. Polyunsaturated fatty acids
   d. Vitamin D

Answers: 1. **(B)** 2. **(A)** 3. **(D)**

REFERENCES:

1. Lawrence S. and Lahteenmaki R. 2014. Public biotech 2013--the numbers. Nature Biotechnology. 32(7):626–32.
2. Martirosyan D.M. and Singh J. 2015. A New Definition of Functional Food by FFC: What Makes a New Definition Unique? Functional Foods in Health and Disease. 5(6):209–23.
3. McConnon A., Cade J. and Pearman A. 2002. Stakeholder interactions and the development of functional foods. Public health nutrition. 5(3):469–77.
4. Wegener C. and Jansen G. 2013. Antioxidants in Different Potato Genotypes: Effect of Drought and Wounding Stress. Agriculture. 3(1):131–46.
5. Kim J., Cha Y.J., Lee K.H. and Park E. 2013. Effect of onion peel extract supplementation on the lipid profile and antioxidative status of healthy young women: a randomized, placebo-controlled, double-blind, crossover trial. Nutrition Research and Practice. 7(5):373.
6. 2011. U.S. Onion Statistics. usda.mannlib.cornell.edu.

7. Bhagwat S.A.,Haytowitz D.B. and Holden J.M. 2014. USDA database for the flavonoid content of selected foods. Release 3.1. 2014.

8. Fares C., Menga V., Martina A., Pellegrini N., Scazzina F. and Torriani S. 2015. Nutritional profile and cooking quality of a new functional pasta naturally enriched in phenolic acids, added with β-glucan and Bacillus coagulans GBI-30, 6086. Journal of Cereal Science. 65(C):260–6.

9. Svoboda P. and Flemr M. 2010. The role of miRNAs and endogenous siRNAs in maternal-to-zygotic reprogramming and the establishment of pluripotency. EMBO reports. 11(8):590–7.

10. Stein A.J., Sachdev H.P.S. and Qaim M. 2008. Genetic Engineering for the Poor: Golden Rice and Public Health in India. World Development. 36(1):144–58.

11. Paine J.A., Shipton C.A., Chaggar S., Howells R.M., Kennedy M.J., Vernon G.,Wright S.Y., Hinchliffe E., Adams J.L., Silverstone A.L. and Drake R. 2005. Improving the nutritional value of Golden Rice through increased pro-vitamin A content. Nature Biotechnology. 23(4):482–7.

12. Meng Z., Meng Z., Zhang R., Liang C., Wan J., Wang Y., Zhai H. and Guo S. 2015. Expression of the Rice Arginase Gene *OsARG* in Cotton Influences the Morphology and Nitrogen Transition of Seedlings. PLoS ONE. 10(11):e0141530.

13. Aldemita R.R., Reaño I., Solis R.O. and Hautca R.A. 2015. Trends in global approvals of biotech crops (1992–2014). GM crops & food. 6(3):150–66.

14. 2011. Approvals of GMOs in the European Union. europabio.org.

15. Blancke S., Van Breusegem F., De Jaeger G., Braeckman J. and Van Montagu M. 2015. Fatal attraction: the intuitive appeal of GMO opposition. Trends in Plant Science. 20(7):414–8.

16. Wesseler J. and Zilberman D. 2014. The economic power of the Golden Rice opposition. Environment and Development Economics. 19(6):724–42.

17. Dubock A. 2014. The politics of Golden Rice. GM Crops & Food. 5(3):210–22.

18. Lowder L.G., Zhang D., Baltes N.J., Paul J.W., Tang X., Zheng X., Voytas D.F., Hsieh T.F., Zhang Y. and Qi Y. 2015. A CRISPR/Cas9 Toolbox for Multiplexed Plant Genome Editing and Transcriptional Regulation. Plant Physiology. 169(2):971–85.

19. Lozano-Juste J. and Cutler S.R. 2014. Plant genome engineering in full bloom. Trends in Plant Science. 19(5):284–7.

20. Osakabe Y. and Osakabe K. 2015. Genome editing with engineered nucleases in plants. Plant and Cell Physiology. 56(3):389–400.

21. Kanchiswamy C.N., Malnoy M., Velasco R., Kim J.S. and Viola R. 2015. Non-GMO genetically edited crop plants. Trends in Biotechnology. 33(9):489–91.

22. Podevin N., Devos Y., Davies H.V. and Nielsen K.M. 2012. Transgenic or not? No simple answer! New biotechnology-based plant breeding techniques and the regulatory landscape. EMBO reports. 13(12):1057–61.

23. Pauwels K., Podevin N., Breyer D., Carroll D. and Herman P. 2014. Engineering nucleases for gene targeting: safety and regulatory considerations. New Biotechnology. 31(1):18–27.

24. Bellou S., Baeshen M.N., Elazzazy A.M., Aggeli D., Sayegh F. and Aggelis G. 2014.

Microalgal lipids biochemistry and biotechnological perspectives. Biotechnology Advances. 32(8):1476–93.

25. Lam M.K. and Lee K.T. 2012. Microalgae biofuels: A critical review of issues, problems and the way forward. Biotechnology Advances. 30(3):673–90.

26. Spolaore P., Joannis-Cassan C., Duran E. and Isambert A. 2006. Commercial applications of microalgae. JBIOSC. 101(2):87–96.

27. Lamers P.P. Janssen M., De Vos R.C.H., Bino R.J. and Wijffels R.H. 2008. Exploring and exploiting carotenoid accumulation in *Dunaliella salina* for cell-factory applications. Trends in Biotechnology. 26(11):631–8.

28. Freitas A.C., Rodrigues D., Rocha-Santos T.A.P., Gomes A.M.P. and Duarte A.C. 2012. Marine biotechnology advances towards applications in new functional foods. Biotechnology Advances. 30(6):1506–15.

29. Brooks G., Franklin S., Avila J. and Decker S.M. 2010. High Protein and High Fiber Algal Food Materials. (12):.

30. 2015. Algae oil: The next big healthy cooking oil? foodnavigator-usa.com. http://www.foodnavigator-usa.com/Suppliers2/Solazyme-algae-oil-The-next-big-healthy-cooking-oil.

31. Clarens A.F., Resurreccion E.P., White M.A. and Colosi L.M. 2010. Environmental Life Cycle Comparison of Algae to Other Bioenergy Feedstocks. Environmental Science & Technology. 44(5):1813–9.

32. Rosenberg J.N., Mathias A., Korth K., Betenbaugh M.J. and Oyler G.A. 2011. Microalgal biomass production and carbon dioxide sequestration from an integrated ethanol biorefinery in Iowa: A technical appraisal and economic feasibility evaluation. Biomass and Bioenergy. 35(9):3865–76.

33. Davis R., Aden A. and Pienkos P.T. 2011. Techno-economic analysis of autotrophic microalgae for fuel production. Applied Energy. 88(10):3524–31.

34. Radakovits R., Jinkerson R.E., Darzins A. and Posewitz M.C. 2010. Genetic engineering of algae for enhanced biofuel production. Eukaryotic Cell. 9(4):486–501.

35. Birkou M., Bokas D. and Aggelis G. 2012. Improving Fatty Acid Composition of Lipids Synthesized by *Brachionus plicatilis* in Large Scale Experiments. Journal of the American Oil Chemists' Society. 89(11):2047–55.

11

Classification of "Healthy" Food by Quantification of Nutrient Content based on Functional and Therapeutic Effect on Human Health

Marisol Ortiz[1] and Danik Martirosyan[2]

Introduction

According to the World Health Organization (WHO), obesity and conditions associated with being overweight are now linked to more deaths worldwide than conditions associated with being underweight, with exception to some areas of Sub-Saharan Africa and Asia [1]. Worldwide, the prevalence of obesity has nearly tripled since 1975 [1]. In 2016, over 1.9 billion adults (18+ years) were overweight (~39% of the population), and of these, 650 million adults were obese (~13% of the population) [1]. Among children and adolescents aged 5 to 19 years, the prevalence of overweight and obesity is alarming. The rates have risen from ~4% in 1975 to over ~18% in 2016 [1].

As the prevalence of obesity has increased, so has the rates for non-communicable diseases (NCDs) such as, cardiovascular diseases, type 2 diabetes, chronic obstructive pulmonary disease, chronic kidney disease, and certain types of cancer, and thus increasing the rates for premature death worldwide [1,2]. Apart from morbidity and mortality in populations, the prevalence of obesity and related NCDs show direct financial burden. According to the Centers for Disease Control and Prevention (CDC), in 2008, medicals costs of obesity in the United States were estimated to be $147 billion [3]. Globally, the economic impact of obesity in 2014 was estimated to be $2.0 trillion dollars or 2.8% of the global gross domestic product (GDP) [4]. In a systematic, meta-analysis review, results up to November 2014 suggested that cardiovascular disease attributed to the highest NCD healthcare expenditure with 12% to 16.5% of costs, and other NCDs ranging between 0.7% and 7.4% depending on the country, region, and type of NCD [5]. In addition, increase in costs was dependently related to severity and total years lived with the disease [5].

If the obesity trend continues to rise exponentially, by 2030 obesity-related medical costs alone could scale up to $48 to $66 billion a year in the United States [6]. Obesity is preventable. Diet and physical activity are important factors in prevention and in reducing the progression of chronic disease. A "healthy" diet is associated with health span and decreased risk of NCDs. Although general patterns delineate what a "healthy" diet should consist of, a wide variety of factors may influence and alter dietary choices. A diet rich in whole foods, primarily composed of plant-based foods carries attributes to a healthier lifestyle when compared to a highly-processed, energy-dense diet. Research suggests that dietary choices are influenced by a variety of factors including marketing and food-labeling, food cost, and food literacy to name a few.

This article provides an overview of the major concepts associated with a "healthy" diet. It highlights emerging scientific evidence in the fields of functional and bioactive food components and their role in health. In addition, this paper discusses food classification, the pros and cons of food labeling and the effect on dietary choices. The aim of this review is to present the need for food concept standardization and quantification of bioactive compounds in foods, both to enhance food and nutrition literacy among the public and to strive to decrease the risk of chronic disease through informed dietary choices.

Diet and Health

Diet and physical activity are main contributors to one's health. Globally, the dramatic rise of chronic diseases can be attributed to a shift to a high-energy dense diet complemented with a sedentary lifestyle. NCDs can be preventable and managed through proper nutrition – "healthy" eating – and exercise. However, what constitutes a "healthy" food may vary from person to person, even among health-care professionals.

Concepts of Food Commonly Associated as "Healthy"

Natural: To date, there is no official definition for the term "natural." In late 2015, the FDA received multiple Citizen Petitions that prompted the agency to release a request for comments on the use of the term on food labels. With more than 7,600 public comments posted, the FDA came with the following definition,

"Nothing artificial or synthetic (including all color additives regardless of source) has been included in, or has been added to, a food that would not normally be expected to be in that food" [7].

However, the FDA claims that this is not a formal definition as it does not address food processing or manufacturing methods, and also the term "natural" is not describing any nutritional or other health benefits [7].

Then USDA identifies the term "natural" in food labeling for meat and poultry products when demonstrating that: "the product does not contain any artificial flavor or flavoring, coloring ingredient, or chemical preservative, or any other artificial or synthetic ingredient; and the product and its ingredients are not more than minimally processed*. Minimal processing may include: (a) those traditional processes used to make food edible or to preserve it or to make it safe for human consumption, . . ., or (b) those physical processes which do not fundamentally alter the raw product and/or which only separate a whole, intact food into component parts" [8]. Moreover, for a product to have a "natural" claim, the USDA requires that the claim is accompanied by a brief statement explaining what is meant by the term natural [8].

Processed*: The term processed includes any food that has been purposely changed from its original state through cooking, canning, freezing, packaging or by changes in nutritional composition with fortifying, preserving or preparation methods [9]. Processed food may be minimally to heavily processed. Minimally processed foods are often simply pre-prepped for convenience (i.e. bagged or cut up vegetables and fruits, and roasted nuts). While among the most heavily processed foods are often pre-made meals such as frozen and microwaveable dinners.

As we can see, the term "natural" has little meaning when it comes to food labeling. No standard definition is established, and thus food manufacturers use the term liberally. While it is unlikely to expect the same from a natural apple as for a natural ice cream, many consumers base shopping preferences to a product so called "natural." This term is highly deceiving to consumers as processed products may still contain potentially damaging ingredients such as high fructose corn syrup and "natural flavors," which, in reality, are flavors produced in the laboratory (Figure 1).

Figure 1. Example of the term "Natural" in a processed product.

Frito-Lay by PepsiCo launched a "Natural" line of chips, which eventually turned into the Pure Deliciousness Simply product line. These products are the "healthy" version as they claim to be Non-GMO, with No artificial ingredients, and made with organic and fewer ingredients.

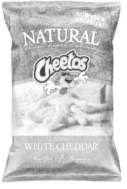

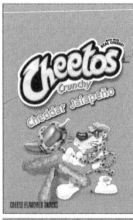

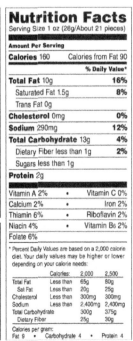

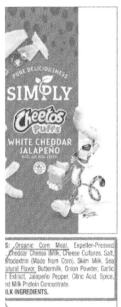

Organic: In comparison to "natural," the term organic is used to describe the way produce is grown, how animals are raised, and in processed foods, the methods of processing. For a food or agricultural product to be labeled as organic, it must be produced through approved methods by the USDA. These methods include integration of cultural, biological, and mechanical practices that promote ecological balance, and conserve biodiversity [10]. In addition, synthetic fertilizers, sewage sludge, irradiation, and genetic engineering are not approved approaches [10].

When it comes to animal products, it refers to the type of feed for the animals and beyond that, to the use of hormones and antibiotics given to raise these animals. For a packaged food to be labeled as organic, it must contain at least 95 percent organically produced raw or processed agricultural ingredients [11]. The remaining ingredients must be organically produced, unless are not commercially available in organic form. Whereas a label stating "made with organic ingredients," the product must contain 70 percent organic ingredients [11].

As to for fish and seafood, the USDA does not currently certify organic aquaculture production. The USDA National Organic Program (NOP) is in the process of developing standards for organic aquaculture practice. However, the proposed standards would only apply to the certification of farmed aquatic animals and their products [12].

Medical: As defined by the Orphan Drug Act, "medical food" is "a food which is formulated to be consumed or administered enterally under the supervision of a physician and which is intended for the specific dietary management of a disease or condition for which distinctive nutritional requirements, based on recognized scientific principles, are established by medical evaluation" [13].

Functional food: The Functional Food Center defines "functional foods" as "Natural or processed foods that contain biologically active compounds; which, in defined, effective non-toxic amounts, provide a clinically proven and documented health benefit utilizing specific biomarkers, for the prevention, management, or treatment of chronic disease or its symptoms" [14].
o A: to manage a disease as a whole
o B: for management of all symptoms
o C: to manage one specific symptom

FOSHU

Japan was the first country to define "Functional food" as "food products fortified with special constituents that possess advantageous physiological effects" [15] And in 1991 the term was changed to "Food for Specified Health Uses" (FOSHU) [16]. The food must satisfy the following three requirements:

- Effectiveness in clinical studies;
- Safety in clinical and non-clinical studies; and
- Determination of active/effective components

Current Dietary Recommendations for Health

USDA 2015-2020 Dietary Guidelines

The USDA has identified three patterns for healthy eating, one of them being the "Healthy U.S. – Style Eating Pattern," which is based on nutrient-dense ways and proportions of foods typically consumed by Americans. This eating pattern is designed to meet the Recommended Dietary Allowances (RDA) and Adequate Intakes for essential nutrients, and outlines the limits for other nutrients or food components set by the Dietary Guidelines [17]. For "healthy" eating, it is recommended to include a mix of foods from the five groups: a variety of vegetables from all five vegetable subgroups (dark green, red and orange, legumes, starchy and other); fruit (including whole fruits and 100% fruit juice); whole grains and limiting the intake of refined grains; dairy, focusing on fat-free and low-fat milk and dairy products; to include a variety of protein foods, both from animal and plant-based sources (seafood, lean meats and poultry, eggs, nuts, seeds and soy products; legumes are listed under the protein group and the vegetable group); and fats that contain a high percentage of monounsaturated and polyunsaturated fats, and that are liquid at room temperature [17]. Moreover, this Pattern remarks the importance to avoid added sugars or to limit to less than 10 percent of daily calories; for fat, the *Dietary Guidelines* recommend to limit saturated fats to less than 10 percent of calories per day and to limit the intake of *trans* fats to as low as possible; and according to the American Heart Association, a healthy eating pattern limits sodium to less than 2,300 mg per day. If alcohol is consumed, only adults of legal drinking age should consume it and in moderation (up to one drink per day for women and up to two drinks per day for men) [17].

The Mediterranean-Style Eating Pattern and the Healthy Vegetarian Eating Pattern are the other two patterns included in the 2015-2020 Dietary Guidelines by the USDA [18, 19]. The Healthy Vegetarian Pattern is an adaptation from the Healthy U.S.-Style Pattern with modifications on amounts from certain food groups to more closely reflect food intake self-reported by vegetarians in the National Health and Nutrition Examination Survey (NHANES) [19]. This Pattern excludes meat, poultry, and seafood, but dairy and eggs are included as were reported to be consumed by the majority of the vegetarians [19]. The pattern may be vegan if eggs are excluded and all dairy choices consist of fortified soy or other plant-based dairy substitutes [19]. All three Patterns are similar in meeting nutrient standards, however, the Healthy Vegetarian Pattern appears to be higher in calcium and fiber and lower in vitamin D due to the differences in the foods included.

Dietary Patterns Associated with "Healthspan"

First, what is healthspan? It is referred to the number of years a person lives free of disease – "healthy." The Mediterranean diet is among one of the most studied diets for its benefit on health and disease prevention and management. It is known that plant-based eating contributes to a healthy lifestyle. A plant-based pattern encourages whole, plant-based foods and discourages animal-based foods, as well as is limited in refined and highly processed foods.

The Longevity Diet and the Fast Mimicking Diet

A more recent dietary pattern, the Longevity Diet by Dr. Valter Longo, has shown to promote a healthy life span with reduced risk for diabetes, cardiovascular disease, Alzheimer's Disease, and cancer [22]. In addition to chronic disease prevention and management, the Longevity Diet has proven to help with weight management and to prevent age-related muscle and bone loss [22]. This diet is the result of over twenty-five years of research and is based on the Five Pillars of Longevity: Juventology/basic research, epidemiology, clinical studies, centenarian studies, and the study of complex systems [22]. To maximize a healthy lifespan while minimizing disease, the Longevity diet emphasizes in eight points: 1) to follow a diet close to 100 percent plant- and fish-based, limiting fish consumption to two or three portions a week; 2) to consume low but sufficient proteins, consume about 0.31 to 0.36 grams of protein per pound of body weight per day, and at age 65 years and older protein intake to be increased slightly; 3) to maximize intake of complex carbohydrates (whole grain, legumes and vegetables) and healthy fats (monounsaturated and polyunsaturated fats) with minimization of unhealthy fats (saturated, hydrogenated, and *trans* fats) and sugars; 4) to follow a diet with high vitamin and mineral content and complete it with a reputable multivitamin and mineral pill, plus an omega-3 fish oil soft gel every two to three days; 5) to include a variety of ingredients in the diet from your ancestry; 6) based on weight, age, and abdominal circumference, to have two or three meals per day plus a low-sugar snack; 7) to confine all eating within a twelve-hour period; and 8) to undergo five days of a fasting-mimicking diet (FMD) every one to six months, this up to age 65 to 70 years depending on weight and frailty.

Fasting or abstention or food has been a tradition for years in many ethnic groups and religions [22]. More research is signaling that fasting, either periodic or intermittent, portrays health benefits. In the book, "The Longevity Diet," Dr. Longo demonstrates through yeast, mice and human studies that fasting has demonstrated to promote stem cell-dependent regeneration in the immune system, nervous system, and pancreas. When the body switches from primarily sugar-burning mode to a fat-burning mode, this occurring during periods of abstention from food, it triggers the activation of "regenerative" programs. Given the health benefits associated with fasting, some programs, such as the Northern California's TrueNorth Health Center and the Buchinger Wilhelmi clinics in Germany, have their patients undergo fasts either of water only (TrueNorth) or deficit to very low calories per day (Buchingger Wilhelmi) [22]. For these types of regimens, it is important that patients convey the fast at a specialized institution and under medical supervision [22]. In contrast to the above programs, the five-day FMD by L-Nutra, can be safely carried out in the outpatient setting as long as the patient receives approval from their doctor with input from a registered dietitian or doctor who specializes in the use of FMD [22]. The effect of FMD on aging and healthy longevity can be explained through the following processes: cells switching to a protected anti-aging mode; by promoting autophagy and replacing damaged cells with functional ones; by activating stem cells in organs and systems; by shifting the body to a fat-burning mode even after reintroduction of a normal diet [22]. Just like animal studies have demonstrated benefits of the FMD, a randomized clinical trial of one hundred subjects carried out at the USC medical center portrayed promising results in the reduction risk for diabetes, cancer, and cardiovascular markers (Table 1).

Table 1. Reduction in risk factors for diabetes, cancer and cardiovascular diseases after three cycles of the FMD (one-hundred subjects randomized controlled trials) [p. 103]	
Weight loss	More than 8 pounds in obese subjects, mostly abdominal fat
Muscle mass	Increased relative to body weight
Glucose	12 mg/dL decrease in subjects with high fasting-glucose (prediabetes) A return to the normal range for subjects with prediabetes No effect in participants with low fasting-glucose
Blood pressure	6 mmHg decrease in subjects with moderately high BP No effect in subjects with low BP
Cholesterol	20 mg/dL decrease in participants with high cholesterol
IGF-1 (associated with a high cancer risk)	55 ng/mL decrease in participants in the higher-risk range
C-reactive protein (CRP; a risk factor for cardiovascular disease)	1.5 mg/dL decrease and, in most cases, a return to normal levels in participants with elevated CRP
Triglycerides	A 25 mg/dL decrease in participants with high triglycerides

In summary, vegetarian or predominately plant-based diets consistently suggest to decrease the risks for NCDs [20-22]. In general, these "diets" or "dietary pattern lifestyles" show that protective effects are related to the higher intake of whole, plant foods (e.g. fruits, vegetables, and complex carbohydrate) with limited intake of animal foods (if any) as well as discouraging added-sugar and highly-refined products. In comparison to animal protein and refined products, plants are unique in composition. Moreover, plants contain micronutrients and bioactive compounds linked with therapeutic effects for better health. It is important to also mention that additionally to a "healthy" diet, physical activity, sleep and other factors comprise a healthful lifestyle.

Bioactive Compounds

In addition to the interest in examining dietary patterns as a whole, there is an increased interest in research to examine the effect of specific nutrients or bioactive compounds on health and disease.

The term "bioactive" is defined by its Greek root for "bio," which is life, and the Latin root of "act," which is the drive or do [23]. Plants are the only natural source of these bioactive compounds. Phytochemicals for example, are bioactive compounds in plants that are responsible for their color, aroma, and taste [24]. Bioactive compounds are classified as either primary or secondary metabolites based on the function and ability to modulate metabolic processes [23]. Amino acids, carbohydrates, and lipids are primary metabolites, and just as for humans, these metabolites or macronutrients are essential for growth and basic metabolism of the organism [23]. In contrast, secondary metabolites are less abundant, with less than 1-5% of the plant's dry weight, and are not necessary for daily function [23]. Yet, the bioactive compounds in secondary metabolites have pharmacological and toxicological effects on humans and animals given their role in protection, attraction, and signaling [23].

Bioactive compounds are further classified as nutritive - such as proteins, carbohydrates, lipids, vitamins, and minerals - and non-nutritive - which are identified for health-promoting benefits. Non-nutritive bioactive compounds include phytochemicals and antioxidants. These compounds have been linked with health promotion and reduction of chronic disease, cancer amongst the most studied NCD linked to intake of phytochemical-rich foods. Even with the evidence on the role of phytochemicals in DNA repair for their antioxidant properties, there is no congruent evidence to date that suggests specific recommendations for intake [24].

Given that bioactive compounds vary in structure, physiological mechanism and concentration dependable in the environment where are sourced, in addition to bioavailability depending on extraction methods and that work synergistically, the specific dosage to impart health benefits remains questionable. However, bioactive compounds in their "natural" state, in food, impart the best benefits.

Determinants to Food Choices

When it comes to eating habits, a variety of factors may influence dietary choices. A number of concepts are used by society to classify food as "healthy" or "unhealthy." Additionally, society is bombarded with non-scientific nutrition information (i.e. fad diets and trends) that may create some dilemma to whether a food or food product is "healthy" or not. Ideally, one should strive to get essential vitamins, minerals and other nutrients mostly from a diet rich in whole foods. Packaged foods, those that are minimally processed, can be part of a healthy diet; however, many packaged foods today are claiming additional health benefits. For example, protein is now being added to many products, from cereals to juices, many products tempt with claims of antioxidants and omega-3s, and probiotics are also a popular ingredient in processed foods. The food industry can influence consumer's food purchasing with all these marketing and labeling techniques. The use of health- and nutrient-claims can dictate the likelihood to select one food over another. When evidence-based nutrition information is not properly communicated and consumers have limited nutrition literacy, it may result in less desirable dietary choices by the public, accompanied by a compromise public health. Food literacy is related to skills and abilities that include knowledge of food, an understanding of the relationship between food and health, the skills needed to make healthy food choices and preparation, and self-efficiency [2].

Label Claims

Food labeling plays an important role when it comes to food choices. Consumers are heavily influenced by the information provided on the front of the package, and all those labels and health claims can be confusing. The Food and Drug Administration is the governing body in the United States that is concerned with all food and drug related products and thus to enforce safety protocols [25]. The FDA requires food labeling for most prepared foods; however, nutritional labeling for raw produce and fish is voluntary [26]. Labels in food and dietary supplements may contain claims under the statute and/or FDA regulations. The FDA categorizes these claims into health claims, nutrient content claims, and structure/function claims.

Health Claims

According to the FDA, a "health claim" has two main components "(1) a substance (whether a food, food component, or dietary ingredient) and (2) a disease or health-related condition." An example would be "adequate calcium throughout life may reduce the risk of osteoporosis."

On September 27, 2016 the FDA announced that a public process to redefine the "healthy" nutrient content claim for food labeling had started [27]. This was meant to help consumers to make quick and easy food choices that align with public health recommendations, as well as to encourage the food industry to develop healthier products [27]. However, food manufactures could continue to use the term "healthy" on foods that met the current regulatory definition as long as certain criteria as described in the guidance document were met [27].

With latest nutrition research and the current dietary recommendations per the 2015-2020 *Dietary Guidelines,* which emphasize in dietary patterns as a whole, the FDA's re-evaluation for "healthy" claims shifted their regulatory views in two areas:

- **Fat**: foods can use the term "healthy" even if they are not necessarily low in fat, as long as the fat profile is predominantly made of mono and polyunsaturated fats [28].
- **Nutrients**: previously, the term "healthy" focused on foods providing a good or excellent source of vitamin A, vitamin C, iron, calcium and dietary fiber, as these were nutrients of public concern. However, concern of nutrient intake has now shifted to potassium and vitamin D, in addition to iron and calcium. For this reason, the claim "healthy" can be used in the label if the food contains at least ten percent of the Daily Value (DV) per reference amount customarily consumed (RACC) or potassium and vitamin D [28].

Nutrient Content Claims

Nutrient content claims are limited to nutrients (Table 2) that are mandated or are voluntarily in the Nutrition Facts and that have an FDA-established Daily Value (DV). Even though these must comply with all FDA definitions and regulations, nutrient content claims can be used in labels without review by the FDA. In contrast, USDA-regulated products must receive USDA approval to place the nutrient content claim on the label. These claims may be used for both conventional foods and dietary supplements.

Table 2. Nutrients that qualify for nutrient content claims:		
Total calories	Niacin	*When threshold levels for fat, cholesterol, saturated fat or sodium are exceeded, the claim must be accompanied with: **SEE NUTRITION PANEL FOR** (NAME OF NUTRIENT) **CONTENT.**
*Total fat	Vitamin B_6	
*Saturated fat	Folate	
*Cholesterol	Vitamin B_{12}	
*Sodium	Biotin	
Potassium	Pantothenic acid	**Although there is no DV for choline or ALA & DHA omega-3 fatty acids and these nutrients are not mandatory or voluntary for Nutrition Facts, these are allowable per FDA to be used in claims.
Dietary fiber	Iodine	
Sugars	Magnesium	
Protein	Zinc	
Vitamin A	Selenium	
Vitamin C	Copper	
Calcium	Manganese	
Iron	Chromium	
Vitamin D	Molybdenum	
Vitamin E	Chloride	
Vitamin K	**Choline	
Thiamin	**ALA & DHA omega-3s	
Riboflavin		

Table 3. Classification for Nutrient Content Claims [29].	
ABSOLUTE NUTRIENT CONTENT CLAIMS are direct statements about the level of a nutrient in the product	
Free	The product's reference amount and labeled serving contains an insignificant* amount of: total fat, saturated fat, cholesterol, sodium, sugars or calories. *Insignificant means that the amount may be rounded to zero, per FDA rounding rules.* Synonyms: *zero, no, without, trivial source of, negligible source of* and *dietary insignificant source of.*
Low	Refers to a product that could be eaten frequently without exceeding the guidelines for: total fat, saturated fat, cholesterol, sodium or calories. Synonyms: *little, few* (for calories), *contains a small amount of* and *low source of. Very low* is only used in respect to sodium levels.

- When using *free* or *low* on a product that has not been specifically processed or altered to qualify for the claim, the manufacturer must indicate that the food inherently qualifies for the claim (e.g., peanut butter, a cholesterol-free food).

- FDA has not defined nutrient content claims for trans-fat, therefore it is not permissible to use the words *free* or *low* (or their synonyms) to describe trans-fat levels (e.g., trans fat free, no trans-fat and zero trans-fat are unauthorized nutrient content claims). However, 0g trans-fat per serving is allowed as a statement of fact.

- FDA has not defined nutrient content claims for carbohydrate; therefore, it is not permissible to use the words *free* or *low* (or their synonyms) to describe carbohydrate levels (e.g., no carbs, carb free and low carb are unauthorized nutrient content claims). However, Xg carb per serving is allowed as a statement of fact as long as it is simply a repeat of information from the Nutrition Facts and does not imply a level.

- FDA has not provided a definition for *low sugar*, therefore this claim cannot be used. However, *sugar free*, *reduced sugar* and *no added sugar* claims are allowed as long as the food includes the required calorie and/or disclosure statements adjacent to the claim.

- If a claim is made about fatty acids or cholesterol, then polyunsaturated fat and monounsaturated fat must be included in the Nutrition Facts (or Supplement Facts) unless the product is fat free. Additionally, specific disclosure about total fat and cholesterol levels must be included directly next to the claim when certain threshold levels are exceeded.

For dietary supplements: Claims for total fat, saturated fat and cholesterol can be made only if the product is greater than 40 calories per serving. Claims for calories can be made only when a similar product exists that contains over 40 calories per serving.

Lean	May be used to describe meat, poultry, seafood and game meat; criteria are different for mixed foods, main dishes and meals. It means: < 10g fat, ≤ 4.5g saturated fat, and < 95mg cholesterol per reference amount or per 100g (whichever is larger).
Extra lean	May be used to describe meat, poultry, seafood and game meat; criteria are different for mixed foods, main dishes and meals. It means: < 5g fat, < 2g saturated fat, and < 95mg cholesterol per reference amount or per 100g (whichever is larger).

Good source	Means the reference amount of a product contains 10-19% of DV for a particular nutrient. Synonyms: *contains* and *provides*.
High	Means the reference amount of a product contains ≥ 20% of DV for a particular nutrient. Synonyms: *excellent source* and *rich in*. • *Good source* and *high* cannot be used to describe nutrients and functional components without an FDA-established DV (i.e. cannot be used to describe carotenoids, flavonoids, etc.). • If a protein claim is made, then the Nutrition Facts (or Supplement Facts) must include the % DV from protein based on specific protein quality factors.
High Potency	Means the vitamin or mineral is present in a product at ≥ 100% of the RDI per reference amount; the nutrient in the claim must be identified. It can also be used to describe a conventional food or dietary supplement when the product contains ≥ 100% RDI for at least two-thirds of vitamins and minerals with DVs present in the product at ≥ 2%
Modified	May be used in statement of identity of a food that bears a relative claim (e.g., "Modified fat cheesecake, contains 35% less fat than our regular cheesecake").
Fiber Source	Is a fiber claim is made and the food does not qualify as a low fat food, then the fiber claim must be accompanied by a disclaimer that discloses the level of total fat per labeled serving.
Antioxidants	The term "antioxidant" can be used in a claim as long as the antioxidant is named, each nutrient must have existing scientific evidence of antioxidant activity, has an FDA-established DV, and qualifies for the *good source, high* or *more* claim (e.g., high in antioxidant vitamin C). • Beta-carotene may be the subject of an antioxidant claim when the level of vitamin A present as beta-carotene in the food is sufficient to qualify for the claim.

ALTERNATIVE NUTRIENT CONTENT CLAIMS compare the level of nutrients of one product to another.

More	Means that the reference of a product (whether altered or not) contains ≥ 10% of the DV of a nutrient than the reference product. It also applies to *fortified, enriched, added,* and *plus* claims but, unlike *more*, these terms can only be used to describe foods that have been altered.
Less	Means that the reference of a product (whether altered or not) contains ≤ 25% of the DV of a nutrient than the reference product. It also applies to *fewer,* which can be used to describe calories.
Reduced	Means that the reference amount of a nutritionally-altered product contains ≤ 25% of a nutrient than the reference product. This definition also applies to *lower*.
Light	Means that the reference amount of a nutritionally-altered product contains 50% less fat or 1/3 fewer calories than the reference product. • For products > 50% calories from fat, the claim must be met on the basis of 50% less fat (not 1/3 fewer calories). For products with < 50% calories from fat, the claim can be met on either the calorie or fat basis. • A *light* claim is not allowed on products when the reference product is low calorie (≤ 40 calories) or low fat (≤ 3g fat), unless the sodium of such a products is reduced by 50%.

According to a meta-analysis and systematic review, findings suggest that health-related and nutrition-related claims increase the likelihood to choose a product compared to an identical product without the claim [30]. However, health-related claims appear to have a larger effect on purchasing and consumption of a food product when compared to a nutrition claim [30]. Given that multiple articles included in the above review were studies in an artificial setting, the authors discuss that further research is needed to conclude the actual effect health- and nutrition-related claims have on real-life dietary choices [30].

Food Classification

When it comes to food classification, it is known that three major components, known as macronutrients, constitute an overall diet. In addition to these three major groups - proteins, carbohydrates and fats - micronutrients, including vitamins and minerals, are essential in nutrition. Food is classified in groups and subgroups based in nutrients and/or other bioactive food components that are known or believed to be important for health [31, 32]. According to Rahman and McCarthy, proper classification of food and terminology used are essential for scientists and engineers for purposes in preservation, packaging, processing, storage, marketing and consumption [33]. In their paper, they identify four classes of food properties: physical and physico-chemical properties, kinetic properties, sensory properties, and health properties [33]. However, they discuss that there is a need to develop rules of classification as well as clear definitions of individual properties as some foods may possess two properties, which make it challenging to clear-cut distinction between the properties [33].

The Use of Databases in Food Classification

Food composition databases are used by scientists and the food industry to categorize foods based on the nutrient or other bioactive components. The selection of nutrients and other food components included are likely to be based on basic need for information, concerns of health problems in the country, the state of current thinking in the nutritional and toxicological sciences, availability of existing data, existence of adequate analytical methods, the feasibility of analytical work, and national and international nutrition labelling regulations [32]. Moreover, database systems may use a concise, comprehensive or reference form of classification [32].

If we take a look into different ways of food classification, for example in studies looking into food purchase patterns, classification varies depending on the country studied and the target population. In a German study, a total of 12 million food purchases from 13,125 households were recorded to look into existing patterns, the level of diet quality and factors associated with the identified patterns in that specific population [34]. The German Food Guide Pyramid was used to classify the scheme of foods [34]. A total of 1954 foods were classified into eighteen groups based on energy and nutrient densities, fiber, fatty acid composition, known preservative effects on the prevalence of chronic diseases [34]. Furthermore, a factor analysis was applied for the identification of food purchase patterns: factor 1) **Natural** included foods that are natural and unprocessed (*healthy foods*); factor 2) **Processed** included mainly combined foods that are industrially processed such as refined grain products, sweets and snacks, low fat milk products, and margarine; and factor 3) **Traditional** was assigned to those that showed higher loadings for all kinds of meat and in the plant-based food group higher loadings appeared predominantly for potatoes [34].

The Role of Food Classification in Diet Quality

As diet quality, in complement to physical activity, are important in disease prevention and management, there is a higher interest in identifying ways to assess "healthy" lifestyle behaviors, especially when it comes to diet quality. "Dietary Quality Indices or Indicators (DQIs) are algorithms aiming to evaluate the overall diet and categorize individuals according to the extent to which their eating behavior is 'healthy'" [35]. DQIs are based on current nutrition knowledge, primarily to assess dietary risk factors for NCDs. Although there exist multiple types of DQIs, the three major categories are: a) nutrient-based indicators; b) food/food group based indicators; and c) combination indexes [35].

As discussed earlier, fruits and vegetables, and whole grains are known to play a role in health and disease prevention and management. DQIs may include these food components as either grouped together or separately. The Healthy Eating Index (HEI), the Diet Quality Index (DQI), the Healthy Diet Indicator (HDI) and the Mediterranean Diet Score (MDS) are the 'original' four diet quality scores, which have been most widely referred to and validated in diet quality research [35]. However, the nutrients included and the scores in diet quality differ in each of these and among other DQIs.

Beyond overall diet quality tools, that focus on specific groups and nutrients, there is a need to provide diet quality assessment tools in food safety to the public. Functional, medicinal and therapeutic food, are terms that have been around for ages. Many civilizations have used "food as medicine," and now with the increasing rates of obesity and NCDs, there is higher interest in identifying the role of bioactive compounds in the prevention and management of disease.

"According to Dr. Martirosyan, two important concepts relating to bioactive compounds are: the amount of bioactive compounds and ratio of bioactive compounds to convert an ordinary food into a functional food" [15]. The current research and scientific evidence for bioactive compounds remains relatively new. Vitamin C in oranges, lycopene in tomatoes, curcumin in turmeric, to name a few, are examples of known active ingredients in these foods that in certain amounts exert health benefits. However, these same foods may contain other 'unknown' bioactive compounds that can either have a health benefit or possess a toxic level when ingested to the therapeutic dosage that the other bioactive compound is recommended for health benefits.

In addition to essential nutrients and compounds found naturally in food that may result in negative impact to health when consumed in inadequate amounts, there are other considerations to take in food consumption and diet quality. With the shifts in farming and food production, there are concerns to food safety. For example, additives, pesticides, other contaminants, and genetically modified foods (GMOs), among others, when consumed in certain amounts have demonstrated detrimental effects on health. A 2014 report on seafood safety by the Environmental Working Group (EWG), explored the controversy between the FDA/Environmental Protection Agency (EPA) guidelines of fish consumption and methylmercury exposure [37]. Per recommendations, fish and seafood consumption is part of a "healthy" diet. As discussed above, food may contain bioactive compounds, in this case – omega-3 fatty acids, which possess health benefits. However, amounts of omega-3 fatty acids and mercury levels differ from one seafood variety to another.

Page | 250

Then, it is important to keep the public informed of the seafood choices and their quantity to keep their intake within a "healthy" diet and safe limits.

A field that is commonly questioned is the impact of organic food vs. conventional food in respect to health. In a comprehensive review, the findings from human studies in regard to organic food consumption remain insufficient to deduct the actual health benefits. There is some evidence suggesting that organic food consumption may reduce risk of allergenic reactions, overweight and obesity, and other NCDs, however, evidence is inconclusive as there is some association between organic food consumption, "healthier" diet (higher fruit and vegetable consumption), as well as other lifestyle behaviors associated. However, at difference to organic foods, conventional foods are exposed to pesticides and other residues that have been encountered to have adverse effects health and increase the risk for disease [1,36].

Given the potential harms from pesticides and residues, through analysis of tests, the EWG's Dirty Dozen and Clean Fifteen (Figure 1) lists are good tools to guide the consumer in produce shopping. The Dirty Dozen highlights the produce with the highest loads of pesticide residues, therefore, it is recommended to buy organic versions of these foods. While the Clean Fifteen is a list of produce least likely to contain traces of pesticides, and thus, conventional produce would be considered safe to consume [37].

Figure 1. EWG's 2017 Shopper's Guide to Pesticide in Produce™	
Dirty Dozen	**Clean Fifteen**
1. Strawberries	1. Sweet corn*
2. Spinach	2. Avocados
3. Nectarines	3. Pineapples
4. Apples	4. Cabbage
5. Peaches	5. Onions
6. Pears	6. Sweet peas frozen
7. Cherries	7. Papayas*
8. Grapes	8. Asparagus
9. Celery	9. Mangos
10. Tomatoes	10. Eggplant
11. Sweet bell peppers	11. Honeydew melon
12. Potatoes	12. Kiwi
	13. Cantaloupe
	14. Cauliflower
	15. Grapefruit
* A small amount of sweet corn, papaya and summer squash sold in the United States is produced from genetically modified seeds. Buy organic varieties of these crops if you want to avoid genetically modified produce.	

What We Propose – Classification of Foods Based on Functional Content and Therapeutic Effect

The term "healthy" is a food descriptor that is open to interpretation, just as the term "natural" is. When it comes to dietary patterns and health, science supports the health benefits of eating predominantly plant-based – including a variety of vegetables, fruits, whole grains, nuts, seeds, and legumes – compared to an eating pattern rich in highly processed, energy dense foods. However, there are exceptions to certain processed and packages foods. As mentioned early in this review, foods be minimally or highly processed. And thus, some processed foods can be part of a healthful lifestyle.

The aim of this review is to address the need of food classification, with special focus in quantifying functional content (either from vitamins, minerals or other bioactive compounds) and its relation to the health and therapeutic effects of food products. As described earlier, *Functional Foods* are "natural or processed foods that contain biologically active compounds; which, in defined, effective non-toxic amounts, provide a clinically proven and documented health benefit utilizing specific biomarkers, for the prevention, management, or treatment of chronic disease or its symptoms" [14]. The Functional Food Center has further classified functional food in three categories: A) manage a single symptom, B) manage multiple symptoms, and C) manage the disease as a whole.

The Code of Federal Regulations by the FDA specifies the requirements for claims, such as for Nutrient Content Claims. The terms *good source*, *high*, and *high potency*, are relevant for our purpose in the classification of foods related to their health effects. Based on the criteria for a product to hold one these nutrient content claims and based on the categories (A, B, C) of functional food by the FFC, then a product can be spotted as "healthy" by the consumer.

The missing piece is to determine and quantify the specific amount needed of that nutrient (vitamin, mineral, or other bioactive compound) for management and treatment of disease. This quantification of dosage of functional nutrients for their therapeutic effects is for scientists to determine by investigation in clinical trials. Then, based on the scientific evidence for the dosage (as quantity) of the specific vitamin, mineral or bioactive compounds that portrays health benefits, a nutrient claim can be further required to specify whereas the product contains X amount of this nutrient to treat or manage X symptoms, XY symptoms, or X disease.

Table 7. Specific Requirement for *Good source*, *High*, and *High Potency* in Nutrient Content Claims.	
Good source	Means the reference amount of a product contains 10-19% of DV for a particular nutrient. Synonyms: *contains* and *provides*.
High	Means the reference amount of a product contains $\geq$ 20% of DV for a particular nutrient. Synonyms: *excellent source* and *rich in*. • *Good source* and *high* cannot be used to describe nutrients and functional components without an FDA-established DV (i.e. cannot be used to describe carotenoids, flavonoids, etc.). • If a protein claim is made, then the Nutrition Facts (or Supplement Facts) must include the % DV from protein based on specific protein quality factors.
High Potency	Means the vitamin or mineral is present in a product at $\geq$ 100% of the RDI per reference amount; the nutrient in the claim must be identified.

> It can also be used to describe a conventional food or dietary supplement when the product contains ≥ 100% RDI for at least two-thirds of vitamins and minerals with DVs present in the product at ≥ 2%.

SUMMARY

➢ According to the Functional Food Center, functional food is defined as "natural or processed foods that contain biologically active compounds; which, in defined, effective non-toxic amounts, provide a clinically proven and documented health benefit utilizing specific biomarkers, for the prevention, management, or treatment of chronic disease or its symptoms."

➢ The USDA Dietary Guidelines 2015-2020 identified three eating patterns for healthy eating: Healthy U.S. Style Eating Pattern, Mediterranean-Style Eating Pattern, and the Healthy Vegetarian Eating Pattern.

➢ Label claims such as health claims and nutrient content claims are important determinants of consumers' food choices.

REVIEW QUESTIONS

1. Any food that has been purposely changed from its original state through cooking, canning, freezing, packaging or by changes in nutritional composition with fortifying, preserving or preparation methods
   a. Organic Food
   b. Natural Food
   c. Processed Food
   d. Functional Food
2. Which of the following about the definition of organic food is false?
   a. Processed foods cannot be organic
   b. It describes how produce is grown
   c. It describes how animals are raised
   d. It describes the methods of processing
3. For a packaged food to be labeled as organic, it must contain
   a. 25 percent organically grown, raw ingredients
   b. 95 percent organically produced raw or processed agricultural ingredients
   c. No processed ingredients
   d. None of the above
4. Which of the following is not one of the three patterns that the USDA has identified for healthy eating?
   a. The Mediterranean-Style Eating Pattern
   b. The Paleo-Style Eating Pattern
   c. The Healthy Vegetarian Eating Pattern
   d. All of the above are identified by the USDA as healthy eating patterns
5. Non-nutritive bioactive compounds include...
   a. Phytochemicals
   b. Antioxidants
   c. Minerals
   d. A & B
6. The FDA says that nutritional labeling for which of the following is voluntary?

    a. Raw produce
    b. Prepared foods
    c. Meat
    d. None of the above

7. Foods can use the term "healthy" if they
    a. Are low in fat
    b. Have no fat
    c. Have mostly mono/polyunsaturated fats
    d. Have no trans fat

8. Which of the following cannot be used to describe the amount of sugar in a food?
    a. Low sugar
    b. Sugar free
    c. No added sugar
    d. Reduced sugar

9. How much of a nutrient must be in a food for the label to call it a "good source"?
    a. 30-39% DV
    b. 50-59% DV
    c. 5-9% DV
    d. 10-19% DV

10. Which of the follow pairs of foods with their bioactive ingredient is correct?
    a. Vitamin C in tomatoes
    b. Lycopene in oranges
    c. Curcumin in turmeric
    d. All the above are correct pairings

Answers: 1. **(C)** 2. **(A)** 3. **(B)** 4. **(B)** 5. **(D)** 6. **(A)** 7. **(C)** 8. **(A)** 9. **(D)** 10. **(C)**

REFERENCES:
1. Obesity and overweight [http://www.who.int/mediacentre/factsheets/fs311/en/]
2. Doustmohammadian A, Omidvar N, Keshavarz-Mohammadi N, Abdollahi M, Amini M, Eini-Zinab H: Developing and validating a scale to measure Food and Nutrition Literacy (FNLIT) in elementary school children in Iran. PLosS ONE 2017, 12(6).
3. Adult Obesity Causes & Consequences [https://www.cdc.gov/obesity/adult/causes.html]
4. Trammel M, Gerdtham UG, Nilsson PM, Saha S: Economic of Obesity: A Systematic Literature Review. Int J Environ Res Public Health 2017, 14:435.
5. Muka T, Imo D, Jaspers L, et al.: The global impact of non-communicable diseases on healthcare spending and national income: a systematic review. Eur J Epidemiol 2015, 30:251-277.
6. Economic Costs [https://www.hsph.harvard.edu/obesity-prevention-source/obesity-consequences/economic/]
7. "Natural" on Food Labeling [https://www.fda.gov/Food/GuidanceRegulation/GuidanceDocumentsRegulatoryInformation/LabelingNutrition/ucm456090.htm]
8. USDA Natural Definition [http://www.redarrowusa.com/_uploads/resources/USDA_Natural_Definition_Statement.pdf]

9. Processed Foods: What's OK and What to Avoid [https://www.eatright.org/food/nutrition/nutrition-facts-and-food-labels/processed-foods-whats-ok-and-what-to-avoid]

10. Organic Production & Handling Standards [https://www.ams.usda.gov/publications/content/organic-production-handling-standards]

11. Subpart D – Labels, Labeling, and Market Information [https://www.ecfr.gov/cgi-bin/text-idx?c=ecfr&sid=c4e0df8f46a4f4b6f56d80be31f95ed3&rgn=div6&view=text&node=7:3.1.1.9.32.4&idno=7#se7.3.205_1300]

12. Organic Aquaculture [https://www.nal.usda.gov/afsic/organic-aquaculture]

13. Frequently Asked Questions About Medical Foods; Second Edition [https://www.fda.gov/downloads/Food/GuidanceRegulation/GuidanceDocumentsRegulatoryInformation/UCM500094.pdf]

14. Welcome to Functional Food Center [http://functionalfoodscenter.net]

15. Martirosyan DM, Singh J: A new definition of functional food by FFC: what makes a new definition unique?. Functional Foods in Health and Disease 2015, 5(6):209-223.

16. Bailey R: Functional Foods in Japan: FOSHU ("Foods for Specified Health Uses") and "Foods with Nutrient Functions Claims." Regulation of Functional Foods and Nutraceuticals: A Global Perspective. 1st edition. Edited by Hasler CM. Iowa: Blackwell Publishing; 2005:247-262.

17. Dietary Guidelines 2015-2020. Chapter 1: Key Elements of Healthy Eating Patterns [https://health.gov/dietaryguidelines/2015/guidelines/chapter-1/a-closer-look-inside-healthy-eating-patterns/]

18. Dietary Guidelines 2015-2020. Appendix 4: USDA Food Patterns: Healthy Mediterranean-Style Eating Pattern [https://health.gov/dietaryguidelines/2015/guidelines/appendix-4/]

19. Dietary Guidelines 2015-2020. Appendix 5: USDA Foods Patterns: Healthy Vegetarian Eating Pattern [https://health.gov/dietaryguidelines/2015/guidelines/appendix-5/]

20. Le LT, Sabate J: Beyond Meatless, the Health Effects of Vegan Diets: Findings from the Adventist Cohorts. Nutrients 2014, 6:2131-2147.

21. Orlich MJ, Fraser GE: Vegetarian diets in the Adventist Health Study 2: a review of initial published findings. Am J Clin Nutr 2014, 100(1): 353S-358S.

22. Longo V: The Longevity Diet. New York: Avery; 2018.

23. Martirosyan DM, Pisarski K: Bioactive Compounds: Their Role in Functional Food and Human Health, Classifications, and Definitions. Functional Foods in Health and Disease 201

24. Thomas R, Butler E, Macchi F, Williams M: Phytochemicals in cancer prevention and management?. BJMP 2015, 8(2): a815.

25. Martirosyan DM, Singharaj B: Health Claims and Functional Food: The Future of Functional Foods under FDA and EFSA Regulation. Functional Foods for Chronic Diseases 2016, 410-424.

26. Labeling & Nutrition [https://www.fda.gov/Food/LabelingNutrition/default.]

27. FDA to Redefine "Healthy" Claim for Food Labeling [https://www.fda.gov/Food/NewsEvents/ConstituentUpdates/ucm520703.htm]

28. Use of the Term "Healthy" in the Labeling of Human Food Products: Guidance for Industry [https://www.fda.gov/downloads/Food/GuidanceRegulation/GuidanceDocumentsRegulatoryInformation/UCM521692.pdf]

29. CFR – Code of Federal Regulations Title 21 [https://www.accessdata.fda.gov/scripts/cdrh/cfdocs/cfcfr/CFRSearch.cfm?fr=101.54]

30. Kaur A, Scarborough P, Rayner M: A systematic review, and meta-analyses, of the impact of health-related claims on dietary choices. Int J Behav Nutr Phys Act 2017, 14(1): 93.

31. Greenfield H, Southgate DAT: Food composition data: Chapter 3: Selection of foods. 2nd edition. Edited by Elsevier Science Publishers. Rome; 2003;33-46.

32. Greenfield H, Southgate DAT: Food composition data: Chapter 4: Selection of nutrients and other components. 2nd edition. Edited by Elsevier Science Publishers. Rome; 2003;47-62.

33. Rahman MS, McCarthy OJ: A classification of food properties. Int J of Food Properties 1999, 2(2): 93-99.

34. Thiele S, Peltner J, Richter A, Mensink GBM: Food purchase patterns: empirical identification and analysis of their association with diet quality, socioeconomic factors, and attitudes. Nutr J 2017, 16:69.

35. Gil A, Martinez de Victoria E, Olza J: Indicators for the evaluation of diet quality. Nutr Hosp 2015, 31(3): 128-144.

36. FIVE THINGS FDA AND EPA DIDN'T TELL YOU ABOUT SEAFOOD SAFETY [https://www.ewg.org/research/five-things-fda-and-epa-didn-t-tell-you-about-seafood-safety#.Wp4JBRiZMnV]

37. EXECUTIVE SUMMARY: EWG's 2017 Shopper's Guide to Pesticides in Produce™ [https://www.ewg.org/foodnews/summary.php#.Wp4IoRiZMnV]

12

FFC's Advancement of Functional Food Definition

Johanna Gur, Marselinny Mawuntu and Danik Martirosyan

Functional Food Center/Functional Food Institute, Dallas, TX 75252, USA

Introduction

In order to create functional food products based on scientific evidence, we must first define functional foods. Previous definitions simply state that functional foods improve health and mitigate disease. However, more refined definitions provide a reason for their efficacy – through the activity of bioactive compounds and the measurement of biomarkers, which are the essential tools for gauging the effectiveness of functional foods. Generally, functional foods are linked to health promotion. The physiological effects of functional food or bioactive compounds may vary, but their categories of action include: physical performance, cognitive, behavioral, and psychological function, organ or system function, and combating chronic disease [1, 2]. Therefore, establishing a formal definition for these foods will help bring legitimate functional foods to the market. The addition of bioactive compounds, or biochemical molecules that improve health through the physiological mechanisms, improves the definition of functional foods. Overall, the advancement of the functional food definition by Functional Food Center (FFC) has grown to provide clarity and a more comprehensive understanding of its meaning.

Previous Definition of Functional Food

Each year since 2004, the Functional Foods Center has held international conferences under the series "Functional Foods for the Prevention and Treatment of Chronic Disease." In December of 2009, the 6th International Conference occurred in Texas Women's University in Denton, TX. The annual conference was entitled, "Functional Foods for Chronic Diseases: Diabetes and Related Disease" [3]. One of the main goals of the 2009 international conference on Functional Food was to initiate the development of a standard definition of functional food. Main conference topics included a presentation on "Functional Food Definition" by Dr. Danik Martirosyan, who suggested the upbringing of a standard definition that was published in the conference proceedings and generally accepted by the audience. That definition is as follows:

"Natural or processed foods that contain known or unknown biologically-active compounds; which, in defined, effective, and non-toxic amounts, provide

a clinically proven and documented health benefit for the prevention, management, or treatment of chronic diseases" [3].

Bioactive Compounds

"Bioactive compounds" are chemical components in functional food that exhibit beneficial biological activities. These bioactive compounds can be considered extra-nutritional constituents that usually occur in small amounts in various food sources. In short, bioactive compounds are beneficial because they act as antioxidants, are chemo- and cardio-preventive, and can even reduce risk or prevent the onset of certain diseases [4]. Scientifically speaking, the term "bioactive" means biologically active [5]. Thus, a bioactive compound is a substance that possesses a biological activity [6]. In various dictionaries of medicine, a bioactive compound is defined by having an effect, causing a reaction, or triggering a response in tissues of the human body [7-9]. Overall, bioactive compounds are considered to be the backbone of functional food effectiveness.

The unique compounds can be categorized into two types of components: extra-, non-nutritional or extra-nutritional constituents. Extra- and non-nutritional components of food are claimed to have beneficial health effects but do not include the essential nutrients. In contrast, extra-nutritional constituents include essential nutrients and typically occur in small food quantities. Additionally, they are studied extensively to evaluate their effects on human health [10-12]. Researchers can perform experiments on these compounds and observe causal relationships between bioactive compounds and overall health outcomes.

When examining bioactive compounds from the aspect of functional foods, food bioactive compounds are primary and secondary metabolites of nutritive and non-nutritive natural components that have the potential to positively affect health [13]. Thus, bioactive compounds can be defined as the inherent, non-nutritive constituents of foods with beneficial promotion on health and/or effects of toxicity when ingested [14]. In other words, different amounts of bioactive compounds can actually be toxic if too much is consumed; bioactive compounds are effective in specific, quantified amounts.

Each bioactive compound has its own unique structure, with physiological mechanisms and concentrations that depend on the environment where it is sourced. Bioavailability varies with the extraction method that is utilized to extract compounds from their source [4]. For example, cooking can alter or eliminate bioactive compounds.

Diet is an essential factor that contributes to health and disease in the normal aging process, and affects reactive oxygen species that, ceteris paribus, cause inflammation and cellular damage leading to CVD, diabetes mellitus, obesity, and Alzheimer disease [15-17]. A variety of nutrition profiles comprising functional foods have been recommended in healthy meal plans to protect and manage type 2 diabetes mellitus, or T2DM, such as a Mediterranean Diet. Nonetheless, a traditional Mediterranean Diet is considered one of the healthiest diets for human longevity based on epidemiological studies associating health risk-reduction with Mediterranean Diet style rather than a single component of the diet [18, 19]. Due to the expanding knowledge and education on bioactive compounds in relation to functional food, FFC strives to exponentiate its resources for general public awareness to combat these chronic diseases.

FFC Functional Food Definition (2017)

The FFC now defines "functional foods" as:

> *"Natural or processed foods that contain biologically active compounds; which, in defined, effective, and non-toxic amounts, provide a clinically proven and documented health benefit utilizing specific biomarkers for the prevention, management, or treatment of chronic disease or its symptoms"* [26].

In prior definitions, the phrase "known or unknown" in regards to biologically active compounds have been used. However, in the current definition, the term "unknown" has been eradicated because there would be no way to quantify the effects of the bioactive compound if the amount was undefined. For that reason, changes had been made accordingly after latest discussion at Harvard Medical School conference in September of 2017 with teaching partners: Dr. Dolores del Castillo, Senior Scientist and Head of Food Bioscience group and Francesco Matrisciano, MD, Ph.D. from Loyola University Department of Molecular Pharmacology and Therapeutics in Loyola University Chicago, IL [26]. This change represents one of the major developments for the current FFC definition for functional foods.

Another change to the previous definition is the addition of "specific biomarkers" as a way to measure disease symptoms. Biomarkers are indicators in the body that give off signals in tissues, organs, or systems. Scientists and researchers utilize the presence of biomarkers in order to determine the efficacy of a biological process in functional foods. To test the effectiveness of a bioactive compound, researchers measure specific biomarkers, to identify changes that occur at the cellular level that can be monitored to identify health or disease. Testing specific and sensitive biomarkers help to identify the health benefits of bioactive compounds in food. There is a plethora of diseases with symptoms that can be characterized through biomarkers; some common ones include: cancer, obesity, cardiovascular disease, diabetes, and emotional and neurological diseases [21].

A final change to the old definition of functional foods is the elaboration of chronic disease "or its symptoms." This signifies that potential signs of a disease are also crucial in treatment of the disease. By including the symptoms of a disease, the definition broadens its scope to include not only the final state of the disease, but all that contributes to this final state. This enables functional foods to be relevant and useful for a larger number of individuals. It is not possible to cure all diseases, with medicine or with food. Those suffering from these kinds of diseases will, with the new definition, be able to turn to functional foods as a source of potential relief of symptoms, thus improving quality of life. Ultimately, the latest FFC definition provides a more comprehensive understanding of functional food and a clearer sense of the organization's vision and purpose for the advancement of functional foods.

Table 1. Functional Food as Defined by Other Organizations (as adapted from "A New Definition of Functional Food by FFC: What Makes a Definition Unique?" *Journal of FFHD*)

Various Definitions of Functional Food	
The Institute of Food Technologists (IFT)	"Foods and food components that provide a health benefit beyond basic nutrition. These substances provide essential nutrients often beyond quantities necessary for normal maintenance, growth, and development, and/or other biologically active components that impact health benefits" [22].
The Institute of Medicine of the U.S. National Academy of Sciences	"Foods that encompass potentially healthful products, including any modified foods or food ingredients that may provide a health benefit beyond the nutrients it contains" [23].
Foods for Special Dietary Use (As defined by the Federal Food, Drug, and Cosmetic Act)	"A particular use for which a food purports or is represented to be used, including to the following: -Supplying a special dietary need that exists by reason of a physiological, pathological, or physical condition -Supplying a vitamin, mineral, or other ingredients for use by humans to supplement the diet by increasing the total dietary intake -Supplying a special dietary need by reason of being a food for us as the sole item of diet" [20].
Food and Drug Administration	Does not provide a legal definition for the term "functional foods," which is currently used as a marketing idiom for the category [24].
American Dietetic Association	Classifies all foods as functional at some physiological level in that food provides nutrient growth, or maintain vital processes [25].
FFC Definition (2014)	"Natural or processed foods that contain known o unknown biologically-active compounds; which, i defined, effective, and non-toxic amounts, provide clinically proven and documented health benefit for th prevention, management, or treatment of chroni diseases" [3].

Components of the New Functional Food Definition

Although a definition is often times interpreted as a whole, dissecting and identifying each segment is vital for quality understanding and explanation to what each sectional part entails.

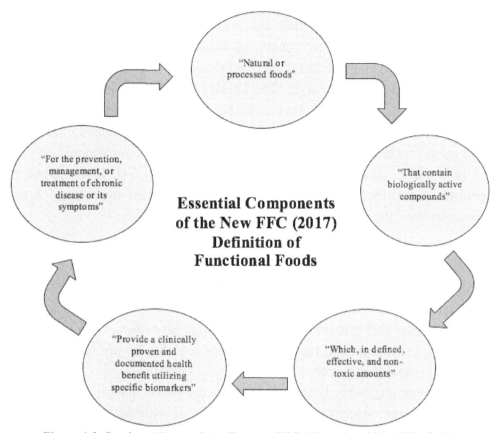

Figure 1.2. Sectional Parts of the Current FFC "Functional Food" Definition

Functional foods are becoming increasingly popular based on their clinically proven health benefits to prevent, manage, and treat chronic diseases. The current definition of functional food has become more precise and specific. In the definition, "natural or processed foods" describes the types of foods dealt with in functional foods. The phrase "that contain biologically active compounds" focuses on the components of these foods have that produce some kind of effect in the body. Moreover, "which, in defined, effective, and non-toxic amounts" concentrates more on the quantity, efficacy, and level of toxicity that these foods possess. The fact that they "provide a clinically proven and documented health benefit utilizing specific biomarkers" means that functional foods allow for successful treatment and there is concrete evidence of the overall impact of their effects. By specifying the use of biomarkers, the definition emphasizes that the "clinically proven health benefits" must be supported by the identification of alterations in the body and signal signs of disease - biomarkers. Lastly, the phrase "for the prevention, management, or treatment of chronic disease or its symptoms" pertains to the three key elements that functional foods aim to achieve: prevent, manage, or treat, not only the disease itself but more concretely, its symptoms. FFC's inclusion of the last two sections of the most recent definition strengthens the notion that it is necessary to provide clinically proven benefits as well as treating the disease as a whole [26].

Current State of Regulations

The discipline of functional food science is an aspect of nutritional science and is centered upon the research and development of these foods by using both a function-driven approach and a lifestyle approach to prevent and manage diseases, like diabetes [27-31]. The primary challenge is that the United States Food and Drug Administration (FDA) does not have a formal definition of functional foods in the United States. Functional foods are regulated by the FDA under the authority of two laws. The Federal Food, Drug, and Cosmetic Act (FD&C) of 1938 requires the regulation of all foods and food additives. The Dietary Supplement Health and Education Act (DSHEA) of 1994 amended the FD&C Act covers diet supplements and ingredients [32, 33].

The current regulations should adequately reflect all foods, including natural, processed, functional and medical. Once the government and scientists agree on what exactly makes food "functional," laws can be enacted that encourage research [33, 34]. If the public is properly educated about functional foods, then they will be able to embrace the concept. A standardized definition gives scientists the credibility needed to educate the public.

Functional Food Regulation

Instead of relying solely on medication to treat diseases, functional food products are an alternative way to combat symptoms and the disease as a whole. Morcover, if functional food is valued by consumers because of its ability to prevent to treat chronic diseases or their symptoms, it would prevent the industry from saturating markets with products that do not have concrete evidence from an empirical standpoint to corroborate their claims [35-37].

When faced with increasing health care costs in the 1980s, Japan's Ministry of Health and Welfare started a regulatory system to approve certain foods with documented health benefits in an effort to improve the health of the nation [38]. At that time, the U.S. did not have a standard definition. Years later, in 1994, the National Academy of Sciences' Food and Nutrition Board in the U.S. defined functional foods as "any modified food or food ingredient that may provide a health benefit beyond the traditional nutrients it contains" [39]. The International Life Sciences Institute defined functional foods as "foods that, by virtue of the presence of physiologically-active components, provide a health benefit beyond basic nutrition" [40]. The American Dietetic Association defined functional foods as foods that are "whole, fortified, enriched, or enhanced" [41]. Although they vary in specificity and cohesion, these definitions are a step towards the regulation of functional foods.

The Japanese Ministry of Health, Labor, and Welfare was the first regulatory agency to acknowledge functional foods as a unique food category [42]. Since then, Japan has been the leader in functional food regulation [43]. Their existing regulations concerning the use of food ingredients are adequate to cover functional food ingredients [44-45]. In the United States, the FDA currently has four categories of claims that food manufacturers can utilize on labels in order to convey health information. These categories include: 1) nutrient content claims, 2) structure/function claims, 3) health claims, and 4) qualified health claims [46]. All of these four claim types are allowed on functional food and regular food labels alike if the claim meets the defined criteria.

Steps to Establish Functional Food as a Separate Category

FFC aims to establish a separate category for the regulation of functional foods, and there are four main steps by which FFC plans to achieve this goal. These four steps will cyclically work to help establish a specific process for regulating functional foods, thus making them safer and more available for public consumption. One step in this processes is educating the public about functional foods. This is the step that FFC focuses on. The primary goal of FFC is to educate physicians, health professionals, researchers, scientists, students, and the general public about the health benefits, current research, and development of functional foods. Since 1998, FFC has worked to accomplish this goal by hosting 25 international conferences around the globe, upholding two peer-reviewed scientific journals, Functional Foods in Health and Disease (FFHD) and Bioactive Compounds in Health and Disease (BCHD), publishing 30 books including 5 textbooks exclusively on functional food science. Educating the public could, in turn, push the government to approve the current, most recent functional food definition as a standard definition for functional food. Simultaneously, FFC is contacting government agencies directly to inquire about the process of approving the definition for standardization and urging them to do so. Ultimately, the organization strives to create standards for the evaluation of functional food products as well as special food labels acceptable for the public. Once the proper regulations for production and labeling are established, we must rely upon the food industry to understand the research that has been conducted and follow the regulations implemented by the government in order to begin standardized production of functional foods for public consumption. The food industry will be responsible for developing labels and health claims for functional food products that are clinically proven by the use of biomarkers. It will be critical for labels to specify "best by" dates that indicates how long bioactive compounds will remain effective. This will not come without benefits for the food industry. Functional foods are an untapped sector of the market in which there is substantial potential for financial gains. Unlike medical foods and nutraceuticals, functional foods will be present in stores and accessible to the general public without the need for a prescription from a doctor. This exponentially increases the availability and will benefit not only the population but the industry producing these products as well.

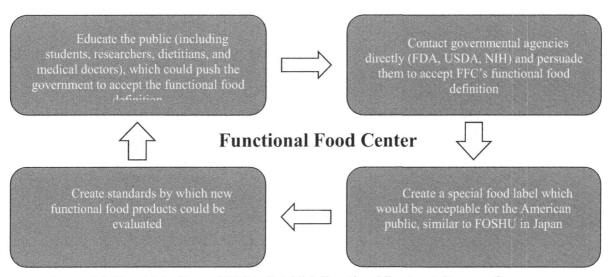

Figure 1.3. Four Main Steps of FFC to Establish Functional Food as A Separate Category

Future Advancements of Functional Food Research

Extensive research is currently directed toward increasing our understanding of functional foods. For example, there have been several reports that have examined the role of antioxidants in reduction of muscle damage since a large increase of oxidative products has been noted in exercised muscles via the biomarker of antioxidant intake [47-51]. In addition, nutrigenomics is an emerging discipline that investigates the interaction between diet and development of diseases that is based on an individual's genetic profile [52]. In February of 2001, the complete sequence of the human genome was announced by Ventor and a group of colleagues [53]. This breakthrough discovery could eventually make it possible to tailor a diet for an individual's specific genetic profile. The extensive personalization abilities of nutrigenomics will have a profound effect on the efforts of future disease prevention [54].

Moreover, another advancement that will greatly influence the future of functional foods is biotechnology. Recent instances of biotechnology-derived crops have great potential to improve the health of many people worldwide through the use of golden rice and iron-enriched rice [55]. These grains can provide enhanced levels of iron and beta-carotene which could, as a result, help prevent iron deficiency anemia and vitamin A deficiency–related blindness in the world. Many other foods enhanced with nutritive or non-nutritive substances may even help to prevent chronic diseases, such as cancer, diabetes, and osteoporosis [56] as well as other diet-related disorders, in the future.

Research suggests that there is significant progress in the field of functional foods. It has been established that nutrient bioavailability within foods is governed by the microstructure and composition of the given food, or otherwise known as the food matrix [59]. Many studies have shown that in the process of functional food development, interactions within this food matrix between nutrients and non-nutrients can vary in nature [60-61]. As a whole, functional food research has greatly progressed over the years and has shown evidence of remarkable changes to overall health. Its advancements will be an ongoing process of remarkable innovations. For these reasons it is especially important that the United States develops a standardized definition for the purpose of regulating functional foods in an effort to stimulate more research in the field.

Evaluating Functional Foods Using FFC's Definition

As the development of functional foods continues to progress, it will be crucial to ensure that the products we are creating and consuming actually are functional foods. FFC's definition of functional foods and the steps required to create new functional food products can be used to retrospectively evaluate scientific evidence in order to decipher whether a product is a functional food.

FFC has used the refined definition of functional foods to outline the steps necessary for the development of functional foods. This process begins by examining the link between a particular food and health benefits. Once a link has been identified, researchers must determine the bioactive compound that is responsible for the observed health benefit. This is accomplished by running in vitro and in vivo studies with non-living and animal specimens. Once a bioactive compound has been identified, researchers will use in vitro and in vivo studies to determine the mechanism of action that by which the bioactive compound imparts health benefits. Through this step, researchers must also establish a daily value that will deliver effective health benefits to the consumer while avoiding toxicity. Once the mechanism and daily value have been determined, the next step is running human studies. Human studies involve administering human-appropriate doses of bioactive compounds and closely monitoring subjects for any adverse side effects. Once human studies determine the proper dosage of bioactive compounds, an appropriate food vehicle must be developed for the bioactive compounds. This food vehicle combined with the bioactive compound is the functional food product.

The remaining steps in the process all have to do with ensuring the proper regulations are met and administering the final product to the public. First, manufacturers must obtain proper labels for functional foods. These labels must include information about daily usage amounts, length of usage, and how long bioactive compounds will remain effective. On labels, manufacturers will need to make health claims that are backed by empirical evidence and closely follow the FDA's health claim regulations. Once the functional food is created and packaged, it must be marketed to the public in a way that adequately educates them about the health benefits of functional food. Once people begin consuming functional foods, researchers can run epidemiological studies to test for overall and long-term effectiveness of functional foods, and use this information to better inform the future research and functional food development.

To determine if a food is a functional food, one can look at the data provided from research studies and walk through each step of the process to create functional foods and the standards detailed in FFC's definition of functional foods to see if requirements are met all the way through. If each standard is met, then that product can be considered a functional food. If any standards are not met, that product cannot be considered a functional food. It is possible that the conclusion will be that there is not enough evidence to determine whether something is a functional food. While this conclusion seems uninformative, it is important because it can be the starting point for more research needed to determine a bioactive compound's potential to be a functional food.

SUMMARY

> Throughout the past decades, FFC has promoted the advancement of functional food research and expanded the scope of its definition of functional food. In order to create functional food products based on scientific evidence, defining them is a crucial first step.

> Previous definitions vaguely state that functional foods improve health and reduce likelihood of disease. However, FFC's current definition provides a clearer sense of what functional foods do by specifying the activity of bioactive compounds and use of biomarkers to determine functional food effectiveness, as well as broadening the scope of their effects from just a disease to a disease *and* its symptoms. FFC's advancing approach accomplishes what they believe to be an attainable standard for developing improved functional foods for a better quality of life.

> Establishing a more formal and standard definition for functional foods will help bring a greater number of legitimate functional foods to the market in order benefit a broader range of individuals. This will create a need for more concrete regulation and evaluation of scientific evidence in regards to functional foods. FFC's definition of functional foods

provides the guidelines necessary to do this. FFC's advancement of the definition will, in turn, create more awareness and understanding of functional foods in today's modern society.

REVIEW QUESTIONS

1. Why was the phrase "known or unknown" bioactive compounds changed to just "biologically active compounds" in the new Functional Food Definition?
    a. Because it sounds more certain
    b. Because there would be no way to quantify the effects of the bioactive compound if the amount was undefined
    c. Because we know the amount of bioactive compounds in all foods we are working with
    d. None of the above
2. What is considered the back bone of functional food effectiveness?
    a. Phytochemicals
    b. Vitamin C
    c. Bioactive compounds
    d. Nutritional claims
3. What Law currently regulates functional foods?
    a. The Federal Food, Drug, and Cosmetic Act (FD&C)
    b. The Dietary Supplement Health and Education Act (DSHEA)
    c. The Functional Food Safety and Efficacy Act (FFSEA)
    d. A & B
    e. All of the above
4. Which step towards making functional foods a separate category is FFC most focused on?
    a. Create standards by which new functional food products could be evaluated
    b. Create a special food label which would be acceptable for the American public, similar to FOSHU in Japan
    c. Educate the public (including students, researchers, dietitians, and medical doctors), which could push the government to accept the functional food definition
    d. Contact governmental agencies directly (FDA, USDA, NIH) and persuade them to accept FFC's functional food definition
5. You can use FFC's definition of functional food and the steps necessary for developing functional foods to
    a. Determine if a functional food is actually a functional food
    b. Determine if consumers will buy a functional food
    c. Determine what kind of functional foods researchers should focus on developing
    d. All of the above

Answers: 1. (**B**) 2. (**C**) 3. (**D**) 4. (**C**) 5. (**A**)

List of Abbreviations: Functional Food Center, FFC; American Dietetic Association, ADA; Academic Society for Functional Foods and Bioactive Compounds, ASFFBC; Cardiovascular

Disease, CVD; Certified Functional Food Scientist, CFFS; Food and Drug Administration, FDA; Institute of Food Technologists, IFS, Mediterranean Diet, MD; Type 2 Diabetes Mellitus, T2DM.

Conflicts of Interest: Authors declare no conflicts of interest.

Authors' Contributions: Danik Martirosyan, PhD. conceived the idea and coordinated the review of the manuscript. Marsie Mawuntu, CFFS is the student intern who contributed to the writing and editing of the full manuscript. Both authors approved the final version before submission.

REFERENCES

1. Dhiman, Anju, Walia, Vaibhav, and Nanda, Arun. "Introduction to the Functional Foods." Introduction to Functional Food Science: Textbook. 2nd ed. Richardson, TX: Functional Food Center, 2014.

2. Westmark, Cara J. "Definition of Functional Food. Healthy, Functional, and Medical Foods. Similarities and Differences between these Categories. Bioactive Food Compounds." Introduction to Functional Food Science: Textbook. 2nd ed. Richardson, TX: Functional Food Center, 2014.

3. Martirosyan, Danik and Prasad, Chandan. Functional Foods for Chronic Diseases: Diabetes and Related Diseases: The 6th International Conference proceedings. 2009.

4. Martirosyan, Danik and Pisarski, Kasia: Bioactive Compounds: Their Role in Functional Food and Human Health, Classifications, and Definition. In "Introduction to Functional Food Science," 3rd edition. Edited by D. Martirosyan, Dallas, TX: Food Science Publisher, 2015.

5. Nahler G; Dictionary of Pharmaceutical Medicine (3rd Ed), B letter, Springer-Verlag Wien, 2013: 19-28.

6. Solomon HK and William WW; Bioactive Food Components, Encyclopedia of Food & Culture (2nd Ed). Acceptance to Food Politics, B Letter, Charles Scribner's Sons, 2003, 1: 201.

7. Kris-Etherton PM and al.; Bioactive compounds in foods: their role in the prevention of cardiovascular disease and cancer. American Journal of Medicine. 2002, 113(Suppl 9B): 71S-88S.

8. Schrezenmeir J et al.; Foreword. British Journal of Nutrition, 2000, 84(S1): 1.

9. Gry J et al.; EuroFIR-BASIS - a combined composition and biological activity database for bioactive compounds in plant-based foods. Trends in Food Science & Technology, 2007, 18(8): 434-444.

10. Cammack R et al.; Oxford Dictionary of Biochemistry and Molecular Biology (2nd Ed). Oxford University Press, 2006: 74-75.

11. Dictionary of Food Science and Technology (2nd Ed). International Food Information Service (IFIS Editor), 2009: 47-48.

12. The American Heritage Medical Dictionary. Houghton Mifflin Company, 2007: 47.

13. Mosby's Dictionary of Medicine, Nursing and Health Professions (9th Ed). Mosby Creator, 2013: 83.

14. Miller-Keane and Marie TO; Miller-Keane Encyclopedia and Dictionary of Medicine, Nursing and Allied Health (7th Ed). Saunders, 2005: 62.

15. Scarmeas N., Stern Y., Tang M.-X., Mayeux R., Luchsinger J.A. Mediterranean diet and risk for Alzheimer's disease. *Ann. Neurol.* 2006; 59:912-921

16. Saura-Calixto F., Goni I. Definition of the Mediterranean diet based on bioactive compounds. *Crit. Rev. Food Sci. Nutr.* 2009; 49:145-152.

17. Salas-Salvado J., Bullo M., Estruch R., Ros E., Covas M.I., Ibarrola-Jurado N., Corella D., Aros F., Gomez-Gracia E., Ruiz-Gutierrez V., et al. Prevention of diabetes with Mediterranean diets: A subgroup analysis of a randomized trial. *Ann. Intern. Med.* 2014; 160:1–10.

18. Salas-Salvado J., Fernandez-Ballart J., Ros E., Martinez-Gonzalez M.A., Fito M., Estruch R., Corella D., Fiol M., Gomez-Gracia E., Aros F., et al. Effect of a Mediterranean diet supplemented with nuts on metabolic syndrome status: One-year results of the PREDIMED randomized trial. *Arch. Intern. Med.* 2008; 168:2449-2458.

19. Trichopoulou A., Costacou T., Bamia C., Trichopoulos D. Adherence to a Mediterranean diet and survival in a Greek population. *N. Engl. J. Med.* 2003; 348:2599-2608.

20. Martirosyan and Singh Jaishree. A New Definition of Functional Food by FFC: What Makes a Definition Unique? *Journal of Functional Foods in Health and Disease.* 2015; 5(6):209-223.

21. Clydesdale, Fergus. "Functional foods: opportunities and challenges." *Food Tech* 58.12 (2004): 35-40.

22. Institute of Food Technologists. Functional foods: Opportunities and challenges. March 2005.

23. Thomas PR, Earl R: Opportunities in the Nutrition and Food Sciences: Research Challenges and the Next Generation of Investigators. Edited by the Institute of Medicine's Food and Nutrition Board (IOM/NAS). Washington, DC: National Academies Press; 1994: 98-142.

24. Danik Martirosyan and Bryan Singharaj. Health Claims and Functional Food: The Future of Functional Foods under FDA and ESFA Regulation. In "Functional Food and Chronic Disease." Edited by D. Martirosyan, Dallas, TX: Food Science Publisher, 2015.

25. American Dietetic Association: Position of the American Dietetic Association: functional foods. *Journal of the American Dietetic Association* 1999, 99: 1278-1285.

26. Functional Food Center. Functional Food Institute. Dallas, TX. Web. 2018. www.functionalfoodscenter.net

27. Bellisle R, Diplock AT, Hornstra G, et al. Functional food science in Europe. *Br J Nutr* 1998;80(suppl): S3–193.

28. Diplock AT, Aggott PJ, Ashwell M, et al. Scientific concepts of functional foods in Europe: consensus document. Br J Nutr 1999; 81(suppl): S1–27

29. Clydesdale F. A proposal for the establishment of scientific criteria for health claims for functional foods. Nutr Rev 1997; 55:413–22.

30. Block G: Micronutrients and cancer: time for actions? *Journal of the National Cancer Institute* 1993, 85: 846-848.

31. Alkhatib, Ahmad, et al. Functional Foods and Lifestyle Approaches for Diabetes Prevention and Management. *Nutrients.* 2017 Dec; 9(12): 1310.

32. Hasler CM: Functional Foods: Benefits, Concerns and Challenges—A Position Paper from the American Council on Science and Health. *The Journal of Nutrition* 2002, 132:3772-3781.

33. Hoy-Rosas J, Arrecis E, Avila M. Central American Food Practices. In Goody C, Drago L. Cultural Food Practices. United States of America. American Dietetic Association; 2010: 54-67.

34. Mahan, L. Kathleen., Escott-Stump Syvlvia., Raymond, Janice L. Krause, Marie V., eds. *Krause's Food & The Nutrition Care Process.* 13th ed. St. Louis, MO. Elsevier/Saunders, 2012.

35. Nelms Marcia, Sucher Kathryn P, Roth Sara, Lacey, eds. *Nutrition Therapy Pathophysiology.* 2nd edition. Belmont, CA. Cengage Learning, 2010.

36. Mazza, G., ed. (1998). *Functional Foods: Biochemical and Processing Aspects.* Lancaster, PA: Technomic Publishing.

37. Wildman, Robert E. C., ed. (2001). *Handbook of Nutraceuticals and Functional Foods.* Boca Raton, FL: CRC Press.

38. Arai, S. (1996) Studies on functional foods in Japan—state of the art. Biosci. Biotechnol. Biochem. 60: 9–15.

39. Committee on Opportunities in the Nutrition and Food Sciences, Food and Nutrition Board, Institute of Medicine (1994) Enhancing the food supply. In: Opportunities in the Nutrition and Food Sciences: Research Challenges and the Next Generation of Investigators (Thomas, P. R. & Earl, R., eds.), pp. 98–142. National Academy Press, Washington, DC.

40. International Life Sciences Institute (1999) Safety assessment and potential health benefits of food components based on selected scientific criteria. ILSI North America Technical Committee on Food Components for Health Promotion. Crit. Rev. Food Sci. Nutr. 39: 203–316.

41. American Dietetic Association (1999) Position of the American Dietetic Association: functional foods. J. Am. Diet. Assoc. 99: 1278–1285.

42. International Life Sciences Institute. Perspectives on ILSI's international activities on functional foods. May 2009.

43. Yamada K, Sato-Mito N, Nagata J, Umegaki K. Health Claim evidence requirements in Japan. *J Nutr.* 2008;138(6): 1192S-1198S.

44. Thompson AK, Moughan PJ. Innovation in the foods industry: Functional foods. *Innov Manage Policy Pract.* 2008;10(1): 61-73.

45. Henry CJ. Functional foods [editorial]. *Eur J Clin Nutr.* 2010;64(7):657-659.

46. US General Accounting Office. Food safety: Improvements needed in overseeing the safety of dietary supplements and "functional foods." July 2000.

47. Aoi W, Naito Y, Takanami Y, Kawai Y, Sakuma K, Ichikawa H, Yoshida N, Yoshikawa T: Oxidative stress and delayed-onset muscle damage after exercise. Free Radic Biol Med. 2004, 37: 480-487.

48. Phillips T, Childs AC, Dreon DM, Phinney S, Leeuwenburgh C: A dietary supplement attenuates IL-6 and CRP after eccentric exercise in untrained males. Med Sci Sports Exerc. 2003, 35: 2032-2037.

49. Takanami Y, Iwane H, Kawai Y, Shimomitsu T: Vitamin E supplementation and endurance exercise. Are there benefits? Sports Med. 2000, 29: 73-83.

50. Kanter MM, Nolte LA, Holloszy JO: Effects of an antioxidant vitamin mixture on lipid peroxidation at rest and postexercise. J Appl Physiol. 1993, 74: 965-969.

51. Aoi W, Naito Y, Sakuma K, Kuchide M, Tokuda H, Maoka T, Toyokuni S, Oka S, Yasuhara M, Yoshikawa T: Astaxanthin limits exercise-induced skeletal and cardiac muscle damage in mice. Antioxid Redox Signal. 2003, 5: 139-144.

52. Fogg-Johnson, N. & Meroli, A. (2000) Nutrigenomics: the next wave in nutrition research. Nutraceuticals World 3: 86–95.

53. The Celera Genomics Sequencing Team (2001) The sequence of the human genome. Science (Washington, DC) 291: 1304–1351.

54. Gura, T. (1999) New genes boost rice nutrients. Science (Washington, DC) 285: 994–5.

55. Institute of Food Technologists (2000) IFT expert report on biotechnology and foods. Food Technol. 54: 61–80.

56. Falk, M. C., Chassy, B. M. Harlander, S. K., Hoban, T. J., 4th, McGloughlin, M. N. & Akhlaghi, A. R. (2002) Food biotechnology: benefits and concerns. J. Nutr. 132: 1384–1390.

57. Shimizu M, Hachimura S. Gut as a target for functional food. Trends Food Sci Technol. 2011;22(12):646-650.

58. Ross S. Functional foods: The Food and Drug Administration perspective. Am J Clin Nutr. 2000;71(6 suppl):1735S-1738S.

59. Hwang J, Sevanian A, Hodis HN, Ursini F. Synergistic inhibition of LDL oxidation by phytoestrogens and ascorbic acid. Free Radic Biol Med. 2000;29(1):79-89.

60. Jeffery E. Component interactions for efficacy of functional foods. J Nutr. 2005;135(5):1223-1225.

61. Yeum KJ, Russell RM, Krinsky NI, Aldini G. Biomarkers of antioxidant capacity in the hydrophilic and lipophilic compartments of human plasma. Arch Biochem Biophys. 2004;430(1):97-103.

Correct Answers:

Chapter 1
1. **(C)** 2. **(B)** 3. **(D)** 4. **(C)** 5. **(D)** 6. **(A)** 7. **(D)** 8. **(D)** 9. **(B)** 10. **(C)**

11. The following term is deemed to be somewhat synonymous with functional food:
    C. Nutraceutical
12. A food in a U.S. supermarket contains a claim that "it supports immune function and healthy cholesterol levels." This claim would be considered a:
    B. Health claim
13. The main difference between functional food and ordinary food is that:
    D. Functional food has some health benefit beyond basic nutrition
14. What is not a part of Hill's criteria?
    C. The result must be widely accepted by the general public
15. What does not affect a bioactive compound's effect on the body?
    D. How long ago the compound has been consumed
16. Indicators in the body that give off signals in tissues, organs, or systems, and are often used to determine the rate or effectiveness of a biological process in its natural state and after functional food administration are called
    A. Biomarkers
17. Strong experimental evidence is backed by
    D. Long term studies with consistent results and little to no adverse side effects
18. Bioavailability varies based on
    D. All of the above
19. All of the following are categories of functional food effects except
    B. Genetic modification
20. Which country is considered the birthplace of functional foods?
    C. Japan

Chapter 2
1. **(F)** 2. **(D)** 3. **(C)** 4. **(B)** 5. **(D)** 6. **(C)** 7. **(A)** 8. **(C)** 9. **(A)** 10. **(D)** 11. **(D)** 12. **(D)** 13. **(C)** 14. **(A)**

15. The definition of Functional Food includes:
    F. All of the above
16. What is true about bioactive compounds?
    D. A and B
17. Supra-physiologic or therapeutic doses of bioactive compounds:
    C. A and B
18. The success of extracting bioactive compounds
    B. Is of utmost importance

19. Functionality of bioactive compounds is obtained when _____ is/are achieved to convert an ordinary food into a functional food.

D. A and B

20. Which of these choices is not a function provided by eggs?

C. Known to prevent the spread of carcinogens

21. _____ produce isothiocyanates.

A. Glucosinolates

22. All of the following are known classifications of bioactive compounds except

C. Beneficiary supplements

23. A health benefit of consuming fiber is

A. The reduction of rates of absorption of glucose

24. Specific protein fragments that have a positive impact on body functions and may ultimately influence human health are known as _____.

D. Bioactive peptides

25. Which of these are toxic compounds found in mushrooms?

D. All of the above

26. Which of these choices is a trait of non-nutritive bioactive compounds?

D. A and C

27. What are nutrient sensors?

C. Specific transcription factors and nuclear proteins that largely determine the amount, timing, and cell specificity of gene expression

28. Which bioactive vitamin plays a significant role in low-density lipoprotein (LDL) levels, "influencing the 'loading' of LDL"?

A. Bioactive vitamin E

Chapter 3

1. **(C)** 2. **(C)** 3. **(D)** 4. **(C)** 5. **(C)** 6. **(A)** 7. **(B)** 8. **(D)** 9. **(D)** 10. **(C)**

11. A selectively fermented ingredient that results in specific changes in the composition and/or activity of the gastrointestinal microbiota

C. Prebiotics

12. The following are all acceptable definitions of dietary supplements except

C. consumed as part of a normal diet and deliver one or more active ingredients

13. Which of the following is not a major challenge that industrialized countries are currently facing in relation to health?

D. Promoting the use of food to generate profit to be used in future treatment of chronic diseases.

14. Inflammation of the joints is known as

C. Arthritis

15. Which of the following could possibly be considered a functional food?

C. Both a and b

16. Oxidation of ____ has a key role in the pathogenesis of atherosclerosis and cardiovascular heart diseases

A. **low-density lipoproteins (LDL)**

17. Which one of the following reasons is a key motivator for the development of functional foods?

    B. The management of the risk of disease

18. How do you make a food product not originally classified as "functional" into such?

    D. Increasing bioavailability or stability of the component known to produce a functional effect

19. Designing and developing functional foods is a scientific challenge that should rely on which of the following?

    D. All of the above

20. Which of the listed foods is not an example of a known functional food?

    C. Becel-margarine

Chapter 4

1. **(A)** 2. **(C)** 3. **(C)** 4. **(D)** 5. **(A)** 6. **(A)** 7. **(D)** 8. **(B)** 9. **(D)** 10. **(D)**

11. Bioactive compounds can be classified into major classes, including:

    A. Lipids

12. _____ has been an essential tool for fingerprinting bioactive compounds in plants, fungi, and marine functional food sources.

    C. HPTLC

13. Why is it difficult to specifically give an estimated dietary intake of most bioactive compounds?

    C. A and B

14. The ____, such as bioavailability, transport, absorption, metabolism, and excretion of bioactive compounds ultimately influence the ____, such as receptor affinity and efficacy, of these compounds for different individuals.

    D. Pharmacokinetics; pharmacodynamics

15. Isolating and purifying bioactive compounds is difficult because.

    A. They are usually found with other compounds bearing different polarities

16. Where does the metabolism of nutrients begin?

    A. Mouth

17. What is not a factor that must be considered when conducting a clinical trial?

    D. None of the above

18. HPLC separates compounds through the usage of

    B. The compounds' different retention rates in certain solvents

19. What is not true about bioactive compounds?

    D. Must be paired with subscribed supplements to take effect

20. In measuring the optimal intake of bioactive compounds in humans, what is an approach that can be considered?

    D. A and B

Chapter 5

1. **(B)** 2. **(D)** 3. **(D)** 4. **(A)** 5. **(C)** 6. **(D)** 7. **(C)** 8. **(B)** 9. **(B)** 10. **(C)**

11. A medical food can be defined by all of the following EXCEPT:

> **B. A change in a person's diet to control chronic diseases**

12. The American Dietetic Association (ADA) subdivides functional foods into four groups:

> **D. Medical foods, modified foods, special diets, conventional foods**

13. food that is produced without using the conventional inputs of modern industrial agriculture, including pesticides, synthetic fertilizers, sewage sludge, genetically modified organisms (GMOs), irradiation or food additives

> **D. Organic food**

14. A lack of consumption of vitamin C is associated with which health effect?

> **A. Scurvy**

15. Which of the following is not an essential amino acid?

> **C. Glycine**

16. What is not true about bioactive compounds?

> **D. Promote health proportional to the amount consumed**

17. Dietary supplements

> **C. May not claim to treat a specific disease or condition**

18. What is a similarity between medical foods and dietary supplements?

> **B. Both are considered functional foods**

19. _____ are organic substances made by plants or animals whereas _____ are inorganic elements that come from the earth.

> **B. Vitamins; minerals**

20. Which of the following statements is true?

> **C. A and B**

Chapter 6

1. **(A)** 2. **(D)** 3. **(C)** 4. **(A)** 5. **(C)**

6. ascorbate is transported to epithelial cells in the body by a transporter called

> **A. SVCT1**

7. Which of the following is not a function of vitamin C in the body?

> **D. support bone growth**

8. Which of the following is not a population that is likely to be at risk of vitamin C deficiency?

> **C. vegetarian**

9. The minimum amount of vitamin C required daily to prevent deficiency is

> **A. 10mg**

10. The cooking method with the least amount of vitamin C loss is

> **C. steaming**

Chapter 7

1. **(B)** 2. **(C)** 3. **(C)** 4. **(B)** 5. **(D)** 6. **(D)** 7. **(B)** 8. **(C)** 9. **(A)** 10. **(D)**

11. A deficiency in all of the following nutrients would be detrimental, except for:

    B. Riboflavin

12. These two minerals decrease absorption of fluoride by forming insoluble complexes.

    C. Calcium and magnesium

13. All of the following are Omega-3 fatty acids, except for:

    C. Linoleic acid (LA)

14. Vitamins can be categorized as fat-soluble and water-soluble. Which of the following vitamins is fat-soluble?

    B. Vitamin D

15. Long periods of insufficient Vitamin C intake can lead to a disease called

    D. Scurvy

16. Which of the following is not a required consideration for selecting food vehicle for fortification?

    D. Highly nutritious

17. Fortification of a food that is consumed regularly by the general population is called

    B. Mass fortification

18. The presence of Vitamin D increases body's absorption of

    C. Calcium

19. The average daily dietary intake level sufficient to meet the nutrient requirement of nearly all healthy individuals in a particular life stage and gender group is known as the

    A. Recommended Dietary Allowance

20. All of the following are common food vehicles for Calcium fortification, except for?

    D. Salt

Chapter 8

1. **(D)** 2. **(B)** 3. **(D)** 4. **(A)** 5. **(B)** 6. **(C)** 7. **(A)** 8. **(A)** 9. **(C)** 10. **(D)**

11. Xerophthalmia, a common cause of childhood blindness, is caused by a dietary deficiency of:

    D. Vitamin A

12. The reason astaxanthin has the ability to pass through the blood retinal barrier is due to:

    B. Esterification

13. Beta-glucan is a soluble fiber that are commonly sourced from all of the following, except for

    D. soybean

14. Omega-3 and Omega-6 fatty acids are essential fatty acids that belong to a group of fatty acids called

    A. Polyunsaturated fatty acids

15. All of the following popular functional food ingredients targeting heart health, except for

    B. Vitamin K

16. Cranberry extract is a functional food ingredient found in the women's health sector that is primarily used to treat

    C. Urinary tract infections

17. Which of the following is not a characteristic of collagen peptides that make it useful for food and beverage applications?

A. High viscosity

18. The leading functional food ingredient in the bone and joint health market, commonly sourced from the outer shells of shrimp, and lobster, and crabs, is called

A. Glucosamine

19. All of the following are examples of prebiotics, except for?

C. Pectin

20. Which of the following is not a challenge for the heart health functional ingredient industry?

D. Low demands for heart health ingredients

Chapter 9

1. **(D)** 2. **(B)** 3. **(D)** 4. **(A)**

5. Nominal measurements used in sensory evaluations:

D. Identify unique attributes with non-ordered or ranked numerical values.

6. The four basic tastes perceived by the human tongue are

B. Bitter, sour, salty, and sweet

7. Which of the following is not an example of an attribute difference test?

D. Duo-trio test

8. When conducting sensory evaluation using a triangle test, the sensory panel used are

A. Trained panelists

Chapter 10

1. **(B)** 2. **(A)** 3. **(D)**

4. The Golden Rice is a genetically modified rice variety that increases the biosynthesis of

B. Beta-carotene

5. Which specific gene was changed to drastically increase the amount of the targeted nutrient in Golden Rice 2 compared to Golden Rice?

A. Phytoene synthase (*psy*) gene from

6. Which of the following is not a functional food ingredient produced by genetically engineering microalgae species?

D. Vitamin D

Chapter 11

1. **(C)** 2. **(A)** 3. **(B)** 4. **(B)** 5. **(D)** 6. **(A)** 7. **(C)** 8. **(A)** 9. **(D)** 10. **(C)**

11. Any food that has been purposely changed from its original state through cooking, canning, freezing, packaging or by changes in nutritional composition with fortifying, preserving or preparation methods

C. Processed Food

12. Which of the following about the definition of organic food is false?

A. Processed foods cannot be organic

13. For a packaged food to be labeled as organic, it must contain

B. 95 percent organically produced raw or processed agricultural ingredients

14. Which of the following is not one of the three patterns that the USDA has identified for healthy eating?

    B. The Paleo-Style Eating Pattern

15. Non-nutritive bioactive compounds include…

    D. A & B

16. The FDA says that nutritional labeling for which of the following is voluntary?

    A. Raw produce

17. Foods can use the term "healthy" if they

    C. Have mostly mono/polyunsaturated fats

18. Which of the following cannot be used to describe the amount of sugar in a food?

    A. Low sugar

19. How much of a nutrient must be in a food for the label to call it a "good source"?

    D. 10-19% DV

20. Which of the follow pairs of foods with their bioactive ingredient is correct?

    B. Curcumin in turmeric

Chapter 12

1. **(B)** 2. **(C)** 3. **(D)** 4. **(C)** 5. **(A)**

1. Why was the phrase "known or unknown" bioactive compounds changed to just "biologically active compounds" in the new Functional Food Definition?

    B. Because there would be no way to quantify the effects of the bioactive compound if the amount was undefined

2. What is considered the back bone of functional food effectiveness?

    C. Bioactive compounds

3. What Law currently regulates functional foods?

    D. A & B

4. Which step towards making functional foods a separate category is FFC most focused on?

    C. Educate the public (including students, researchers, dietitians, and medical doctors), which could push the government to accept the functional food definition

5. You can use FFC's definition of functional food and the steps necessary for developing functional foods to

    A. Determine if a functional food is actually a functional food

GLOSSARY

Absolute Intake: The absolute intake of a bioactive compound is often determined by gathering data on the flavonoid content of foods and then calculating the amount ingested by humans. In order to determine the absolute intake levels of bioactive compounds, accurate and comprehensive food composition tables are necessary.

Active Pharmaceutical Ingredients (APIs): Central ingredient in a pharmaceutical

Adequate Intake (AL): The recommended average daily intake level based on observed or experimentally determined approximations, when the RDA cannot be established, and scientific evidence is not available

Adipocytokines: Biologically active molecules produced by adipocytes

Adipogenesis: A differentiation of adipogenic precursor cells (i.e., preadipocytes) into adipocytes

Age-related macular-degeneration (AMD): disease that blurs the sharp, central vision you need for "straight-ahead" activities such as reading, sewing, and driving. AMD affects the macula, the part of the eye that allows you to see fine detail

Alzheimer's Disease (AD): A form of dementia and the most frequent neurodegenerative disorder associated with aging

Amino Acids: A bioactive compound. Examples include isoleucine, lysine, leucine, methionine, phenylalanine, threonine, tyrptophan, valine and histidine.

Angiotensin Converting Enzyme (ACE): Located in many tissues and plays an important role in blood pressure regulation and hypertension. Flavonoids suppress effects of ACE.

Anthocyanins: Anthocyanins are powerful antioxidants that support healthy blood pressure, improved memory and lower risks of cancer and heart disease. They also give fruits and vegetables their red, blue, or purple coloration.

Antioxidants: Natural antioxidants occur in all parts of higher plants, including seeds. Antioxidants are known to decrease the risk of degenerative diseases.

Arachidonic Acid (AA): The most important long-chain fatty acid of the ω6 series. Contributes to the conversion of linoleic acid

Association Colloids: Micelles, vesicles and microemulsions are some of the most common types of self-assembled structures in food materials

ATP-Binding Cassette (ABC): Expressed in the mucosal cells and the canalicular membrane; they resecrete sterols (especially absorbed plant sterols) back into the intestinal lumen and from the liver into bile

Autophagy: Crucial for protection from cancers, infections, inflammation, autoimmunity, metabolic diseases, neurodegenerative disorders, and cardiovascular and pulmonary diseases. Autophagy, including aggrephagy, xenophagy, mitophagy, and lipophagy, is an intracellular cleaning system including regenerating metabolic precursors, contributing to cellular and tissue homeostasis by degrading long-lived proteins, protein aggregates, and defective organelles

Avidin: An egg-white glycoprotein resistant to pancreatic proteases

Beta-glucans: Branched polymers of glucose that form a highly viscous mixture in solution. They occur naturally as cell wall components in grains like oats, barley, rye and wheat

Bioactive Compound: Essential and non-essential compounds that occur in nature, are part of the food chain, and can be shown to have an effect on human health. Dietary sources include fruits, vegetables, and whole grains

Bioavailability: The proportion of an ingested nutrient in a food that is absorbed and utilized through normal metabolic pathways. In other words, how well the human body absorbs and utilizes nutrients

Biomarkers: indicators in the body that give off signals in tissues, organs, or systems. Scientists often use biomarkers to determine the rate or effectiveness of a biological process in its natural state and after functional food administration

Biopolymers: May be present as individual molecules, or they may be present as supra-molecular structures where they are associated with one or more molecules of the same or different kind

Biotechnology: Biotechnology-derived crops, including golden rice and iron-enriched rice, have tremendous potential to improve the health of millions worldwide. They are genetically engineered to provide enhanced levels of iron and β-carotene which could, in turn, help prevent iron deficiency anemia and vitamin A deficiency–related blindness worldwide

Body Mass Index (BMI): Strongly associated with dietary glycemic load and risk of coronary heart disease, as well as stroke among overweight and obese women

Bolus: Food that has been chewed and mixed in the mouth with saliva, and then passes down through the esophagus and into the stomach

Butyrate: Produced by resistant starches and non-digestible oligosaccharides fermented in the large intestine. Thought to be protective against colon cancer

Calcitriol: The active form of vitamin D; has a significant effect on adipocytes and obesity

Cardiovascular Disease (CVD): Degenerative disease pertaining to the heart; it has been shown that people consuming healthy diets, living active lifestyles, not smoking and not indulging in excessive alcohol consumption tend to have a reduced risk of CVD

Caries: Also known as cavities or tooth decay; a low consumption of dietary sugars has been reported to be seen in populations with low caries experience

Carotenoids: Lipid-soluble plant pigments consisting of oxygenated or non-oxygenated hydrocarbon chains with a minimum of 40 carbons and an extensive conjugated double bond system. Examples include beta-carotene, lutein and lycopene

Catabolisms: Examples include glycolysis and fatty acid oxidation

Cellulose: The major component of a plant cell wall and constitutes of a linear chain consisting of several thousand glucose units linked with β-1 and 4 glucosidic bonds

Chyme: The mass produced when the bolus reaches the stomach, mixes with gastric juices, and becomes reduced in size

Cinnamon: A spice from the genus Cinnamomum reported to reduce inflammation and enhance memory, and also has antidiabetic effects

Conjugated Linoleic Acids (CLAs): Found in animal products such as milk and meat and their products; is considered a functional food with many health benefits including preventing diabetes, obesity, atherosclerosis, and carcinogenesis, in addition to modulating immune function

Consumer Testing: Consumer tests are otherwise called the affective test when a large array of specific and sensitive tools fit in this category

Coriander Seeds: A spice used for glycemic control and management of diabetic complications

Coronary Heart Disease (CHD): Occurs when the heart's blood supply is blocked or interrupted by a build-up of fatty substances (atheroma) in the coronary arteries which supply blood to the heart

Cumin: A spice which, taken daily, reduces the fasting blood sugar level and also lowers the dosage of insulin needed

Curry Leaf: Extensively used for food flavoring in curries and chutneys in India, and are traditionally consumed by diabetics in India

Cytochrome P450: Superfamily enzymes found in both mitochondria and microsomal ER fractions, with most abundance in the liver where they are primarily responsible for detoxifying xenoboitics

Cytokines: Free radicals scavengers

Diabetes: Increased insulin resistance and decreased insulin secretion are two major characteristics

Dietary Fibers: Non-digestible polysaccharides. Facilitates the formation of a complex matrix which "traps" nutrients and contributes to delayed gastric emptying, which can also act to attenuate blood glucose concentrations

Dietary Supplement: A product intended to supplement a diet that contains one or more of the following dietary ingredients: a vitamin, a mineral, an herb or other botanical organism, an amino acid, a dietary substance used to increase the total daily intake, or a concentrate, metabolite, constituent, extract, or a combination of these ingredients. Functional foods are not considered dietary supplements

Directed Self-Assembly: Unlike spontaneous self-assembled systems, components do not form spontaneously even if they are all mixed together. The phenomenon of directed self-assembly requires optimum control of conditions such as order of mixing, temperature-time, pH-time, or ionic strength-time profiles

Dyspepsia: A medical condition typically characterized by chronic or recurrent pain in the upper abdomen, upper abdominal fullness, and feeling of satiety much earlier than expected with eating

Esterification: A process involves the condensation of ferulic acid, fatty acid or sugar molecules with the hydroxyl (OH^-) group on C-3 of the phytosterols

Fenugreek Seeds: Commonly used in India and other countries as a condiment, is an excellent source of dietary fiber; hence, advantageous in the context of diabetes

Fibroblast: Often cultured using 96 microwell plates. Depending on the type of medium that will enhance the cell growth, preparation involves ensuring the proper pH of the medium, as well as the addition of any necessary supplements or antibiotics

Fish Oil: Contain omega-3 fatty acids which may have a beneficial effect on cardiovascular health. About 2-4 grams of fish oil should be consumed per day

Fluoride: A trace mineral in the human body that makes bones stronger by replacing a part of the hydroxyapatite crystal with fluorapatite. Fluoride deficiency causes dental caries, whereas high exposure results in dental fluorosis

Folic Acid: Vitamin B9, involved in the synthesis of S-adenosylmethionine the metabolism of nucleic acids. It is also involved in the synthesis of amino acids as a coenzyme. Deficiency of folate causes folate-deficient erythropoesis, and meaining. Also, DNA synthesis is impaired and neutrophils hypersegmentation occurs. If there is a deficiency in pregnant women, the baby can have neural tube defects such as spina bifida or anencephaly

Food allergies: medical conditions in which one's immune system reacts abnormally to the ingestion of particular foods

Food Fortification: Is in the modified food categories of functional foods; defined as the addition of one or more essential nutrients (forticant) to a particular food (food vehicle), whether or not it is normally contained in the food

Food Vehicles: Are sought to protect bioactive ingredients added to food while controlling and targeting their release as they pass through the human GIT

French Paradox: The French population had curiously lower cardiovascular problems than the USA population and other countries in Europe in spite of their high consumption in saturated and trans-fatty acids. This was explained by their possible daily wine consumption

Functional Food: Natural or processed foods that contains known or unknown biologically-active compounds; which, in defined amounts, provide a clinically proven and documented health benefit for the prevention, management, or treatment of chronic disease.

Gastroesophageal Reflux Disease (GERD): Gastroesophageal acid, which can be introduced in the oral cavity from reflux in people

Genetically Modified Organism (GMO): Food produced using the conventional inputs of modern industrial agriculture including pesticides, synthetic fertilizers, and sewage sludge

Generally Recognized as Safe (GRAS): GRAS is a term that states which substances are safe to use as food additives by experts and published scientific evidence. The FDA has published a GRAS substance list that categorizes using three terms, namely: substances generally recognized as safe, direct food substances affirmed as generally recognized as safe, and indirect food substances affirmed as generally recognized as safe

Ginseng: A perennial plant found in the Northern Hemisphere. It has a long history of use in Chinese traditional medicine. It has been considered a folk remedy for tension and fatigue for years. It also has a reputation as an aphrodisiac and stimulant. In recent years, ginseng has been used in energy drinks, teas and special coffee (page 413).

Glucosinolates: Present in cruciferous vegetables, and activators of liver detoxification enzymes. These chemicals are responsible for the pungent aroma and bitter flavor of cruciferous vegetables

Glutamic Acid: Important in long-term potentiation as neurotransmitters and critical in the functions of learning and memory

Glycine: An amino acid and an inhibitory neurotransmitter in the brain and spinal cord

Hemicelluloses: Polysaccharides found in the plant cell wall

Hepcidin: An antimicrobial peptide made in the liver; a negative regulator of iron trafficking

Hormone Replacement Therapy (HRT): Uses phytoestrogens to have beneficial effects on the cardiovascular system and may even alleviate menopausal symptoms

Hypertension: One of the major risk factors for cardiovascular disease and stroke

Inflammatory Bowel Disease (IBD): A chronic inflammatory disorder caused by deregulated immune responses in a genetically predisposed individual

In Vitro Studies: inanimate lab-based studies

In Vivo Studies: involve living subjects, such as animals or humans

Insoluble Fiber: Include cellulose and other hemicelluloses. Most soluble fibers reduce plasma total and LDL cholesterol concentrations

Iodine Deficiency: A worldwide disorder that results in impaired synthesis of the thyroid hormones, thereby causing not only goiter but retarding growth, physical and mental development, and functional and developmental abnormalities

Isoflavones: Could protect against heart diseases and improve mineral (calcium) absorption (page 37).

Lactic Acid Bacteria (LAB): Produce organic acids, predominantly lactate and acetate, which create an acidic environment inhibitory to pathogens

Lignin: Forms the woody part of the plant. It is comprised of a group of non-carbohydrate dietary fibers containing about 40 oxygenated phenylpropane units, including coniferyl, sinapyl and p-coumaryl alcohols

Limonoids: Terpenes present in citrus fruit. Limonoids are unique highly oxygenated triterpenoid compounds, long recognized as significant biologically active natural compounds

Lipids: Found in oily fish, nuts, and vegetables. Foods that contain some form of fat

Liposome: Artificial vesicles formed by one or more concentric lipid bilayers separated by water compartments

Lycopene: A red pigment found in tomatoes, watermelon, pink grapefruit and papaya; is the most potent antioxidant of the estimated 600 naturally occurring carotenoids

Medical Foods: Specially formulated, regulated products for the dietary management of specific diseases, not meant to prevent or cure illnesses

Mediterranean Diet: Typically, rich in flavonoids from fruits and vegetables and wine. Has been associated with a lower risk of developing Alzheimer's and mild cognitive impairment and conversion of such impairment to Alzheimer's

Metabolic Syndrome: Clustering of risk factors such as hypertension, elevated blood glucose, elevated triglyceride, low high density lipoprotein (HDL) cholesterol, and abdominal or central obesity

Microflora: Commensal bacteria naturally present in the colon, existing in a homeostatic environment in the intestinal mucosa

Minerals: Inorganic elements that come from the earth

Multilayer Emulsion: Formed by adding polyelectrolytes to an emulsion containing oppositely charged droplets, so that they adsorb and form a coating

Nominal: the measurement that identifies unique attributes with non-ordered or ranked numerical values

Non-Alcoholic Fatty Liver Disease (NAFLD): Encompasses a wide spectrum of liver damage, ranging from simple steatosis to non-alcoholic steatohepatitis (NASH), advanced fibrosis, and cirrhosis. NAFLD is not only associated with insulin resistance, but also associated with other features of the metabolic syndrome

Non-Hodgkin Lymphoma (NHL): A heterogenous group of malignancies that arises primarily from lymphoid tissue throughout the body. Greater risks have been associated with immune suppression and infections, but the causes of NHL are not clearly established

Nutraceutical: A food (or part of a food) that provides medical or health benefits, including the prevention and/or treatment of a disease

Oligofructose: A subgroup of inulin, consisting of polymers with a degree of polymerization (DP) ≤ 10

Omega-3-Fatty Acids: Polyunsaturated fatty acids with a double bond at the 3rd carbon atom from the end of the carbon chain. Omega-3 fatty acids are an example of an essential nutrient not synthesized by humans and must be acquired through diet

Omega-6-Fatty Acids: Polyunsaturated fatty acids, found in soybean, corn, sunflower, canola, and cottonseed oils. It is now recognized that diets high in omega-6 fatty acids and low in omega-3 fatty acids may exacerbate several chronic diseases

Osteoporosis: Affecting the bones and joints, and recognized as a condition affecting mostly women and the elderly; however, this disorder is increasingly affecting a wider population including men and young adults

Oral Health: A state of being free from chronic mouth and facial pain, oral and throat cancer, oral sores, birth defects such as cleft lip and palate, periodontal (gum) disease, tooth decay and tooth loss, and other diseases and disorders that affect the oral cavity. Risk factors for oral diseases include unhealthy diet, tobacco use, harmful alcohol use, and poor oral hygiene

Ordinal: the measurement where the attributes are ordered but the *differences between levels are not equal*

Oxysterols: Derived from either enzymatic or non-enzymatic hemolytic reactions; are cytotoxic to both biomembranes and cellular functions

Pectin: Plant cell wall components and are also present as intercellular cementing substances

Pharmacodynamics: Interactions with receptors

Pharmacokinetics: Include the mechanisms of absorption, distribution, the chemical changes of the substance/drug in the body by metabolic enzymes and the excretion of the metabolites of the drug/substance

Phase Separation: Is a common phenomenon which may occur when two different materials are mixed; can be used to create new structures and systems

Phospholipids (PL): Form the lipid bilayer, serving as anchors of membrane proteins

Phytochemicals: Plant metabolites critical for plant survival and functions

Phytoestrogens: Non-steroidal phytochemicals quite similar in structure and function to gonadal estrogen hormones

Phytosterols: The plant equivalent of mammalian cholesterol found in nuts, seeds and legumes

Pinoresinol: The precursor to the antioxidant sesamin in the seeds of sesame

Polyphenols: A group of dietary antioxidants found naturally in fruits and vegetables

Prebiotics: A selectively fermented ingredient that results in specific changes in the composition and/or activity of the gastrointestinal microbiota, thus conferring health benefits upon the host

Prebiotic Index: Assesses the effectiveness of a prebiotic based on changes in the population of four types of bacteria: *Bacteroides*, *Bifidobacteria*, *Clostridia* and *Lactobacilli*. The prebiotic index of a substrate is defined as: Prebiotic Index (PI) = (Bif/Total) - (Bac/Total) + (Lac/Total) - (Clos/Total)

Proanthocyanidins: Polyphenolic compounds that can be found in the plant physiology of several plant species, and are mainly concentrated in tree bark and the outer skin of seeds

Probiotics: Live microorganisms that confer a health benefit on the host when administered in adequate amounts. The probiotic arsenal includes multiple mechanisms for preventing infection, enhancing the immune system, and providing increased nutritional value to food

Prostate Cancer (PCA): Aging and oxidative stress are prime factors in the promotion/progression of malignancy, green tea may prevent prostate cancer

Protein-Energy Malnutrition (PEM): Nutritional deficiencies in proteins, minerals and vitamins

Pyroptosis: Inflammatory cell death

Ratio: the measurement where the attributes are ordered and the *differences are equal, as well as the fact that there is a true zero*

Reactive Oxygen Species (ROS): Involved in the pathogenesis of both acute and chronic heart diseases as a result of cumulative oxidative stress

Recommended Dietary Allowance (RDA): The average daily dietary intake level sufficient to meet the nutrient requirement of nearly all healthy individuals in a particular life stage and gender group

Relative intake: the amount of a bioactive compound an individual consumes compared to the amount of other nutrients an individual consumes

Resveratrol: A polyphenol compound commonly found in grapes and most berries. These bioactive compounds have demonstrated efficacy in a variety of ways, including acting as anti-inflammatories, anti-oxidants, anti-tumors, anti-platelet aggregators, anti-aging compounds, and anti-atherogenics

Retinoids: vitamin A compounds together with their metabolites and synthetic derivatives that exhibit the same properties

Sensory Analysis: A scientific measurement that analyzes and measures human responses to the characteristics of food and drink

Sensory Cells: cells in taste buds that are connected to many different nerve fibers. They are renewed once a week and transmit information based on the intensity of stimulus and the brain translates the nervous electrical impulses into sensation, which is recognized as taste

Serine: Important in many aspects of neural metabolism. It is a primary donor of one carbon unit to biosynthesis in the nervous system

Sesamin: From the sesame seed, has *in vitro* antioxidant properties that stabilize sesame oil against turning rancid during commercial storage

Short-Chain Fatty Acids (SCFAs): Have been shown to have various potential physiological benefits. These include the inhibition of the proliferation of pathogenic species such as *Salmonella*, decrease in colonic and fecal pH, and provide metabolite and energy sources for colonocytes

Solid Lipid Particle (SLP) Emulsion: Usually involves homogenizing an oil and water phase in the presence of a hydrophilic emulsifier at a temperature above the melting point of the lipid phase

Spontaneous Self-Assemblies: Resulting in micelles, vesicles, fibers, tubes and liquid crystals under appropriate conditions (these structures form since spontaneous self-assembly reduces the free energy of the system)

St. John's Wort: A member of the hypericum perforatum species. It is widely used as an herbal remedy for depression. It is believed that its effect on mood comes from inhibition of the reuptake of neurotransmitters and a very mild monoamine-oxidase inhibitor effect

Supra-Molecular Structures: Biopolymers associated with one or more molecules of the same or different kind

Synbiotics: A combination of probiotics and prebiotics administered together

Taurine: Commonly associated with many areas of neurotransmission, but the effect of taurine in the human nervous system is unclear. Taurine supplements have been touted to enhance memory and are often used in energy drinks

Terpenoids: The largest class of phytonutrients in green foods and grains. These compounds are found in higher plants, mosses, liverworts, algae and lichens, as well as in insects, microbes or marine organisms

Thrombosis: The formation or presence of a blood clot within a blood vessel

Tolerable Upper Intake Level (UL): The highest average level of daily intake likely to pose no risk of adverse health effects for almost all people in the general population [1]. The ULs are presented in Table 1-10

Toxic Levels: when compounds are consumed at toxic levels, they switch from being beneficial antioxidants, to harmful pro-oxidants

Traditional Chinese Medicine (TCM): A particularly well-known and well-established example of how food is looked at beyond its simple nutritional value in this area of the world. It represents a functional food tradition that incorporates aspects of natural science (e.g. chemistry), social science (e.g. food and health history) and human science (e.g. nature philosophy)

Trypsin: A pancreatic enzyme that has been associated with efforts toward production, characterization and identification of many known peptides

Tryptophan: The precursor of several important compounds active in the human nervous system. It is found in a variety of plant and animal resources

Turmeric: An important spice widely cultivated and consumed in India; may possess beneficial anti-diabetic influences in a limited number of studies

Tyrosine: Synthesized from phenylalanine in the human body and available in popular supplements. In nature, tyrosine is found in milk, lima beans, pumpkin seeds, soy products and bananas

Viscosity: A fluid's resistance to flow

Vitamins: Organic substances made by plants or animals, whereas minerals are inorganic elements from the earth

Vitamin A: Carotenoids, associated with a lower risk of age-related macular degeneration

Vitamin C: A vitamin thought to boost immunity, deficiency can lead to scurvy

Vitamin D: Beneficial to bones and joints. Deficiency causes a reduction in the absorption of calcium and results in osteoporosis affecting elderly women

Vitamin E: An antioxidant found in vegetable oils, nuts, and the germ portion of grains

AUTHOR INDEX

Abugri DA	81
Dhiman A	67
Gur J	257
Holmes M	167
John SG	167
Johnson M	81
Kahraman O	147
Martirosyan DM	6, 25, 127, 228, 239, 257
Mawuntu M	257
Nanda A	67
Ortiz M	239
Pacier C	127
Pisarski K	25
Reynolds T	228
Sreelatha S	219
Walia V	67
Westmark CJ	113

Basic Principles of Functional Foods Science

Textbook
First Edition

Edited by Danik M. Martirosyan, PhD

Editorial Assistants: Johanna Gur, Jacky Zong

Made in the USA
Monee, IL
13 February 2023

27647314R00162